# Non-Migraine Primary Headaches in Medicine

AF400165

Paolo Martelletti

Editor

# Non-Migraine Primary Headaches in Medicine

A Machine-Generated Overview of Current Research

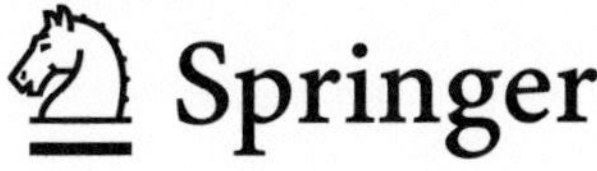 Springer

*Editor*
Paolo Martelletti 
Department of Clinical and Molecular Medicine
Sapienza University of Rome
Rome, Italy

ISBN 978-3-031-20896-6     ISBN 978-3-031-20894-2   (eBook)
https://doi.org/10.1007/978-3-031-20894-2

© The Editor(s) (if applicable) and The Author(s), under exclusive license to Springer Nature Switzerland AG 2023
This work is subject to copyright. All rights are solely and exclusively licensed by the Publisher, whether the whole or part of the material is concerned, specifically the rights of translation, reprinting, reuse of illustrations, recitation, broadcasting, reproduction on microfilms or in any other physical way, and transmission or information storage and retrieval, electronic adaptation, computer software, or by similar or dissimilar methodology now known or hereafter developed.
The use of general descriptive names, registered names, trademarks, service marks, etc. in this publication does not imply, even in the absence of a specific statement, that such names are exempt from the relevant protective laws and regulations and therefore free for general use.
The publisher, the authors, and the editors are safe to assume that the advice and information in this book are believed to be true and accurate at the date of publication. Neither the publisher nor the authors or the editors give a warranty, expressed or implied, with respect to the material contained herein or for any errors or omissions that may have been made. The publisher remains neutral with regard to jurisdictional claims in published maps and institutional affiliations.

This Springer imprint is published by the registered company Springer Nature Switzerland AG
The registered company address is: Gewerbestrasse 11, 6330 Cham, Switzerland

# Preface

It is well established in all the international scientific literature that headache disorders are among the most prevalent and disabling conditions worldwide. The Global Burden of Diseases, gathering many important epidemiological studies, has confirmed the evidence of the high prevalence of tension-type headache, with a moderate level of caused disability, and the low prevalence of trigeminal autonomic cephalalgias which cause a very high disability, and the others non-migraine headache disorders for their potential risk caused by an incorrect diagnostic definition among primary and secondary forms.

The help of Artificial Intelligence in finding, capturing and structuring what the most recent publications have highlighted in these non-migraine forms of primary headache is the fundamental passage of this book.

It is aimed at all those who want to directly consult the original source of the literature to make informed clinical decisions reaching the exact publication needed. It is a new way of approaching the culture of headaches by skipping the interpretations and filters of the authors, providing everything that is necessary for a clinical decision that is informed from a diagnostic and therapeutic point of view. The correctness of the original information will allow both the headache expert and any clinician to reduce the diagnostic errors that can often lead to the risks of analgesics abuse and delays, sometimes even life-threatening.

This volume, like the previous one on migraine, is dedicated to physicians facing in their daily clinical practice the non-migraine headache forms, to PhD students, to residents aiming to add value to the management of underestimated tension-type headache, to improve the immediate definition of trigeminal autonomic cephalalgias and other non-migraine primary headache disorders.

Department of Clinical and Molecular Medicine                    Paolo Martelletti
Sapienza University of Rome
Rome, Italy

# Contents


**1  Tension-Type Headache** . . . . . . . . . . . . . . . . . . . . . . . . . . . . . . . . . . 1

**2  Trigeminal Autonomic Cephalalgias** . . . . . . . . . . . . . . . . . . . . . . . . 131

**3  Other Non-migraine Primary Headache Disorders** . . . . . . . . . . . . . 321

# Chapter 1
# Tension-Type Headache

## 1.1 Introduction

Tension-type headache is the second most common cause of chronic pain in the Global Burden of Disease, affecting an estimated population of nearly 900 million new cases per year. The estimated prevalence of tension-type headache is enormous, with a very high variability from 10% up to 86% in young subjects. The global prevalence of the chronic form is equally important because it covers about two 3% of the global population. Despite such an important epidemiological economic impact, tension-type headache causes less disability than migraine. In terms of years of life lived with disabilities the comorbidities of tension-type headache are often similar to those of migraine such as anxiety, depression, sleep disturbances and other pain disorders including migraine itself. The physiopathology of the tension-type headache is mainly based on genetic factors, myofascial mechanisms and chronicization mechanisms such as sensitization, therefore peripheral mechanisms and vascular factors are mostly unimportant. The central factors are important in the transformation from the episodic form to the chronic one. Unfortunately, the non-exact definition of the pathophysiology and the moderate burden impact and even a modest economic impact has left the tension-type headache, from a therapeutic point of view, still with old generation drugs, with no new compounds dedicated to this pathology for many decades. However, being a pathology with a great impact in the general population, it is useful to know the most important lines of research and any updates also in the field of complementary medicine that can guide the clinician in his/her daily practice.

© The Author(s), under exclusive license to Springer Nature Switzerland AG 2023
P. Martelletti (ed.), *Non-Migraine Primary Headaches in Medicine*,
https://doi.org/10.1007/978-3-031-20894-2_1

1

## 1.2   Machine-Generated Summaries

Machine generated keywords: tth, migraine tth, tensiontype, tensiontype headache, burden, child, gbd, country, global, sleep, manual, muscle, adolescent, tension, tth migraine.

### *Public Health*

Machine generated keywords: gbd, burden, global, country, burden disease, burden headache, tth, adolescent, participant, migraine tth, epidemiological, global burden, live disability, million, health.

### *The Global Prevalence of Headache: An Update, with Analysis of the Influences of Methodological Factors on Prevalence Estimates*

DOI: https://doi.org/10.1186/s10194-022-01402-2

**Abstract-Summary**

According to the Global Burden of Disease (GBD) study, headache disorders are among the most prevalent and disabling conditions worldwide.

GBD builds on epidemiological studies (published and unpublished) which are notable for wide variations in both their methodologies and their prevalence estimates.

Our first aim was to update the documentation of headache epidemiological studies, summarizing global prevalence estimates for all headache, migraine, tension-type headache (TTH) and headache on $\geq 15$ days/month (H15+), comparing these with GBD estimates and exploring time trends and geographical variations.

Our second aim was to analyse how methodological factors influenced prevalence estimates.

From 357 publications, the vast majority from high-income countries, the estimated global prevalence of active headache disorder was 52.0% (95% CI 48.9–55.4), of migraine 14.0% (12.9–15.2), of TTH 26.0% (22.7–29.5) and of H15+ 4.6% (3.9–5.5).

Methodological factors contributing to variation, were publication year, sample size, inclusion of probable diagnoses, sub-population sampling (e.g., of health-care personnel), sampling method (random or not), screening question (neutral, or qualified in severity or presumed cause) and scope of enquiry (headache disorders only or multiple other conditions).

With these taken into account, migraine prevalence estimates increased over the years, while estimates for all headache types varied between world regions.

The review confirms GBD in finding that headache disorders remain highly prevalent worldwide, and it identifies methodological factors explaining some of the large variation between study findings.

These variations render uncertain both the increase in migraine prevalence estimates over time, and the geographical differences.

Extended:

Future studies should not assess prevalence alone but include data allowing TIS to be estimated, preferably among the various age and gender subgroups.

## Introduction

Through the Global Burden of Disease (GBD) study, headache disorders are revealed as one of the major public-health concerns globally and in all countries and world regions [1].

For the various disorders it considers, GBD uses multiple data sources (epidemiological studies, health registers, official statistics, hospital data, etc.) to make best-informed estimates of prevalence and burden.

They included criteria for judging the quality of studies from their reported methodology, and some adjustments to prevalence estimates were based upon these in the most detailed analysis of headache data, from GBD 2016 [1].

We reviewed all published studies of the prevalence and burden of headache [2].

We update that review, and the documentation of headache epidemiological studies, summarizing global prevalence estimates for headache, migraine, tension-type headache (TTH) and headache on $\geq 15$ days/month (H15+), comparing these with GBD estimates and exploring time trends and geographical variations.

## Methods

To geographical origin and publication year, we extracted data related to the quality criteria [3]: those describing the population of interest (the general population or a specified sub-population), sampling method (randomness and representativeness), size of sample, participating proportion, methods of data collection (access to and engagement with participants) and validation of diagnostic questions.

For MLR analyses we dichotomized the quality measures [3] that were not interval or ordinal variables: population of interest (unselected [general] population of a country, community or tribe, or pupils of obligatory schools, versus selected sub-populations [e.g., university students, factory/workplace employees, minorities, etc.], or unstipulated [additionally, we registered whether selected subpopulations were health-care personnel such as medical students, hospital employees, neurologists, etc.]); sample representativeness of the population of interest (random sampling versus non-random sampling or failed attempt to secure randomness); access to and engagement with participants (face-to-face or telephone interview versus unsupervised questionnaire completion or unstipulated); validation of diagnostic questions (effort at validating versus none or unstipulated); application of ICHD criteria and distinction between definite and probable diagnoses versus not or unstipulated.

## Results

Studies with mid-range age values below 10 or above 65 years reported lower migraine prevalences in both males and females, and studies with values below 10 years reported lower TTH prevalences in both genders.

In studies estimating prevalences of an active headache disorder and of specific headache types, there were clear positive correlations between them: for headache with migraine ($r = 0.46$, $p < 0.01$, 142 studies), with TTH ($r = 0.48$, $p < 0.01$, 84 studies) and with H15+ ($r = 0.45$, $p < 0.01$, 42 studies), for migraine with TTH ($0.36$, $p < 0.0000$, 105 studies) and with H15+ ($0.45$, $p < 0.01$, 43 studies), and for TTH with H15+ ($0.37$, $p = 0.2$, 43 studies).

## Discussion

It is uncertain whether or to what extent these differences over time and place are real: overall, the MLR analyses show that the present models explain relatively little of the large variations in prevalence estimates between studies (for migraine less than 30%, and even less for other headache types, possibly because of fewer studies).

In the MLR analyses, publication year appeared important as a factor explaining variation in migraine prevalence estimates (6.4% of variation in Model 2, higher estimates associated with more recent publication), but it played no role in other headache types.

The negative association of prevalence estimates of all headache, migraine and H15+ with number of study participants (Model 2: 3.2%, 1.6% and 12.5% of variations respectively) may indicate that smaller studies can afford more sensitive methods (personal interview, face to face or by phone) to detect cases.

## Conclusions

While this review updates our earlier documentation of headache epidemiological studies [2], it also highlights the dependence of prevalence estimates on a small number of methodological factors (and relative independence of others that might be expected to be influential).

Future prevalence estimates from all parts of the world will be derived from studies performed in a relatively standardized way, in accordance with published recommendations.

Future studies should not assess prevalence alone but include data allowing TIS to be estimated, preferably among the various age and gender subgroups.

## Acknowledgement

*A machine generated summary based on the work of Stovner, Lars Jacob; Hagen, Knut; Linde, Mattias; Steiner, Timothy J. 2022 in The Journal of Headache and Pain.*

# Incidence, Prevalence and Disability Associated with Neurological Disorders in Italy Between 1990 and 2019: An Analysis Based on the Global Burden of Disease Study 2019

DOI: https://doi.org/10.1007/s00415-021-10774-5

**Abstract-Summary**

Neurological conditions are highly prevalent and disabling, in particular in the elderly.

The Italian population has witnessed sharp ageing and we can thus expect a rising trend in the incidence, prevalence and disability of these conditions.

We relied on the Global Burden of Disease 2019 study to extract Italian data on incidence, prevalence and years lived with a disability (YLDs) referred to a broad set of neurological disorders including, brain and nervous system cancers, stroke, encephalitis, meningitis, tetanus, traumatic brain injury, and spinal cord injury.

The most prevalent conditions were tension-type headache, migraine, and dementias, whereas the most disabling were migraine, dementias and traumatic brain injury.

YLDs associated with neurological conditions increased by 22.5%, but decreased by 2.3% in age-standardized rates.

The increase in YLDs associated with neurological conditions is mostly due to population ageing and growth: nevertheless, lived disability and, as a consequence, impact on health systems has increased.

Extended:

The Italian population comprised 60.6 million in 2019, with a life expectancy at birth of 83.1 years (ranking third at European level) and 71.0 years of healthy life expectancy years (ranking sixth at European level) [4].

The most prevalent conditions in 2019 were migraine and TTH, with 12.5 and 23.2 million prevalent cases (28.5 million cases when combined), and an increase of 8.2% and 12.8% compared to 1990.

**Introduction**

The authors of this manuscript evidenced a consistently increasing trend for number of prevalent cases and disability, in addition to burden, for the selected neurological diseases, and hypothesized that the same indices are reasonably expected to further on increase in reason of population ageing and growth: however, no direct information was referred to YLDs associated with neurological disease by country.

The aims of this article are, therefore, the following: to describe the incidence, prevalence and YLDs associated with a broad group of neurological disorders in Italy, and their variation between 1990 and 2019; to address the trends for those NCDs with typical onset in young to adult age (e.g. headache disorders) and for those with typical onset in old age (e.g. Alzheimer's disease and other dementias), as well as for neurological injuries and for communicable neurological diseases; to compare estimates referred to Italy to those of other Western Europe countries.

## Methods

This broad group of neurological conditions included both level 3 and level 4 conditions as presented in the GBD, specifically as follows: a) A set of level 3 NCDs, namely Alzheimer's disease and other dementias, brain and nervous system cancers, epilepsy, MND, MS, PD and stroke, as well as two level-4 ones, namely migraine and TTH.

Non-fatal outcomes for the individual disorders included in this residual category need to be approximated by assuming the same YLDs/YLLs ratios estimated for the main fatal neurological disorders, which can be a precise approach for those conditions associated to relevant mortality (e.g. Huntington's disease), but not for those associated to little or no mortality (e.g. myasthenia gravis).

Changes over the period were also analysed at the group level, i.e. young to adult-age onset NCDs, older age onset NCDs, neurological injuries, and communicable neurological diseases.

## Results

With regard to incidence, a consistent decrease both for counts and age-standardized rates was observed for stroke, meningitis, tetanus and TBI, whereas a consistent increase both for counts and age-standardized rates was observed for TTH, MS, dementias and MND.

As for prevalence, a consistent decrease both for counts and age-standardized rates was observed for meningitis and tetanus, whereas a consistent increase both for counts and age-standardized rates was observed for migraine, TTH, MS and MND.

For PD, stroke, TBI and SCI the trend was increasing when counts were taken into account, and decreasing in age-standardized rates; for migraine, TTH and dementias and brain and nervous system cancers the trend was increasing when counts were taken into account, and stable in age-standardized rates; finally, for encephalitis, the trend was decreasing in age-standardized rates, and stable in counts.

## Discussion

There has been a dramatic increase in the counts and age-standardized rates of incidence and prevalence of some conditions with typical onset in old age, in particular for Alzheimer disease and other dementias, brain and nervous system cancers and MND.

The increase in YLDs was due to a clear epidemiological change mostly for young to adult-onset conditions, for which age-standardized YLD rates increased by 5.0%, whereas for old-age onset disease the variation herein observed was mostly an effect of population ageing and growth as age-standardized YLDs rates decreased by 13.7%.

Incidence, prevalence and YLDs associated with Alzheimer's disease and other dementias have more than doubled in Italy over the 1990–2019 period, but not in terms of age-standardized rates, where only for incidence a minor increase was found, suggesting that such an increase is a consequence of population ageing.

**Conclusions**

We reported information on incidence, prevalence and disability associated with neurological disorders in Italy relying on the GBD 2019 estimates.

Our results show that headache disorders are still the most prevalent and disabling conditions, and that epidemiological patterns have changed between 1990 and 2019.

Our work pinpoints a worrisome rise in incidence and prevalence for conditions with typical onset in older ages, particularly dementias and PD as an effect of population ageing; for MND, on the contrary, estimates suggest a consistent increase which cannot be explained by population ageing only, but also as an effect of prolonged survival.

The increase is mostly due to population ageing and growth, with the only exceptions of MND and MS (for which classification changes and the inclusion of less severe varieties can be also implicated), and points out the increased survival for many of these conditions.

**Acknowledgement**

*A machine generated summary based on the work of Raggi, Alberto; Monasta, Lorenzo; Beghi, Ettore; Caso, Valeria; Castelpietra, Giulio; Mondello, Stefania; Giussani, Giorgia; Logroscino, Giancarlo; Magnani, Francesca Giulia; Piccininni, Marco; Pupillo, Elisabetta; Ricci, Stefano; Ronfani, Luca; Santalucia, Paola; Sattin, Davide; Schiavolin, Silvia; Toppo, Claudia; Traini, Eugenio; Steinmetz, Jaimie; Nichols, Emma; Ma, Rui; Vos, Theo; Feigin, Valery; Leonardi, Matilde. 2021 in Journal of Neurology.*

## Burden of Tension-Type Headache in the Middle East and North Africa Region, 1990–2019

DOI: https://doi.org/10.1186/s10194-022-01445-5

**Abstract-Summary**

As there is a gap in the literature regarding the disease burden attributable to TTH in the Middle East and North Africa (MENA) region, the aim of the present study was to report the epidemiological indicators of TTH in MENA, from 1990 to 2019, by sex, age and socio-demographic index (SDI).

In 2019, the age-standardised point prevalence and annual incidence rates for TTH in the MENA region were 24504.5 and 8680.1 per 100000, respectively, which represents a 2.0% and a 0.9% increase over 1990–2019, respectively.

The age-standardised YLD rate of TTH in this region in 2019 was estimated to be 68.1 per 100000 population, which has increased 1.0% since 1990.

Iran [29640.4] had the highest age-standardised point prevalence rate for TTH, while Turkey [21726.3] had the lowest.

In 2019, the regional point prevalence of TTH was highest in the 35–39 and 70–74 age groups, for males and females, respectively.

While the prevalence of TTH in the MENA region increased from 1990 to 2019, the incidence rate did not change.

The burden of TTH in MENA was higher than at the global level for both sexes and all age groups.

Extended:

In 2019, the national age-standardised point prevalence of TTH ranged from 21726.3 to 29640.4 cases per 100000 population, among the countries that comprise the MENA region.

In 2019, the national age-standardised YLD rate of TTH ranged from 62.0 to 77.6 cases per 100000 population among the MENA countries.

In 2019, the regional point prevalence of TTH was highest in the 35–39 and 70–74 age groups, for males and females, respectively.

The age-standardised YLD rates due to TTH were higher in the MENA region than the corresponding global rates for both sexes and across all age groups.

Future high quality epidemiological studies at the national and subnational levels, which are calibrated to the local settings in MENA, are needed to strengthen the certainty and validity of the estimated burden.

## Introduction

According to the Global Burden of Disease (GBD) study 2016, about 1.89 billion people suffer from TTH [1].

According to the GBD 2016, more than 175 million people in the MENA region had TTHs, and the mean burden of this disease was more than 777 thousand YLDs [1].

A number of studies have reported the prevalence of this disorder at the global level, but these studies do not provide detailed information regarding each individual region or the countries within these regions.

Although epidemiological studies should be regularly updated, and despite the importance of headache disorders for public health, there has been no comprehensive study investigating the burden of TTH within the MENA region.

Using data from the GBD study 2019, the present study reported the point prevalence, annual incidence and YLDs of TTH in the MENA region from 1990 to 2019, by sex, age and socio-demographic index (SDI).

## Methods

If studies reported the prevalence for wide age groups by sex (e.g., among 20–55 year old males and 20–55 year old females), or by specific age groups with the two sexes combined (e.g., prevalence in 15–30 year olds, for males and females together), age-specific estimates were split by sex using the sex ratio reported and the bounds of uncertainty.

Those studies that only reported definite TTH were also adjusted to the total TTH category, in order to better inform the model.

Following this, those studies that reported both definite and total TTH were added to the regression models, by sex, in order to produce age- and sex-specific adjustments.

In GBD 2019, data from the meta-analysis Lifting the Burden was used to provide the symptomatic time for TTH, as well as estimates for probable, definite, and total TTH.

**Results**

In 2019, the national age-standardised point prevalence of TTH ranged from 21726.3 to 29640.4 cases per 100000 population, among the countries that comprise the MENA region.

Iran [29640.4 (26202.1–32949.4)], Egypt [26290.9 (22878.1–29775.3)] and Bahrain [23716.0 (20422.0–27274.1)] had the three highest age-standardised point prevalences of TTH in 2019.

The national age-standardised incidence rates of TTH in 2019 ranged from 8197.3 to 9837.5 cases per 100000 population.

In 2019, the national age-standardised YLD rate of TTH ranged from 62.0 to 77.6 cases per 100000 population among the MENA countries.

In 2019, the regional point prevalence of TTH was highest in the 35–39 and 70–74 age groups, for males and females, respectively.

There was an increase in the regional YLD rate of TTH for females up to the 65–69 age group, followed by a decrease.

**Discussion**

We found the burden attributable to TTH in the MENA region was larger than the corresponding global burden for both sexes and in all age groups.

According to reports from the GBD 2016 and 2017 studies, the age-standardised point prevalence of TTH has decreased since 1990 [1, 5].

At regional level, the GBD 2016 study reported an 8.5% reduction in the age-standardised point prevalence of TTH in the MENA region since 1990 [1].

The age-standardised YLD rates due to TTH were higher in the MENA region than the corresponding global rates for both sexes and across all age groups.

Another recent study came to the conclusion that psychological comorbidities, such as depression, were the cause of the larger burden of TTH among females [6].

**Conclusion**

The present study has shown that TTH causes a large burden in the MENA region, in terms of disabilities and loss of health, and that the burden in MENA is higher than the global level for both sexes and all age groups.

Future high quality epidemiological studies at the national and subnational levels, which are calibrated to the local settings in MENA, are needed to strengthen the certainty and validity of the estimated burden.

**Acknowledgement**

*A machine generated summary based on the work of Safiri, Saeid; Kolahi, Ali-Asghar; Noori, Maryam; Nejadghaderi, Seyed Aria; Aslani, Armin; Sullman, Mark J. M.; Farhoudi, Mehdi; Araj-Khodaei, Mostafa; Collins, Gary S.; Kaufman, Jay S.; Gharagozli, Kurosh. 2022 in The Journal of Headache and Pain.*

# The Burden of Headache Disorders in the Eastern Mediterranean Region, 1990–2016: Findings from the Global Burden of Disease Study 2016

DOI: https://doi.org/10.1186/s10194-019-0990-3

## Abstract-Summary

Using the findings of the Global Burden of Disease Study (GBD), we report the burden of primary headache disorders in the Eastern Mediterranean Region (EMR) from 1990 to 2016.

Years lived with disability (YLDs) were calculated by multiplying prevalence and disability weight (DW) of migraine and tension-type headache (TTH).

During the same period, age-standardised YLD rates of migraine and TTH in EMR increased by 0.7% and 2.5%, respectively, in comparison to a small decrease in the global rates (0.2% decrease in migraine and TTH).

The age-standardised YLD rates of both headache disorders were higher in women with female to male ratio of 1.69 for migraine and 1.38 for TTH.

All countries of the EMR except for Somalia and Djibouti had higher age-standardised YLD rates for migraine and TTH in compare to the global rates.

Libya and Saudi Arabia had the highest increase in age-standardised YLD rates of migraine and TTH, respectively.

The findings of this study show that primary headache disorders are a major and a growing cause of disability in EMR.

Extended:

During the same period, the relative contribution of migraine YLDs and TTH YLDs to the overall YLDs in EMR increased from 6.0% (95% UI 4.3–7.8) to 6.7% (95% UI 4.9–8.5) and from 1.00% (95% UI 0.75–1.30) to 1.16% (95% UI 0.86–1.49), respectively.

During the same period, age-standardised YLD rates of migraine remained generally unchanged in EMR countries.

## Introduction

GBD 2016, provided more accurate estimations of prevalence and burden of headache by countries, regions, and super regions [7].

According to GBD 2016, prevalence of headache disorders was variable across different geographic regions.

Although prevalence of headache is an important epidemiologic measure, the burden of disability related to headache, as measured by YLD, is more informative for health policy making.

GBD 2016 emphasized that primary headache disorders are an important health priority.

Estimating the burden of headache is the first step to implement further measures to reduce its burden such as educating health care providers, developing primary care management, and allocating resources.

We reported the prevalence and burden of primary headache disorders (including migraine and TTH) in Eastern Mediterranean Region (EMR) countries from 1990 to 2016 using data and methods of the Global Burden of Diseases, Injuries, and Risk Factors Study 2016.

**Methods**

The Global Burden of Diseases, Injuries, and Risk Factors Study 2016 (GBD 2016) is a standardised analytical method that used all eligible sources to estimate the epidemiological data, including prevalence, mortality, years of life lost (YLL), YLDs, and disability-adjusted life years (DALYs), for 328 causes by sex, age, and location from 1990 to 2016.

In the previous GBD iteration (GBD 2015), in addition to migraine and TTH, medication overuse headache (MOH) was also included as a separate disorder.

We presented numbers and rates of prevalence and YLDs of migraine and TTH in 2016 and the changes from 1990 to 2016 for all EMR countries.

From the EMR, data sources from Iran [8–10], Pakistan [11], Tunisia [12], and UAE [13] for migraine, and data sources from Iran [8, 10, 14], Pakistan [11], and Qatar [15] for TTH were used in GBD 2016; however, data inputs from all over the world were used to model the burden of migraine and TTH in EMR countries.

**Results**

In the EMR, female to male ratio of age-standardised YLDs were 1.69 for migraine and 1.38 for TTH.

From 1990 to 2016, age-standardised YLD rates of migraine and TTH remained generally unchanged.

Comparing the overall all-age YLD rates of migraine and TTH combined, Kuwait had the highest and Djibouti had the lowest YLD rates.

During the same period, age-standardised YLD rates of migraine remained generally unchanged in EMR countries.

The ratio of observed to expected age-standardised YLD rate for migraine ranged from 0.82 in Djibouti to 1.31 in Palestine.

Similar to migraine, age-standardised YLD rates of TTH showed an overall consistency between 1990 and 2016 in EMR countries.

Observed to expected age-standardised YLD rate ratio for TTH ranged from 0.85 in Djibouti to 1.42 in Iran.

**Discussion**

Our study provides a comprehensive assessment of the values and trends of prevalence and burden of primary headache disorders in EMR countries and their trends from 1990 to 2016.

Risk factors for progression of episodic migraine to chronic migraine can explain a part of the higher burden of headache in the EMR.

Given the limited data sources from the EMR countries, the role of risk factors of chronic migraine in higher burden of headache in the EMR should be interpreted cautiously.

The significant and increasing non-fatal burden of headache inform policy makers and health care providers of EMR countries that primary headache should be a health care priority, and intervention strategies focusing on improvement of diagnosis and treatment of headache must be implemented.

Although we estimated prevalence and YLDs of the primary headache disorders with considerable burden (including migraine, TTH, and MOH—as a sequel of the first two syndromes), we could not include all primary headache disorders classified in ICD-10 classification [16].

## Conclusion

Findings from this study show that primary headache disorders are a large cause of disability in the EMR.

Our findings inform policy makers of the EMR countries that headache is a health care priority, and preventive and management interventions must be implemented to address the growing burden of headache in this region.

More studies are needed to provide more accurate data on the prevalence and severity of primary headache disorders in EMR as well as more efficient preventive and management methods to reduce the burden of headache.

## Acknowledgement

*A machine generated summary based on the work of Vosoughi, Kia; Stovner, Lars Jacob; Steiner, Timothy J.; Moradi-Lakeh, Maziar; Fereshtehnejad, Seyed-Mohammad; Farzadfar, Farshad; Heydarpour, Pouria; Malekzadeh, Reza; Naghavi, Mohsen; Sahraian, Mohammad Ali; Sepanlou, Sadaf G.; Tehrani-Banihashemi, Arash; Majdzadeh, Reza; Feigin, Valery L.; Vos, Theo; Mokdad, Ali H.; Murray, Christopher J. L. 2019 in The Journal of Headache and Pain.*

# One-Quarter of Individuals with Weekly Headache Have Never Consulted a Medical Doctor: A Danish Nationwide Cross-Sectional Survey

DOI: https://doi.org/10.1186/s10194-022-01460-6

## Abstract-Summary

Among the causes are poor or disorganized provision of headache services, but reluctance to seek healthcare has frequently been identified as a significant barrier.

We conducted a national survey of people with headache to assess the extent of this problem in Denmark, a country with well organized, highly resourced, and readily accessible services.

We conducted a nationwide cross-sectional survey of adults ≥18 years old in Denmark reporting at least one headache day in the last year.

Of the respondents, 54.2% reported headache at least once a week, 33.4% reported headache a couple of times a month, and 12.4% reported headache a couple of times a year.

Two-thirds of respondents (66.6%) reported that headache limited their social lives occasionally or frequently.

Most respondents (86.8%) reported going to work or attending educational activities occasionally or more frequently even though they had headache.

Half of the respondents (49.5%) experienced lack of understanding of their headaches from people occasionally or more frequently.

Further studies are needed to investigate and clarify why even people with the highest burden are hesitant to seek and make use of widely available headache services.

Extended:

We conducted a national survey of people with headache to assess the extent of this problem in Denmark, a country with well organized, highly resourced, and readily accessible services.

**Key Messages**

In Denmark it is evident that many people, even among those with the highest headache-attributed burden, are hesitant to make use of headache services that offer mitigation of symptoms and their consequences of disability, lost productivity, and economic losses.

It is insufficient merely to make headache services available: public education—in when, how and when not to use these services—is also needed if they are to reach all (or even the majority) of those who would benefit.

**Introduction**

Headache disorders are a leading cause of disability, directly affecting more than 1 billion people across all regions of the world [17].

In Denmark, headache disorders are responsible for more than one-third of all disability-adjusted life years (DALYs) due to neurological disorders according to the Global Burden of Disease study [18].

Because the most common headache disorders, tension-type headache and migraine, are highly prevalent during the most productive years of life [17, 19, 20], the impacts and importance of this disability burden are magnified.

We conducted a national survey of people with headache to assess the extent of this problem in Denmark, a country with well organized, highly resourced, and readily accessible services.

**Methods**

Consent of participants was presumed from their participation following explanation of the nature and purpose of the survey (the latter broadly expressed as an assessment of life with headache and its impacts).

Eligible participants were those meeting the age criterion and reporting at least one headache day in the last year.

Social life: Does your headache disorder limit your social life? (Never, rarely, occasionally, often, very often).

Social support: Do you experience a lack of understanding of your headache from people around you? (Never, rarely, occasionally, often, very often).

We used descriptive statistics to present survey demographics and headache-attributed burden, calculating means and standard deviations (SDs) for continuous outcomes and proportions (%) for binary and multinomial outcomes.

The strength of the association between headache-attributed burden (at least once a week, a couple of times a month, a couple of times a year) and survey outcomes of 'Does your headache limit your social life?'.

## Results

Of the 6567 respondents, 3558 (54.2%) reported headache at least once a week, 2195 (33.4%) reported headache a couple of times a month, and 814 (12.4%) reported headache a couple of times a year.

There was a strong positive correlation between headache-attributed burden and limitation of social life (G = 0.576, p < 0.0001).

This was frequency-dependent: of respondents with weekly or monthly headache, almost all (90.7% and 91.0%, respectively) reported doing so, but fewer, although still more than half (56.3%) of those with yearly headache did so.

There was a strong positive correlation between headache-attributed burden and lack of social support (G = 0.448, p < 0.0001).

## Discussion

In this national survey of people with headache in Denmark, a high-income country with readily accessible services, we identified a low healthcare utilization rate.

Utilization rate among the general Danish population with headache is almost certainly lower—and perhaps much lower—than in our sample.

Headache-attributed burden was strongly associated with a negative impact on social life, higher rates of presenteeism, and lack of understanding from those around them.

While other countries in the study reported higher rates, there were still substantial proportions of people with headache who did not seek headache care [21, 22].

Clinical, social, and political/economical barriers hinder people with headache from accessing healthcare services who would otherwise benefit from them [17, 23].

These are people with a lower probability of having headache, or, if they do, of having a high attributable burden.

## Conclusions

In Denmark it is evident that many people, even among those with the highest headache-attributed burden, are hesitant to make use of headache services that offer mitigation of symptoms and their consequences of disability, lost productivity, and economic losses.

In Denmark, a high-income country with headache services that are free, easily accessible and among the best in the world, the main drivers must be found elsewhere.

What is clear meanwhile is that it is insufficient merely to make headache services available: public education—in when, how and when not to use these services—is also needed if they are to reach all (or even the majority) of those who would benefit [24].

**Acknowledgement**
*A machine generated summary based on the work of Do, Thien Phu; Stefansen, Simon; Dømgaard, Mikala; Steiner, Timothy J.; Ashina, Messoud. 2022 in The Journal of Headache and Pain.*

## A Prospective Real-World Study Exploring Associations Between Passively Collected Tracker Data and Headache Burden Among Individuals with Tension-Type Headache and Migraine

DOI: https://doi.org/10.1007/s40122-021-00336-y

**Abstract-Summary**
We explored the associations between passively collected activity data, headache burden, and quality of life in headache sufferers.

Data from wearable activity tracking devices and daily short questionnaires were collected over 12 weeks to assess occurrence of headache, activity, quality of life and self-rated health.

Behaviors inferred from activity tracker data suggested that individuals slept more, had reduced physical activity, and had lower maximum heart rate on days with headache.

As headache-specific impact on quality of life increased, activity and maximum heart rate decreased and sleep increased.

Headache days with higher self-rated health were associated with less napping, higher step count and maximum heart rate, correlating with increased activity.

This study adds to existing evidence that activity trackers can be used to quantify headache burden in real-world settings and aid in understanding symptom management.

Extended:

This study adds support and expands the existing knowledge of the links between physical activity and both migraine and TTH.

The data obtained in this study can be used to help develop new metrics that can be used in future research, and to increase understanding of the diversity in self-treatment patterns outside primary care.

## Introduction

There is a relative lack of prospective and real-world data on primary headache disorders, although recent studies indicate that stress, sleep, and daily physical activity may be linked to headache [25–27].

The widespread use of commercially available, wearable activity tracking devices presents a unique opportunity to understand daily activity among headache sufferers in an unobtrusive and less burdensome manner.

This prospective, observational, exploratory study paired passively collected activity data from wearable tracking devices with online questionnaires to understand the impact of headache on daily activities and quality of life (QoL) among frequent headache sufferers, and understand how they self-manage their symptoms in real-world settings.

## Methods

The primary objective was to understand the day-level association between passively collected activity data features and (1) headache occurrence on a given day (i.e., days with headache), and (2) QoL, as measured by impact on daily life and self-rated health on days with headache.

In the primary objective analysis, 14 passively collected activity features related to sleep (i.e., naps, total time spent asleep, and sleep from the night before), steps (e.g., total number of steps that day), and heart rate (e.g., resting heart rate) were assessed individually as outcomes, with day with or without headache as a binary predictor, using linear and logistic mixed-effects models with random intercepts to account for intra-individual correlations.

## Results

On days when a headache occurred, participants in Analysis Population 1 were more likely to nap (OR 1.35; 95% CI 1.23, 1.48; q < 0.001) and to sleep more hours ($\beta$ = 0.07; 95% CI 0.03, 0.11; q = 0.002).

Participants were on average less active on days with headache than on days without headache (19.9% of the day spent inactive vs. 20.4% of the day, respectively; q < 0.001) and took fewer steps (9413 vs. 9656 steps, respectively; q < 0.001).

On days with headache with greater impact, participants were less active (9685 steps on days with 'no impact' of headache vs. 7966 steps on days with 'a great deal of impact' of headache).

There were no differences between users of prescription medication and participants who did not use it in terms of demographics, comorbidities, headache type and intensity, or tracker-based activity levels (data not shown).

## Discussion

The aims of this study were to analyze the impact of headache on passively collected tracker-based activity variables, to explore their associations with QoL in individuals suffering from frequent episodic primary headache, and to understand headache-related treatment preferences and decisions.

Previous studies also showed that the overall perception of QoL, health, and physical activity were significantly lower among migraine sufferers compared with other headache types, emphasizing that migraine burden is, in general, underestimated and poorly managed [28–33].

The particular strengths of this study stem from its practical design, the use of passive data collection from activity trackers, the inclusion of headache sufferers from the wider community, i.e., those who do not usually seek treatment in primary care, and analysis of daily diaries of participant-reported outcomes.

## Conclusion

The findings provide preliminary evidence that activity trackers are useful tools for quantifying headache burden among individuals with frequent headaches in real-world settings.

The data obtained in this study can be used to help develop new metrics that can be used in future research, and to increase understanding of the diversity in self-treatment patterns outside primary care.

## Acknowledgement

*A machine generated summary based on the work of Cerrada, Christian J.; Min, Jae S.; Constantin, Luminita; Hitier, Simon; Igracki Turudic, Iva; Amand-Bourdon, Caroline; Stewart, Andrew; Ebel-Bitoun, Caty; Goadsby, Peter J. 2021 in Pain and Therapy.*

# *Prevalence and Burden of Headache in Children and Adolescents in Austria: A Nationwide Study in a Representative Sample of Pupils Aged 10–18 Years*

DOI: https://doi.org/10.1186/s10194-019-1050-8

## Abstract-Summary

Headache disorders are highly prevalent worldwide, but not so well investigated in children and adolescents as in adults: few studies have included representative nationwide samples.

In a representative sample of children and adolescents in Austria, we estimated the prevalence and attributable burden of headache disorders, including the new diagnostic category of "undifferentiated headache" (UdH) defined as mild headache lasting less than 1 hour.

Within the context of a broader national mental health survey, children and adolescents aged 10–18 years were recruited from purposively selected schools.

Prevalence and attributable burden of all headache, UdH, migraine (definite plus probable), tension-type headache (TTH: definite plus probable) and headache on ≥15 days/month (H15+) were assessed using the Headache-Attributed Restriction, Disability, Social Handicap and Impaired Participation (HARDSHIP) questionnaire for children and adolescents.

The 1-year prevalence of headache was 75.7%, increasing with age and higher in girls (82.1%) than in boys (67.7%; p < 0.001).

UdH, migraine, TTH and H15+ were reported by 26.1%, 24.2%, 21.6% and 3.0% of participants.

HrQoL was reduced for all headache types except UdH. Participants in single parent or patchwork families had a higher probability of migraine (respectively, OR 1.5, p < 0.001; OR 1.5, p < 0.01).

Headache disorders are both very common and highly burdensome in children and adolescents in Austria.

This study contributes to the global atlas of headache disorders in these age groups, and corroborates and adds knowledge of the new yet common and important diagnostic category of UdH. The findings call for action in national and international health policies, and for further epidemiological research.

Extended:

Headache disorders are very common in children and adolescents in Austria, as they are in other countries worldwide.

## Background

Two reviews have estimated the overall mean prevalence of headache in children and adolescents at 54.4–58.4%, with 7.7–9.1% migraine [34, 35].

While a few earlier epidemiological studies had reported unclassifiable headaches, with an average prevalence of about 20% [36–38], most were silent on what appears to be a substantial proportion of affected children and adolescents.

The authors recommended inclusion of UdH in epidemiological studies not only to report the whole spectrum of headache disorders but also to give a full account of headache-attributed burden.

To redress this, and to contribute to the global atlas of headache disorders in children and adolescents, we performed this epidemiological study in a representative national sample of children and adolescents in Austria.

This study assessed prevalence and burden of, and use of acute medication for, headache overall and each of the common specific headache disorders.

## Methods

Burden questions referred to the numbers of days missed from school, leaving school early or with impaired everyday activities due to headache, within the previous 4 weeks.

To participants reporting headache on <15 days/month we applied diagnostic criteria, in order, for definite migraine, definite TTH, probable migraine and probable TTH.

We enquired into gender, school grade, socioeconomic status (SES) of the family, migration background, family constellation and place of residence.

Prevalence estimates (%) for any headache and for each headache type were calculated for the total sample and for each gender and school grade.

In these regression models, all sociodemographic variables (gender, school grade, SES, family constellation, place of residence and migration background) were entered simultaneously, and only main effects were analyzed.

We analyzed impact of headache type on HrQoL, school attendance, school performance and everyday activities, as well as differences regarding medication use, using general linear models.

## Results

Some of these sociodemographic characteristics were more associated with specific headache types.

With regard to overall model fit, the sociodemographic characteristics included in the logistic regression models significantly predicted headache type (in all cases, $p < 0.001$), whereas the explained variance was low (Nagelkerke $R^2 = 0.018$–$0.037$).

Higher school grades were associated with migraine and TTH; older participants had a higher probability of these headache types.

During the preceding 4 weeks, 15.6% of participants with headache missed at least one whole school day because of headache, while 11.7% left school early at least once; 41.9% reported at least 1 day on which they were unable to do other activities they had wanted to.

HrQoL scores were reduced in participants with any headache compared with those with no headache on overall KIDSCREEN-10 score and on scores for self-perception, parent-relations and home life, and school environment (all $p < 0.001$).

## Discussion

Headache prevalence was higher than reported in earlier reviews [34, 35], but comparable to those from a nationwide study in Turkey also applying the Child and Adolescent HARDSHIP questionnaire (bearing in mind that the Turkish study included 6–18-year-olds) [37].

Although the proportions reporting missed daily activities, school days or lessons were lowest in UdH compared with other headache types, they were still noteworthy (27%, 11%, 8%), clear evidence that the burden of headache is substantially underestimated if UdH is not included.

Among children and adolescents, headache prevalence has, with similar consistency, been reported to increase with age [34, 36, 39, 40].

We found the same, overall and for all headache types except for H15+ and, of course, UdH. Children and adolescents with divorced parents and those living with a single parent have earlier reported higher prevalences of headache [41–43].

One study showed a correlation between migration background of the family and prevalence of headache in children [44].

As UdH is expected to be an immature form of headache with a higher prevalence in younger children, the prevalence of UdH might increase with the inclusion of younger children.

## Conclusion

Headache disorders are very common in children and adolescents in Austria, as they are in other countries worldwide.

This study confirms that UdH, a new diagnostic category, is very common in children and adolescents, while supporting the hypothesis that UdH may be a precursor or immature form of migraine or TTH.

Our results contribute to the global atlas of headache disorders in children and adolescents, and reconfirm that headache disorders are highly relevant to health policy.

## Acknowledgement

*A machine generated summary based on the work of Philipp, Julia; Zeiler, Michael; Wöber, Christian; Wagner, Gudrun; Karwautz, Andreas F. K.; Steiner, Timothy J.; Wöber-Bingöl, Çiçek. 2019 in The Journal of Headache and Pain.*

# Epidemiological and Clinical Characteristics of Primary Headaches in Adolescent Population: Is There a Relationship with the Way of Life?

DOI: https://doi.org/10.1007/s13760-019-01220-5

## Abstract-Summary

The headache in the adolescent population is one of the most common conditions that doctors deal with.

The aim of the study was to investigate the frequency, as well as different epidemiological and clinical characteristics, of primary headaches in adolescents.

An epidemiological study was conducted on 1800 adolescents of both sexes based on a questionnaire consisting of 65 questions referring to sociodemographic and clinical characteristics of headaches.

Based on the questionnaire information, the examinees were divided into four groups: adolescents with migraine, tension-type and mixed headache and the fourth group were examinees without headaches.

The most common primary headache is tension-type headache.

There were significantly more headaches among adolescents who had their own computer and who spent more than 2 h using it.

Primary headaches in adolescent population occur frequently and despite numerous studies, they are still not taken seriously enough.

Extended:

Based on the data from the questionnaire, 1800 respondents were divided into four groups: (A) adolescents with tension-type headache characteristics, (B) adolescents with migraine headache characteristics, (C) adolescents with likely mixed migraine and tension-type headaches, and (D) adolescents without headaches.

Based on the aforementioned questionnaire, the data on the incidence of headache in adolescents, the year of commencement of headaches, the distribution of the type of headaches by age and sex, the influence of social status, dietary and other habits of the respondents and sociodemographic characteristics on the occurrence of headaches were obtained.

The most common headaches in adolescence are migraine and tension-type headaches that, according to the ICHD-III-beta, fall into primary headaches [45–47].

## Introduction

Paediatric headaches are one of the most common neurological problems in children and adolescents [48].

The most common headaches in adolescence are migraine and tension-type headaches that, according to the ICHD-III-beta, fall into primary headaches [45–47].

Most studies on primary headaches have been conducted on adults, and adolescence is significantly different from adulthood with regard to psychological, physical and other changes [49].

Epidemiological research conducted in Croatia on 1876 adolescents investigated tension-type and migraine headaches.

The prevalence of headaches in this study was 38.3% for tension-type and 12.8% for migraine headaches [50].

Headaches in children and adolescents differ from adult headaches in their clinical characteristics and risk factors, and they have a very significant psychosocial background.

Stress has been identified as the most common factor, triggering tension-type and migraine headaches, but often it is ignored by the stressful background.

## Methods

The criteria for the inclusion of patients in the research were adolescents of the age group of 13–19 years who duly filled out the required questionnaires and had parental approval to participate in the research.

Based on the data from the questionnaire, 1800 respondents were divided into four groups: (A) adolescents with tension-type headache characteristics, (B) adolescents with migraine headache characteristics, (C) adolescents with likely mixed migraine and tension-type headaches, and (D) adolescents without headaches.

A similar questionnaire was also used in the study of the frequency of primary headaches in adolescents in Zagreb, Croatia [51, 52].

Based on the aforementioned questionnaire, the data on the incidence of headache in adolescents, the year of commencement of headaches, the distribution of the type of headaches by age and sex, the influence of social status, dietary and other habits of the respondents and sociodemographic characteristics on the occurrence of headaches were obtained.

## Results

High school students in 86.8% of respondents have tension-type headaches, with migraine and mixed headaches being more common in vocational schools.

More migraine headaches were found in the sample of pupils walking to school, mixed headaches dominated in those who were riding the bus, and in those who were driven by parents, the highest percentage was with tension-type headaches.

Those who travel more than half an hour to school were most commonly found with migraine, while subjects who travel to school for less than half an hour had tension-type and mixed headaches most frequently.

The respondents who spend less than 2 h daily with a PC, suffered from migraine the most, those who are more than 2 h daily with a PC are most commonly affected by mixed headaches, while those who only occasionally use PCs are most often suffering from tension-type headaches.

## Discussion

Among those with headache, tension-type headaches are most commonly found in elementary school students, while in high school students, migraine and mixed headache were most common.

High school students in 86.8% of respondents had tension-type headaches, and in vocational schools the migraine and mixed headaches were more common.

By dividing headaches into tension-type, migraine and mixed headaches, and comparing with regard to having one's own room, a PC, the way of transportation to school, and the time it takes to get to school, we obtained statistically significant differences.

Tension-type headaches occur more often in respondents who are driven to school by parents or travel to school for less than half an hour, as well in children watching TV for more than 2 h, children who occasionally use a PC, those who never use it, or use it for more than 2 h daily.

## Acknowledgement

*A machine generated summary based on the work of Mlinarevic-Polic, Ines; Kuzman, Zdravko; Aleric, Ivan; Katalinic, Darko; Vcev, Aleksandar; Duranovic, Vlasta. 2019 in Acta Neurologica Belgica.*

# The Epidemiology of Headache Disorders: A Face-to-Face Interview of Participants in HUNT4

DOI: https://doi.org/10.1186/s10194-018-0854-2

## Abstract-Summary

The primary aim of this cross-sectional population-based study was to evaluate the 1-year prevalence of common headache disorders by a face-to-face interview.

There were 71.6% (95% CI 65.7–77.4) who reported headache during the last year, and 18.5% (95% CI 13.5–23.6) had suffered from headache in the same period.

The 1-year prevalence of tension-type headache (TTH) was 43.1% (95% CI 36.7–49.5), of idiopathic stabbing headache 34.1% (27.9–40.2), and of definite migraine 18.1% (95% CI 13.1–23.1).

A total of 7.6% (95% CI 4.0–10.7%) had migraine with coexisting TTH.

Lifetime prevalence of migraine was 32.8% (95% CI 26.7–38.8).

In this population-based cross-sectional headache study performed by a face-to-face interview, the 1-year prevalence of TTH was 43.1% and of idiopathic stabbing headache 34.1%.

Extended:

The 1-year prevalence of tension-type headache was 43.1% (95% CI 36.7–49.5), 40.1% (336.7–49.5) had episodic TTH and 3.0% (05% CI 0.8–5.2) chronic TTH.

The 1-year prevalence of idiopathic stabbing headache was 34.1% (27.9–40.2), whereof 4.7% (95% CI 2.0–7.5) reported attacks with idiopathic stabbing headache at least on a weekly basis.

A total of 33.2% fulfilled the DSM-V diagnosis of insomnia, and 54.3% suffered from chronic musculoskeletal pain during the last year.

A total of 120 participants were 60 years or older.

A total of 18.1% had active migraine (18.1%), whereas the lifetime prevalence of migraine was 32.8%.

## Background

This is, however, time-consuming and costly, therefore relatively few large population-based studies have used a face-to-face interview approach [53–61].

Most large-scale population-based studies have used telephone interview by lay interviewers, a self-administrated questionnaire, or a combination of a screening questionnaire and an interview by a physician [3, 62].

We have done two face-to-face headache interviews in the general population to validate questionnaire-based diagnosis with diagnosis made by a headache specialist [58, 63].

The aim of the present study was to estimate the 1-year prevalence of common headache types by using a face-to-face interview in a random sample of participants in a large-scale population-based study.

## Methods

All inhabitants aged 20 years or more in Nord-Trøndelag county of Norway have been or will be invited to participate in the adult version of HUNT4 in the period between September 2017 and March 2019, whereas adolescents aged 13–19 will be invited to Young-HUNT4.

Individuals living in the town Stjørdal were consecutively invited to participate in HUNT4 in the period between September 4th, 2017 and February 22th 2018.

A random sample of adults living in Stjørdal who had participated in HUNT4 and answered both the first and the second questionnaire received a written invitation.

The invitation letter informed about an initial interview focusing on sleep and pain and to have ambulatory PSG and measurements of pain thresholds performed later.

In the interview, we focused on those who answered "yes" to the question "Have you had a headache during the last 12 months?"

## Results

As demonstrated, 71.6% (95% CI 65.7–77.4) reported that they had had headache during the past year, whereas 18.5% (13.5–23.6) stated that they had suffered from headache.

The 1-year prevalence of tension-type headache was 43.1% (95% CI 36.7–49.5), 40.1% (336.7–49.5) had episodic TTH and 3.0% (05% CI 0.8–5.2) chronic TTH.

The 1-year prevalence of idiopathic stabbing headache was 34.1% (27.9–40.2), whereof 4.7% (95% CI 2.0–7.5) reported attacks with idiopathic stabbing headache at least on a weekly basis.

Headache yesterday was reported by 12.1% (95% CI 7.9–16.3), 15.1% (95% CI 9.4–20.9) among women and 6.3% among men (95% CI 0.8–11.7), and 5.6% (95% CI 2.6–8.6) reported headache during the interview.

**Discussion**

In this population-based cross-sectional study evaluating 1-year prevalence of headache disorders by a face-to-face interview, TTH was most common (43.1%), followed by idiopathic stabbing headache (34.1%) and migraine (18.1%).

Relatively few population-based studies have estimated 1-year prevalence of headache using a face-to-face interview performed by medical doctors with special interest and competence in headache [53–61].

We have previously performed interviews of a random sample of 297 participants of HUNT3, reporting higher 1-year prevalence of TTH (51.9%), but almost similar prevalence of idiopathic stabbing headache (35.0%) and migraine (17.2%) [58].

With a high proportion of elderly participants, cervicogenic headache was common with a total 1-year prevalence of 3.9%.

The present study did not estimate the 1-year prevalence of very rare headache diagnoses very precisely.

**Conclusions**

In this cross-sectional study evaluating 1-year prevalence of headache by a face-to-face interview, 43.1% had TTH, and 34.1% idiopathic stabbing headache.

A total of 18.1% had active migraine (18.1%), whereas the lifetime prevalence of migraine was 32.8%.

**Acknowledgement**

*A machine generated summary based on the work of Hagen, Knut; Åsberg, Anders Nikolai; Uhlig, Benjamin L.; Tronvik, Erling; Brenner, Eiliv; Stjern, Marit; Helde, Grethe; Gravdahl, Gøril Bruvik; Sand, Trond. 2018 in The Journal of Headache and Pain.*

## *Proposing a Measurement Model of REBT and Applying it to the Assessment of Well-Being and Happiness in Patients with Tension-Type Headaches*

DOI: https://doi.org/10.1007/s10942-021-00413-3

**Abstract-Summary**

The current research investigates how irrational cognitions, according to the theory of Rational Emotive Behaviour Therapy (tREBT), are associated with DAS.

We determine how tREBT predicts well-being and happiness outcomes of people experiencing tension-type headaches through DAS.

This research aims to advance understanding of the psychological factors associated with tension-type headaches, and our measurement model of tREBT may help reverse declining research interest.

Across two studies, using physicians and family members as third-party assessors of patients with tension-type headaches, we use HMLP to show how irrational cognitions are expressed through DAS in the prediction of patient well-being and happiness.

Our results provide a new understanding of cognitions associated with tREBT, a measurement model of tREBT, and we identify cognitions associated with tension-type headaches.

We conclude that learning and cognitive processes related to the development and maintenance of irrational beliefs are important in the prediction of the severity of tension-type headaches and their well-being outcomes.

Extended:

Across two studies, we apply the theory of Rational Emotive behaviour Therapy (tREBT; Ellis, 64) to predict third-party rated well-being and happiness in people suffering from tension-type headaches.

These results indicate the relationship between low rationality and well-being is fully expressed through DAS and support H2.

## Introduction

Across two studies, we apply the theory of Rational Emotive behaviour Therapy (tREBT; Ellis, 64) to predict third-party rated well-being and happiness in people suffering from tension-type headaches.

Using these constructs, HMLP provides empirically tested paths from low sensation seeking to low rationality and therefore can explain the cognitive processes underlying tREBT.

We test: HMLP pathways from low sensation seeking to low rationality will predict low well-being and happiness of people experiencing tension-type headaches (excluding paths through low conscientiousness).

Consistent therefore with tREBT and what is known about psychological factors associated with tension-type headaches (as introduced previously), we propose: Low rationality will predict low well-being and happiness of people experiencing tension-type headaches through DAS.

In Study 2, we use tREBT (measured as HMLP) to predict a close family members' third-party ratings of well-being and happiness in people experiencing tension-type headaches.

## Study 1: Predicting Physician Ratings of Well-Being in People Experiencing Tension-Type Headaches

We then chose five questions which provided (a) a good correlation with all eight scales of the SF–36 (lowest correlation was with physical role, $r = 0.22$, $p < 0.01$ and highest correlation was with vitality was $r = 0.56$, $p < 0.001$) and (b) a very high correlation with mental health ($r = 0.80$, $p < 0.001$) which we regarded as a key component of well-being.

HADS consists of 14 items, seven for depression and seven for anxiety subscales.

An example item for the anxiety subscale is "I feel tense and wound up" and for the depression subscale "I still enjoy the things I used to enjoy".

The internal consistency of the HADS in Montazeri and others [64] was reported as 0.78 for anxiety and 0.86 for depression.

## Results

Mastery and rationality are significantly negatively correlated with low physician rating of well-being.

Low rationality is highly correlated with DAS.

Paths from low sensation seeking to low rationality are all significant, except from low deep learning to low conscientiousness and from low conscientiousness to low rationality.

H1a was rejected and H1b was supported with a significant indirect effect from low sensation seeking to well-being ($p < 0.05$) and with good goodness of fit indices ($\chi^2 = 2.35$, df = 6, p = 0.89; Bollen-Stine bootstrap: p = 0.91; GFI = 0.99; AGFI = 0.96; CFI = 1.00; RMSEA = 0.00).

The direct path from low rationality to well-being is now no longer significant.

## [Section 4]

Third-party ratings of happiness and well-being were collected from an attending close family member (usually sister, brother or mother) or occasional friend who accompanied the patient.

Happiness Measure (Eysenck happiness questionnaire; Eysenck [65]).

This measure includes 39 items with a four-point response category was used (1 = very low to 4 = very high).

The happiness measure was adapted for third-party ratings.

## Results

With significant indirect pathways from low sensation seeking to low happiness ($p < 0.01$) and good goodness of fit ($\chi^2 = 37.73$ (df = 19) p = 0.006; Bollen-Stine bootstrap p = 0.07; GFI = 0.94; AGFI = 0.86; CFI = 0.97; RMSEA = 0.09) results provide support for H2.

Despite a significant relationship between low rationality and low well-being, and significant overall indirect effects from low sensation seeking to low well-being ($p < 0.01$), there was once again poor support for H1a as the path from low deep learning through low conscientiousness to low rationality was not significant ($\chi^2 = 26.29$ (df = 13) p = 0.02; Bollen-Stine bootstrap p = 0.04; GFI = 0.95; AGFI = 0.86; CFI = 0.96; RMSEA = 0.09).

## Discussion

Our results support Ellis' [66] central propositions associated with tREBT by empirically identifying mechanisms from undirected initial impulses to low rationality as important predictors of DAS and tension-type headaches.

Our results identify important psychological factors related to improving health outcomes of people with tension-type headaches.

General support for H1b provides evidence of indirect paths from sensation seeking to low rationality and on to outcomes of tension-type headaches associated with well-being and happiness.

From a "failed" mechanism of functional learning in which initial impulses of low sensation seeking (i.e. low curiosity and exploration) are related to low higher order cognitions culminating in low rationality and poor outcomes associated with tension-type headaches.

Our results emphasize the usefulness of tREBT to the understanding of outcomes associated with tension-type headaches and provide suggestions for intervention.

**Acknowledgement**
*A machine generated summary based on the work of Izadikhah, Zahra; Jackson, Chris J.; Mohammadi, Zahra; Najafi, Mohammad Reza. 2021 in Journal of Rational-Emotive & Cognitive-Behavior Therapy.*

## *Mechanisms*

Machine generated keywords: tth, muscle, tth migraine, pressure pain, value, serum, trigger point, pericranial, peripheral, tensiontype headache, tenderness, migraine, pressure, sensitization, emotional.

## *Tension-Type Headache*

DOI: https://doi.org/10.1038/s41572-021-00257-2

**Abstract-Summary**
Pharmacological therapy is the mainstay of clinical management and can be divided into acute and preventive treatments.

Simple analgesics have evidence-based effectiveness and are widely regarded as first-line medications for the acute treatment of TTH.

Preventive treatment should be considered in individuals with frequent episodic and chronic TTH, and if simple analgesics are ineffective, poorly tolerated or contraindicated.

Recommended preventive treatments include amitriptyline, venlafaxine and mirtazapine, as well as some selected non-pharmacological therapies.

**Introduction**
A. Frequency: at least 10 headache episodes occurring on average <1 day/month (that is, <12 days/year) B. Duration: 30 min to 7 days frequent ETTH Meeting the following criteria A and B, in addition to criteria C–E, below.

A. Frequency: at least 10 headache episodes occurring on average 1–14 days/month for >3 months ($\geq$12 and <180 days/year) B. Duration: 30 min to 7 days CTTH Meeting the following criteria A and B, in addition to criteria C–E, below.

A. Frequency: headache occurring on $\geq$15 days/month on average for >3 months ($\geq$180 days/year) B. Duration: hours to days, or unremitting C. At least two of the following four characteristics: 1.

Neither moderate or severe nausea nor vomiting E. Not better accounted for by another ICHD-3 diagnosis. CTTH, chronic tension-type headache; ETTH, episodic tension-type headache; ICHD-3, International Classification of Headache Disorders, 3rd edition.

## Epidemiology

The estimated 1-year prevalence of TTH in population studies was 10.8% in China [67], 36.1% in Jordan [68], 38.3% in the USA [69], ~80% in European studies and 86.6% in Denmark [53, 70].

One study in rural Tanzania found a very low prevalence for TTH of 0.04% in individuals 0–10 years of age and 1.3% in people 11–20 years of age [71].

The 2017 GBD study found a global prevalence of TTH in individuals aged 5–9, 10–14 and 15–19 of 12.1%, 35.7% and 35.8% in women/girls and 11.7%, 34.5%, and 34.0% in men/boys, respectively [72].

In a Danish study, poor prognosis of TTH (defined as ≥180 days with TTH per year at follow-up due either to increased frequency from ETTH at baseline into CTTH or to persistent CTTH) was associated with baseline CTTH, coexisting migraine, being unmarried and sleeping problems [73].

One population-based study found that 83% of people with migraine within the past year also had TTH [53].

## Mechanisms/Pathophysiology

A few studies have reported increased levels of substances involved in pain and inflammation, such as IL-6, bradykinin and serotonin in the blood and myofascial trigger points of patients with TTH [74, 75].

These findings could be explained by the vasodilator activity of CGRP and NO, or by impaired sympathetic function; however, although increased NO levels have been found in patients with CTTH, further studies are needed to clarify the role of CGRP and the sympathetic system in TTH pathophysiology [76].

Pain perception studies support the presence of hyperalgesia (increased sensitivity to painful stimuli) and allodynia (pain elicited by stimuli that are normally not painful) in patients with frequent ETTH or CTTH [77–83].

In patients with TTH and migraine, the presence of back pain was associated with increased central sensitization and muscular tenderness compared with individuals without headache [77].

Fibromyalgia is also an important comorbidity of TTH, with a twofold increased prevalence in patients with CTTH compared with those with ETTH, implying a shared mechanism between the two conditions, such as central sensitization [84].

## Diagnosis, Screening and Prevention

TTH should be suspected in any individual who reports recurrent headache of mild or moderate intensity.

Diagnostic headache diaries are the best available assessment tool for TTH and can be used to support diagnosis and guide clinical decision-making.

The benefits of headache diaries are multifold and include better differentiation of ETTH from CTTH compared with clinical evaluation alone.

A wide range of headache disorders can mimic the clinical features of TTH [85]; careful exclusion of these disorders relies on a thorough review of medical history and an adequate physical examination.

It is very common for individuals with chronic migraine to experience at least some headache days with clinical features that fulfil the diagnostic criteria for TTH.

No biomarkers can differentiate between TTH, migraine and other headache disorders, therefore, clinicians can benefit from the use of diagnostic headache diaries, in which clinical features are prospectively recorded.

## Management

An observational clinic-based study found that patients using prophylactic amitriptyline for TTH had higher headache frequency, higher headache burden, worse sleep quality and more severe depression than those who did not receive medicinal prevention, because patients with these particular features considered themselves to benefit more [86].

In those with MOH and TTH, the key elements of management may include patient education and cognitive behavioural approaches both to educate the patient and to help manage anxiety, management of risk factors for MOH (such as high frequency of headache attacks, comorbidity with anxiety disorders and depression, and the use of specific medications for acute treatment) [87], withdrawal of overused medications and prophylactic treatment along with management of the potential comorbidities [88, 89].

There is moderate evidence that myofascial trigger point dry needling is effective in patients with chronic TTH (in terms of a reduction in headache intensity, frequency and duration, or improvement in functional and sensory outcomes) [90, 91].

## Quality of Life

In a population study from Denmark, using the SF-12 survey, both PCS and MCS scores were lower for individuals with coexistent headache (TTH and migraine), followed by pure TTH and pure migraine than for those without headache when adjusted for age, sex and education level [92].

Patients with CTTH had numerically lower SF-36 scores in six out of eight domains than those with migraine, indicating worse HRQOL, in a large study in an outpatient tertiary headache clinic in Taiwan [93].

In a small study with 25 patients with CTTH referred from a neurology clinic, anxiety had a mediating effect and depression had a modulating effect between headache frequency and intensity, and reduced QOL (mental health and social functioning) measured with SF-36 (ref [94]).

In another small study of 89 patients with TTH, depression scores positively correlated with poor QOL in patients with CTTH.

## Outlook

Katie MacDonald, Alliance for Headache Disorders Advocacy Future epidemiological studies should use rigorous methodology, and better and uniform definitions of TTH, including the use of ICHD criteria.

Epidemiological studies should also quantify indirect consequences of TTH to provide accurate total cost estimates, which may include effect on family life (for example, partner relationships and childcare) and career potential (such as sick days and productivity losses at work).

Further research, including larger samples of patients with TTH, is also needed to better elucidate the role of vascular inputs in TTH pathophysiology.

Similar to migraine, there is a growing urge to identify reliable serum and clinical biomarkers useful to diagnose primary headaches including TTH, monitor their activity and determine the response to treatment.

Prospective daily headache diary studies in patients with TTH are needed for better characterization of the disease and identification of clinical biomarkers, and would also be valuable in ascertaining how often patients with CTTH have a secondary diagnosis of MOH.

**Acknowledgement**
*A machine generated summary based on the work of Ashina, Sait; Mitsikostas, Dimos D.; Lee, Mi Ji; Yamani, Nooshin; Wang, Shuu-Jiun; Messina, Roberta; Ashina, Håkan; Buse, Dawn C.; Pozo-Rosich, Patricia; Jensen, Rigmor H.; Diener, Hans-Christoph; Lipton, Richard B. 2021 in Nature Reviews Disease Primers.*

# *Current Understanding of the Pathophysiology and Approach to Tension-Type Headache*

DOI: https://doi.org/10.1007/s11910-021-01138-7

## Abstract-Summary
Description of headache dates back thousands of years, and to date, tension-type headache (TTH) remains the most common form of headache.

We will review the history and current understanding of the pathophysiology of TTH and discuss the recommended clinical evaluation and management for this syndrome.

Despite being the most prevalent headache disorder, TTH pathophysiology remains poorly understood.

Patients with TTH tend to have muscles that are harder, more tender to palpation, and may have more frequent trigger points of tenderness than patients without headache.

An approach to TTH has been outlined including historical context, evolution over time, and the best evidence regarding our current understanding of the complex pathophysiology and treatment of this disease.

## Introduction and Historical Background
TTH was historically attributed to emotional conflict/anxiety precipitating sustained contraction of skeletal muscles in the head and neck with resultant head pain [95, 96].

Given sustained muscle contraction as a defining feature, Langemark and Olesen conducted a blinded, controlled study that demonstrated increased pericranial muscle tenderness to manual palpation in patients with muscle contraction headache [97].

New classification and diagnostic criteria were published by the International Headache Society, adopting the term tension-type headache (TTH) with division based on frequency (episodic and chronic forms) as well as the presence or absence of an associated disorder of the pericranial muscles.

The long-accepted concept of sustained muscle contraction as a defining feature of TTH was called into question after multiple EMG studies yielded conflicting results.

The International Classification of Headache Disorders, 2nd edition retained the distinction of with or without pericranial tenderness but removed criteria of increased EMG activity of pericranial muscles.

## Epidemiology

TTH is the most common headache disorder, with a reported global annual prevalence of 26–38% [1, 2, 98] or nearly 2 billion people with TTH [1].

TTH was the third most prevalent disorder when hundreds of disorders were assessed by the Global Burden of Disease study in 2016 [1].

The annual prevalence of chronic TTH has been most consistently reported as 2–3% [69, 99, 100].

In one study of patients with episodic TTH, lost workdays were reported in 8.3% of patients, with reduced effectiveness at work, home, or school in 43.6% of patients [69].

In chronic TTH, the individual impact is higher, with 11.8% of patients reporting lost workdays, missing an annual average of 27.4 days each [69].

In the Global Burden of Disease study, TTH burden was calculated by considering prevalence, average time with headache, and suspected severity of disability from disease and then reported as disability-adjusted-life-years.

## Pathophysiology

Patients who had developed chronic TTH over the course of the study demonstrated decreased pain detection thresholds in follow-up, whereas patients who developed frequent episodic TTH demonstrated increased pericranial muscle tenderness, but no change in their pain detection threshold [101].

An effort to understand this increased tenderness and lowered pain threshold has led to observations that support not only the role of peripheral nociception but a possible role of central modulation, with studies of chronic TTH patients demonstrating decreased pressure pain thresholds at sites distant from the pericranial region [82, 102–105].

It has been proposed that the reduced pain threshold and tenderness experienced by chronic TTH patients may be related not only to peripheral sensitization at the level of the myofascial nociceptors, but also to sensitization of second order neurons at the level of the spinal trigeminal nucleus and dorsal horn, or even sensitization of supraspinal structures such as the somatosensory cortex, thalamus, limbic system, or motor cortex [19].

**Diagnosis and Differential Diagnosis**

Migraine has many overlapping diagnostic criteria with TTH, with potential differentiating factors including possible presence of aura (not present in all patients with migraine); aggravation by routine physical activity; and more frequent accompanying symptoms including nausea, vomiting, photophobia, phonophobia, and osmophobia.

Osmophobia appears to be more specific for migraine than photophobia or phonophobia alone and, therefore, can be a distinguishing feature when present [106].

The diagnostic criteria for chronic migraine include the presence of possible tension-type-like headaches as long as the majority of headache days have features consistent with migraine [107].

**History, Examination, and Evaluation**

Additional evaluation is required for any red flags in the headache history, such as an onset of headache after age 50, rapid rise to peak of pain (thunderclap), progressively worsening headache, systemic symptoms (fever/chills, night sweats), unintentional weight loss, focal neurologic symptoms, and exacerbation by position (lying down or standing up) or Valsalva maneuver.

Frequency of acute analgesic use is also an important factor to consider in assessment of TTH, as medication-overuse headache may be concomitantly diagnosed.

Medication-overuse headache is defined as taking any combination of pain medicines (triptan, opioid, combination-analgesics, or multiple analgesics) more than 9 days per month.

When acute analgesics are being overused, pre-existing TTH could be exacerbated, and a subsequent decrease in analgesic use may improve headache.

Examination in the setting of suspected TTH should additionally include manual palpation of the pericranial muscles to assess for tenderness.

While palpating pericranial muscles, evaluation for tender points should also be performed.

**Treatment of TTH**

In a Cochrane review on the possible use of selective serotonin reuptake inhibitors (SSRIs) and serotonin-norepinephrine reuptake inhibitors (SNRIs) for prevention of TTH, these antidepressants were found to demonstrate similar reductions in headache frequency to amitriptyline; however, this reduction was not clearly better than placebo [108].

Mirtazapine 15–30 mg daily demonstrated a reduced area under the headache curve of 34% including reduction in headache frequency, duration and intensity when compared to placebo in a randomized double-blind placebo-controlled trial [109].

One study randomized patients with TTH to receive either an antidepressant (amitriptyline at 50–100 mg daily or nortriptyline at 50–75 mg daily), stress management, a combination of antidepressant plus stress management, or placebo.

Within the non-pharmacologic treatments, EMG-guided biofeedback may be considered a first-line option based on meta-analysis data which demonstrated decreased headache frequency and less analgesic medication use [110].

**Prognosis**

They examined 146 patients with TTH, including frequent episodic TTH (they defined as 15–179 headache days per year) and chronic TTH (defined as $\geq 180$ headache days per year) and found that 45% of patients improved by follow-up to infrequent TTH (1–14 headache days per year) or no headache days (remission).

A subset of patients (16%) had a poor outcome at follow-up ($\geq 180$ headache days per year).

Predictive factors for poor outcome were chronic TTH at baseline, coexisting migraine, not being married, and sleeping difficulty.

**Conclusion**

TTH is the most prevalent headache disorder with significant societal burden.

Diagnosis is clinical, based on headache characteristics and frequency, but TTH may present similarly to many other types of headache.

Given rather non-specific features, detailed history and examination should be performed to rule out alternative causes of headache.

Increased pericranial muscle tenderness and a decreased pressure pain threshold have been consistently observed in patients with chronic TTH.

**Acknowledgement**

*A machine generated summary based on the work of Steel, Stephanie J.; Robertson, Carrie E.; Whealy, Mark A. 2021 in Current Neurology and Neuroscience Reports.*


# *Understanding the Interaction Between Clinical, Emotional and Psychophysical Outcomes Underlying Tension-Type Headache: A Network Analysis Approach*

DOI: https://doi.org/10.1007/s00415-022-11039-5


**Abstract-Summary**

The current study aimed to quantify potential multivariate relationships between headache-related, psychophysical, psychological and health-related variables in patients with TTH using network analysis.

Demographic (age, height, weight), headache-related (intensity, frequency, duration, and headache-related disability), psychological and emotional (Hospital Anxiety and Depression Scale, Pittsburgh Sleep Quality Index), psycho-physical (pressure pain thresholds [PPTs] and myofascial trigger points) and health-related variables (SF-36 questionnaire) were collected in 169 TTH patients.

Network connectivity analysis was unsupervised conducted to quantify the adjusted correlations between the modelled variables and to assess their centrality indices (i.e., the connectivity with other symptoms in the network and the importance in the modelled network).

The connectivity network showed local associations between psychophysical and headache-related variables.

This is the first study applying a network analysis to understand the connections between headache-related, psychophysical, psychological and health-related variables in TTH.

Current findings support a model on how the variables are connected, albeit in separate clusters.

Extended:

These findings support that management of patients with TTH should include multimodal therapeutic approaches targeting all the aspects identified in the clusters.

## Introduction

Supporting these associations, some previous studies have reported different interactions and mediation effects between headache features, emotional/psychological, and psychophysical variables in people with TTH [111, 112].

Network analysis can provide a method to identify the most important variables in the associated complex network, which could be used to potentially design better therapeutic strategies [113].

From a network perspective, TTH can be viewed as a complex condition sustained by mutual interactions between clinical, emotional/psychological, and physiological systems.

Network analysis has previously been used to better understand the complexity of chronic pain syndromes [114, 115], but so far, no study has applied network analysis in TTH research.

The main objectives of the present study were: (1) to apply a network connectivity analysis including demographic, clinical, emotional/psychological and psychophysical variables in individuals with TTH; and (2) to illustrate the potential of a network analysis for understanding underlying features of TTH, generating new research questions, and improving options for developing more targeted treatment strategies.

## Methods

After conducting an exploratory data analysis on the dataset, missing values were found in 25 variables divided into 5 attributes: sociodemographic (sex, age); psychological/emotional (anxiety, depression, sleep quality, mental health, emotional role); headache-related (years with pain, disability, and headache intensity, duration and frequency); health-related quality of life (physical and social function, physical role, general health, vitality and bodily pain) and psycho-physical (active and latents TrPs and PPTs).

Nodes with high strength centrality could be potentially good therapeutic targets since a change in their value can have a strong and direct influence on the other nodes in the network without considering the mediating role of other nodes [116].

Closeness centrality, which is defined as the inverse sum of the distances of the shortest paths (inverse of the absolute value of the edge's weight) of the target node from all other nodes in the network [116].

## Results

The variability associated with the weight of each edge is shown graphically in Suppl.

Of the utility of this figure, the non-overlap of the 95% CI of the edge between PPTs at the hand and tibialis anterior locations (nodes 11 and 12) with the 95% CI of the edge between headache frequency and emotional burden due to headache disability (nodes 6 and 13) indicates that the strength of the former is greater than the latter.

Other nodes with higher centrality were vitality (strength centrality) or headache intensity (closeness and betweeness centrality centralities).

## Discussion

This study applied network connectivity analysis to understand the multivariate interaction between headache-related, psychological, health-related or psycho-physical variables in TTH.

Consistent with modern theories on TTH features, the identified network supports a complex model where headache-related, psychological, health-related, and psycho-physical variables interact but also grouped in different clusters.

Mood disorders seem to play a key role in TTH, so if clinicians want to influence other variables, e.g., those related to headache or quality of life, the best variable to focus treatment on would be depressive levels.

The results further reinforce theories suggesting that management of patients with TTH should include multimodal therapeutic approaches targeting headache-related pain and function (i.e., physical therapy approaches), psychological aspects (i.e., cognitive behavior, relaxation interventions), health-related (i.e., exercise programs) and also psychophysical pain mechanisms (i.e., pain neuroscience education programs) [117].

## Conclusion

The application of network connectivity analysis in a sample of patients with TTH revealed a model where headache-related, psychological, health-related, and psycho-physical variables interact but grouped in different clusters, with small associations between them.

These findings support that management of patients with TTH should include multimodal therapeutic approaches targeting all the aspects identified in the clusters.

## Acknowledgement

*A machine generated summary based on the work of Fernández-de-las-Peñas, César; Palacios-Ceña, María; Valera-Calero, Juan A.; Cuadrado, Maria L.; Guerrero-Peral, Angel; Pareja, Juan A.; Arendt-Nielsen, Lars; Varol, Umut. 2022 in Journal of Neurology.*

# Brain Excitability in Tension-Type Headache: A Separate Entity from Migraine?

DOI: https://doi.org/10.1007/s11916-020-00916-1

## Abstract-Summary

There has been many studies linked migraine to a brain excitability disorder.

This review summarized earlier studies on brain excitability of TTH and discuss if TTH is a separate clinical entity from migraine as suggested by the diagnostic criteria.

Studies on brain excitability of TTH yielded negative findings or a common change shared with migraine.

Future studies using strict diagnostic criteria to avoid the unwanted interference from migraine comorbidity may help decipher the "true" pathophysiology of TTH, which may pave the way to a TTH-specific brain signature and treatment.

## Introduction

Tension-type headache (TTH) is the most common primary headache worldwide.

The global age-standardized prevalence for TTH is 26.1% overall, 30.8% for women, and 21.4% for men, which is higher than migraine, the other common form of primary headache (14.4% overall; 18.9% for women and 9.8% for men) [1].

Common migraine-associated symptoms, including nausea and vomiting, are usually absent in TTH, although mild photo- or phonophobia may be present [107].

TTH, like migraine, can evolve from its episodic form to a chronic condition (chronic TTH, defined as $\geq 15$ headache days/month) [118, 119].

## Pathophysiology of TTH: Peripheral or Central?

Among the various approaches used to explore the mechanisms of TTH, pertinent studies have mainly focused on two areas: peripheral factors (e.g., electromyography (EMG)) and brain excitability (e.g., brainstem reflexes, electroencephalography (EEG), evoked potential (EP), and event-related potential (ERP) studies).

The peripheral mechanism of TTH remains inconclusive because of the heterogeneous findings obtained from earlier EMG studies.

Studies in the central mechanism or brain excitability of TTH have revealed a relatively congruent finding.

We evaluate earlier data on the brain excitability change in patients with episodic and chronic TTH, discuss the caveat of these studies, and summarize our recent findings obtained from magnetoencephalography (MEG).

## Brain Excitability Studies in TTH

As for the R3 response, a study in patients with chronic TTH and CM showed a reduced threshold to elicit R3 response of BR in both headache patients (vs. controls), but no difference between chronic TTH and CM was observed [120].

An earlier EEG study compared photic driving responses by using discriminant analysis and artificial neural network classifiers showed an increased amplitude of the first harmonic response to flash stimulation at 15–27 Hz in patients with TTH (n = 64) and migraine without aura (n = 64) vs. controls (n = 51) [121].

The other VEP study investigated the low-frequency VEP habituation and the arousal-related personality trait in patients with migraine (n = 22), episodic TTH (n = 13), chronic TTH (n = 20), and controls (n = 26) [122].

**Scope for the Future**

In view of somatosensory cortex excitability, our study [123] has provided evidence that TTH and migraine are different clinical entities.

Our companion brain MRI study on the "strict-criteria" TTH [124] also showed TTH and migraine are separate headache disorders with different characteristics in relation to gray matter changes.

In line, some comparative studies also showed that patients with TTH and those with migraine differed in pressure pain threshold [125], habituation of blink reflex [126], laser-evoked potentials [127], and temporal discrimination thresholds [128].

Most of the earlier studies in TTH did not find any significant brain excitability change.

These findings suggest that patients with TTH might be inherent with an impaired central inhibition in pathophysiology rather than an excitability change secondary to allostatic load caused by the headache.

To confirm the causal relationship of the aberrant brain excitability in TTH pathophysiology, future longitudinal studies are mandatory.

**Conclusions**

Most earlier studies on brain excitability of TTH yielded negative findings or a common change shared with migraine.

Our recent study on patients with strict-criteria TTH has demonstrated a TTH-specific brain excitability change that can be distinguished from migraine and controls.

We expect more longitudinal studies using the strict-criteria to avoid migraine comorbidity can disentangle TTH-migraine interrelationship and pave the way to TTH-specific brain signature and treatment.

**Acknowledgement**

*A machine generated summary based on the work of Chen, Wei-Ta; Hsiao, Fu-Jung; Wang, Shuu-Jiun. 2020 in Current Pain and Headache Reports.*

## *Pressure Pain Thresholds over the Cranio-Cervical Region in Headache: A Systematic Review and Meta-Analysis*

DOI: https://doi.org/10.1186/s10194-018-0833-7

**Abstract-Summary**

A systematic review was conducted to assess the current scientific literature describing pressure pain threshold (PPT) values over the cranio-cervical region in patients with migraine, tension-type headache (TTH), and cervicogenic headache (CeH).

The search strategy included the following keywords: migraine, TTH, CeH, PPT and algometry.

Mean PPT values of several sites measured in the cranio-cervical region in patients with migraine, chronic TTH and CeH scored lower values compared to controls.

The trapezius muscle (midpoint between vertebrae C7 and acromion) was the most frequently targeted site and showed significantly lower PPT values in adults with migraine (pooled standardized mean difference kPa: 1.26 [95% CI −1.71, −0.81]) and chronic TTH (pooled standardized mean difference kPa: −2.00 [95% CI −2.93, −1.08]).

Most studies found no association between PPT values and headache characteristics such as frequency, duration or intensity.

Further standardization of PPT measurement in the cranio-cervical region is recommended.

Extended:

Most studies found no significant association of headache characteristics (frequency, intensity, duration) with PPT values within the different types of headache.

## Review

PPT represent the sensitivity of tissues and depending on the site of measurement (cervico-cephalic and/or extra-cervico-cephalic region) where these PPT are decreased, they are supposed to reflect signs of sensitization of the trigemino-cervical nucleus caudalis [120, 129, 130].

People with headache can be expected to have lower PPT values in the cranio-cervical region.

To date, no aggregated evidence on the association between PPT values in the cranio-cervical region and headache is available.

Physical- and manual therapy interventions are predominantly directed to the cranio-cervical region in order to reduce headaches [131].

Providing clinicians who administer such interventions with reference PPT values in the cranio-cervical region may assist them in their evaluation of PPT values.

The question of this review is whether PPT values in the cranio-cervical region in participants with migraine, TTH and CeH are decreased compared to healthy controls.

## Methods

This limitation of the search period was to ensure the inclusion of studies that were published after the publication of the updated and more detailed classification of headaches, especially TTH (ICHD II, 2004).

Two reviewers (RC, WDH) independently screened the titles and abstracts of the citations generated by the literature search.

The following inclusion criteria were applied to decide if papers would be included for further evaluation: (a) headaches were classified as migraine, TTH or CeH, (b) pain threshold measurements (algometry) were applied in the cranio-cervical region, (c) scores on PPT were available, (d) research involved humans, (e) were case-control studies, and (f) research was published after 2004.

These five selected criteria items were, independently, scored by two reviewers (RC, WD) as either "positive", "negative" or "unclear", in case an item was inadequately reported upon.

In case pooling of data was considered we assessed the following sources: classification of headache, age, site of measurement, and measurement units.

## Results

Mean PPT scores of a combination of measurements on the splenius muscle, trapezius muscle, temporalis muscle, and index finger in migraine were described in two studies by Engstrom and others in which one study reported significant lower values between not sleep-related migraine versus controls (kPa: 519, sd 125 vs kPa: 661, sd 249, p = 0.05, 16, 18).

Three studies reported PPT values in the cranio-cervical region in participants with CeH. Zito and others found no between-group differences in PPT scores at the C2–3 zygapophyseal joint, but significantly lower PPTs in the area over the transverse process of C4 in comparison to the control group (p 0.05) [132].

Participants with chronic TTH show significant lower PPT values at three different sites in the neck region (1) the suboccipital muscle insertions, (2).

## Discussion

It is noteworthy that in four out of five studies the suboccipital region reported significantly lower PPT in chronic TTH and migraine.

This limitation can be considered as a weakness of this study because this paper covers not all available evidence on PPT measurement over the cranio-cervical region.

The validity of the reported results on PPT values in the selected studies therefore depends partly on the reliability of measurement.

Although the performance of the PPT measurement was comparable across the studies there was a great variety of sites measured in the cranio-cervical region.

Some studies reported sum scores, i.e. average mean scores of the PPT of multiple sites in the cranio-cervical region or cranio-cervical sites in combination with extra-cephalic sites.

All studies show lower, but not in all studies significantly lower, PPT values in the cranio-cervical region in patients with headache versus controls.

## Conclusion

We conclude that the PPT values of the trapezius muscle are significantly lower in migraine and chronic TTH compared to controls.

No significant associations were reported between PPT values in the cranio-cervical sites and headache characteristics such as frequency, duration or intensity.

The increased sensitivity of cranio-cervical sites supports the neurophysiological model of sensitization in migraine and chronic TTH.

## Acknowledgement

*A machine generated summary based on the work of Castien, René F.; van der Wouden, Johannes C.; De Hertogh, Willem. 2018 in The Journal of Headache and Pain.*

# Myofascial Trigger Points in Migraine and Tension-Type Headache

DOI: https://doi.org/10.1186/s10194-018-0913-8

## Abstract-Summary

It has been suggested that myofascial trigger points take part in chronic pain conditions including primary headache disorders.

The aim of this narrative review is to present an overview of the current imaging modalities used for the detection of myofascial trigger points and to review studies of myofascial trigger points in migraine and tension-type headache.

Different modalities have been used to assess myofascial trigger points including ultrasound, microdialysis, electromyography, infrared thermography, and magnetic resonance imaging.

Active myofascial trigger points are prevalent in migraine patients.

Whether myofascial trigger points contribute to an increased migraine burden in terms of frequency and intensity is unclear.

Active myofascial trigger points are prevalent in tension-type headache coherent with the hypothesis that peripheral mechanisms are involved in the pathophysiology of this headache disorder.

Active myofascial trigger points in pericranial muscles in tension-type headache patients are correlated with generalized lower pain pressure thresholds indicating they may contribute to a central sensitization.

The number of active myofascial trigger points is higher in adults compared with adolescents regardless of no significant association with headache parameters.

Myofascial trigger points are prevalent in both migraine and tension-type headache, but the role they play in the pathophysiology of each disorder and to which degree is unclarified.

Extended:

The aim of this narrative review is to present an up-to-date overview on MTrPs in general and then in migraine and TTH, respectively.

## Background

Tenderness in pericranial myofascial tissue is correlated with the intensity and frequency of headache in TTH [133–140], and studies show increased muscle stiffness in TTH patients [135, 136].

Myofascial structures may be associated with TTH pathophysiology.

While attempts have been made to visualize MTrPs [137], the gold standard for detection of MTrPs has been unchanged since the 1950s [137] and remains to be by way of palpation of the affected muscles.

MTrPs have come to play a central role in the diagnosis and treatment of myofascial pain syndrome [138].

MTrPs have been proposed to take part in primary headache disorders and other chronic pain conditions [139].

The aim of this narrative review is to present an up-to-date overview on MTrPs in general and then in migraine and TTH, respectively.

**Review**

Subjects with active MTrPs in the trapezius muscle showed increased concentrations of all substances compared to the other groups.

Studies show that there is a significantly higher prevalence of active MTrPs in migraine patients compared to healthy controls [140–142].

Studies show that active MTrPs are correlated with the intensity, duration and frequency of headache episodes in TTH [143, 144].

In a different study, active MTrPs in the right upper trapezius muscle and left sternocleidomastoid muscle was correlated with a greater headache intensity and duration [145].

Chronic TTH patients with active MTrPs in the analyzed muscles had a greater forward head position than those subjects only with latent MTrPs [143, 145].

The same group found that chronic TTH patients with bilateral active MTrPs in the trapezius muscles have a significantly lower pain pressure threshold compared to patients with only unilateral active MTrPs [146].

**Discussion**

Active MTrPs affect the electrical activity at rest and during muscle contraction in EMG studies [147–150].

Although there are currently no studies investigating if it is possible to identify MTrPs with ultrasound without prior manual palpation.

Future studies should investigate if ultrasound is comparable with manual palpation in identifying MTrPs.

Studies show a high occurrence of active and latent MTrPs [140, 141, 151–153] and correlation between neck mobility and MTrPs in migraine patients [141, 142, 152, 153].

Palpation of MTrPs may provoke a migraine attack in some patients [140, 154] but needs further confirmation in placebo-controlled studies.

This calls for therapeutic studies targeting patients with a high degree of MTrPs, but this is only speculative at this point.

There are many overlapping findings in studies of MTrPs in migraine or TTH.

Palpation of MTrPs can, in some cases, provoke an attack in migraine patients, while palpation of MTrPs in TTH can provoke pain resembling the usual headache pattern of patients.

**Conclusion**

MTrPs are very frequent in both migraine patients [140, 141, 151–153] and TTH patients [79, 143, 144, 155–160] compared to healthy controls.

Active MTrPs are especially interesting as these are rarely found in control groups.

The results of the provocation and intervention studies support the hypothesis of a trigemino-cervical-complex pathophysiology model in both migraine [79, 140, 154–165] and TTH [157, 158, 160].

Whether MTrPs contribute to an increased disease burden in migraine is uncertain [140, 151, 152] and needs further exploration [161, 163].

**Acknowledgement**
*A machine generated summary based on the work of Do, Thien Phu; Heldarskard, Gerda Ferja; Kolding, Lærke Tørring; Hvedstrup, Jeppe; Schytz, Henrik Winther. 2018 in The Journal of Headache and Pain.*

# Comparison of Gray Matter Volume Between Migraine and "Strict-Criteria" Tension-Type Headache

DOI: https://doi.org/10.1186/s10194-018-0834-6

**Abstract-Summary**
Changes in gray matter (GM) volume associated with headache diagnosis (TTH vs. migraine) and frequency (episodic vs. chronic) were examined using voxel-based morphometry.

The correlation with headache profile and the discriminative ability between TTH and migraine were also investigated for these GM changes.

With controls (n = 43), the patients with TTH (25 episodic and 24 chronic) exhibited a GM volume increase in the anterior cingulate cortex, supramarginal gyrus, temporal pole, lateral occipital cortex, and caudate.

The patients with migraine (31 episodic and 25 chronic) conversely exhibited a GM volume decrease in the orbitofrontal cortex.

A voxel-wise 2 × 2 factorial analysis further revealed the substantial effects of headache types and frequency in the comparison of GM volume between TTH and migraine.

The migraine group (vs. TTH) had a GM decrease in the superior and middle frontal gyri, cerebellum, dorsal striatum, and precuneus.

In receiver operating characteristic analysis, the GM volumes of the left superior frontal gyrus and right cerebellum V combined had good discriminative ability for distinguishing TTH and migraine (area under the curve = 0.806).

TTH and migraine are separate headache disorders with different characteristics in relation to GM changes.

The major morphological difference between the two types of headaches is the relative GM decrease of the prefrontal and cerebellar regions in migraine, which may reflect a higher allostatic load associated with this disabling headache.

Extended:

TTH and migraine thus seem more inter-related than would be suggested by their diagnostic criteria.

**Background**
Tension-type headache (TTH) and migraine are both common headache disorders.

In the Spectrum Study, 37% of patients initially diagnosed with TTH were later revealed to have migraine or migrainous headache [166].

A study reported normal interictal plasma levels of calcitonin gene-related peptide (CGRP) in patients with chronic TTH; however, in the patient subgroup with pulsating pain quality, the CGRP level was higher, as in the group of patients with interictal migraine [167].

Some studies on quantitative sensory testing [125], brainstem excitability [126], laser evoked potentials [168], and temporal discrimination thresholds [169] have congruently revealed different somatosensory information processing between TTH and migraine, although migraine comorbidity was not deliberately excluded in patients with TTH.

The present study thus hypothesized that TTH and migraine are different in brain morphology, which may reflect their distinct symptomatology, sensory processing, and disease burden.

Few studies have compared the brain morphological differences between TTH and migraine.

## Methods

Preprocessed whole-brain GM tissue segments and the mean GM volumes of specific ROIs were used to address the following three research questions: To determine the GM volume difference between controls and patients with TTH, or migraine, a statistical design of voxel-wise single-factor three-level (TTH, migraine, and controls) analysis of covariance (ANCOVA) was employed, with age, sex, and BDI entered as nuisance variables.

A voxel-wise $2 \times 2$ factorial design with the factors TYPE (TTH vs. migraine) and FREQUENCY (episodic vs. chronic headache) was used to examine the main effects of TYPE and FREQUENCY and their interaction.

The GM volumes indicating group differences between headache diagnoses (TTH vs. migraine) were further analyzed using a logistic regression model which adjusted for age, sex, and BDI to confirm the significance of the headache type prediction (TTH vs. migraine).

## Results

In patients with TTH, GM volume was increased in the right caudate, temporal pole, left anterior cingulate cortex, supramarginal gyrus, and lateral occipital cortex.

In the effect of headache type (TTH vs. migraine), GM volume was lower for the migraine group in the bilateral putamen, cerebellum, right caudate, putamen, precuneus, middle frontal gyrus, and left superior frontal gyrus.

Regarding the effect of headache frequency (episodic vs. chronic), GM volume was lower for the chronic group (TTH and migraine combined) in the bilateral insula, right anterior cingulate cortex, and cerebellum.

GM volume of the right lateral occipital cortex was lower in episodic TTH compared with episodic migraine.

A logistic regression model was employed to assess whether the GM volume differences between TTH and migraine could predict headache types (TTH vs. migraine).

## Discussion

We determined that TTH and migraine differed in brain morphology because (1) the GM volume of specific brain regions were increased (anterior cingulate cortex, supramarginal gyrus, temporal pole, lateral occipital cortex, and caudate) in patients with TTH whereas decreased (orbitofrontal cortex) in patients with migraine compared with healthy controls; (2) a direct comparison of GM volume between both headache disorders revealed a lower GM volume in the superior and middle frontal gyri, cerebellum, dorsal striatum (putamen and caudate), and precuneus in patients with migraine; (3) the GM of the left superior frontal gyrus and right cerebellum V together demonstrated good discriminative ability for TTH and migraine in the ROC analysis.

The present findings of GM change in TTH and migraine (vs. controls) and the GM difference between both types of headaches mostly involved brain regions of the pain processing network, which suggested these plastic changes may reflect the allostatic load in response to headache pain [170].

## Conclusions

TTH and migraine are separate headache disorders with different characteristics of GM change.

The major morphological difference between the two types of headaches is a relative GM decrease in the prefrontal and cerebellar regions in migraine, which may reflect a higher allostatic load associated with this disabling headache.

These GM changes remain undetermined in the neurobiological mechanism, temporal stability, and causal relationship with headache phenotypes.

## Acknowledgement

*A machine generated summary based on the work of Chen, Wei-Ta; Chou, Kun-Hsien; Lee, Pei-Lin; Hsiao, Fu-Jung; Niddam, David M.; Lai, Kuan-Lin; Fuh, Jong-Ling; Lin, Ching-Po; Wang, Shuu-Jiun. 2018 in The Journal of Headache and Pain.*

# *Salivary Inflammatory Markers in Tension Type Headache and Migraine: The SalHead Cohort Study*

DOI: https://doi.org/10.1007/s10072-019-04151-4

## Abstract-Summary

To investigate the possible association between salivary CRP, IL-1β, and IL-6 levels, depression/anxiety and migraine, and tension type headache (TTH) in saliva of these patients.

Salivary IL-6, IL-1β, and CRP were collected in distinct time points as A: headache-free period, B: during headache, C: 1 day after headache attack, and measured by using ELISA kits.

No significant differences were found in time variation of CRP, IL-1β, and IL-6 levels between migraine and TTH (p > 0.05).

IL1-β had the highest discriminative value between headache patients and controls compared with CRP and IL-6.

CRP and IL-6 were correlated with lower symptom scores of anxiety and depression prior or immediately after the headache period in patients groups.

Extended:
No significant differences were found at any time point.

Future studies investigating possible correlations between migraine, TTH, and other cytokine levels in saliva of a large series of patients would be useful in verifying this relationship.

Future studies should adopt a noninvasive sampling method such as saliva collection to overcome the issue of small sample size and increase the number of time points of sampling.

## Introduction

Serum levels of IL-1$\beta$ were significantly elevated in patients with chronic TTH, which contribute to central sensitization and enhanced general hyperalgesia [171].

Both serum and CSF levels of IL-6 were elevated in individuals with the episodic/chronic forms of TTH and migraine [172].

No study to date has evaluated whether the increase of these salivary proinflammatory cytokines in TTH and migraine could be secondary to psychiatric comorbidities.

No research has been conducted as yet with a view to comparing the salivary levels of CRP, IL-1$\beta$, and IL-6 in patients with TTH and migraine versus age-matched controls.

The primary aim of this study was to establish whether attacks of migraine and TTH are associated with changes in the concentration of inflammatory markers.

The secondary objective was to investigate whether cytokines levels in TTH and migraine could be influenced by psychiatric comorbidities such as depression and anxiety.

## Materials and Methods

The main exclusion criteria were (1) abnormal plasma hs-CRP, IL-1$\beta$, and IL-6 levels (>10 mg/L); (2) smoking cigarettes >1 pack/day; (3) current pregnancy, lactation, or hormonal contraceptive use; (4) alcohol or substance abuse; (5) drug use such as antiplatelet agents, anticoagulants, statins, or hormonal drugs; (6) headache patients with recent history of a disease with known elevated levels of inflammatory markers; (7) patients under anti-inflammatory therapy; (8) other primary or secondary headaches; (9) major psychiatric disease; and (10) oral health problems.

All headache sufferers were instructed to collect salivary headache-free baseline samples at the time of study screening when they had been free of headache for at least 48 h (time point A).

They collected additional samples during moderate/severe headache (time point B), and at self-defined resolution phase, 24 h of their headache attack (time point C).

Healthy control subjects were instructed to collect samples at the time of study screening (time point D).

## Results

In both TTH and migraine sufferers, IL-1$\beta$ was found to significantly decrease from time point A to time point B, while from time point B to time point C, a significant increase was recorded.

Repeated measures analysis of variance showed no significant differences in time variation of CRP, IL-β, and IL-6 levels between subjects with migraine and those with TTH (p > 0.05).

CRP levels at time point A were negatively correlated with HAM-A and BDI scores.

IL-6 measured at time point A was negatively correlated with BDI scores.

## Discussion

The main findings of this study were as follows: (1) IL-1β was found to significantly decrease from time point A to time point B, while a significant increase was recorded from time point B to time point C. (2) All headache sufferers had greater IL-1β levels at time point B as compared with controls at time point D. (3) No significant differences were found in time variation of CRP, IL-1β, and IL-6 levels between migraine and TTH. (4) CRP was negatively correlated with HAM-A and BDI scores. (5) IL-6 measured at time point A was negatively correlated with BDI scores. (6) IL1-β had the highest discriminative value between headache patients and controls compared with CRP and IL-6.

A further novel finding of this study is that it demonstrates increased salivary IL-1β levels in both migraineurs and TTH subjects during the headache period.

## Conclusions

Migraineurs had elevated IL-1β levels in saliva compared with controls.

Higher levels of CRP and Il-6 were correlated with lower symptom scores of anxiety and depression prior or immediately after the headache period.

Future studies should adopt a noninvasive sampling method such as saliva collection to overcome the issue of small sample size and increase the number of time points of sampling.

## Acknowledgement

*A machine generated summary based on the work of Bougea, Anastasia; Spantideas, Nikolaos; Galanis, Petros; Katsika, Paraskevi; Boufidou, Fotini; Voskou, Panagiota; Vamvakaris, Ioannis; Anagnostou, Evangelos; Nikolaou, Xrysa; Kararizou, Evangelia. 2019 in Neurological Sciences.*

# The Association Between Serum Vitamin B₁₂ Deficiency and Tension-Type Headache in Turkish Children

DOI: https://doi.org/10.1007/s10072-018-3286-5

## Abstract-Summary

This study aimed to determine the relationship between serum vitamin $B_{12}$ level and tension-type headache.

The serum vitamin $B_{12}$ levels in the headache and control groups were $273.01 \pm 76.77$ and $316.22 \pm 74.53$ pg/ml, with the difference determined as statistically significant ($p = 0.003$).

The serum vitamin $B_{12}$ level in the children with tension-type headache was significantly lower than that in the control group.

Of the study, it was concluded that there may be an association between vitamin $B_{12}$ level and tension-type headache.

Extended:

The serum vitamin $B_{12}$ level was evaluated by the electrochemiluminescence (ECLIA) procedure.

## Introduction

Tension-type headache is also the most frequently reported primary headache syndrome in school children and adolescents with a prevalence of 7.8–57.5% [38, 173–176].

Although the exact pathogenesis of tension-type headache has not yet been fully clarified, both muscular and psychogenic factors are thought to be associated with tension-type headache [177].

Recent studies have revealed a remarkable association of depression and anxiety with tension-type headache, especially in girls [178–181].

There is current debate as to whether a comprehensive diet regulating the number of core constituents of nutrients such as vitamins, iron, proteins, carbohydrates, and fats may be effective in the therapy of headache [182–184].

The purpose of this study was to measure serum vitamin $B_{12}$ levels in children with tension-type headache and through comparison with healthy control subjects, to determine whether there is an association of vitamin $B_{12}$ deficiency with tension-type headache.

## Material and Methods

The study included patients aged <18 years with complaints of headache ongoing for at least 6 months.

Full blood count, biochemical tests, and vitamin $B_{12}$ levels were examined for all the patients selected for inclusion in the study.

Children were excluded if they had secondary headache with specific pathology detected on brain MRI and EEG, migraine type headache, or if antidepressant treatment was initiated for any psychiatric disorder, if they were taking nutritional support as medication or vitamin supplements or if folate deficiency was determined.

Serum vitamin $B_{12}$ level <200 pg/ml was defined as deficient, and <160 pg/ml as severely deficient as described in previously published studies [185, 186].

For children determined with severe vitamin $B_{12}$ deficiency, treatment was started with intramuscular cyanocobalamin at a test dose (for the first 2 days) of 10 µg/day.

For cases determined as deficient in vitamin $B_{12}$, treatment with cyanocobalamin was started at 100 µg/day.

## Results

The study groups comprised 75 patients (40 females, 35 males) with headache and a control group of 49 healthy children (25 females, 24 males).

The mean serum vitamin $B_{12}$ level was 273.01 ± 76.77 pg/mL in the headache group and 316.22 ± 74.53 pg/mL in the control group.

The minimum and maximum levels of serum vitamin $B_{12}$ in the headache group were 133 and 482 pg/mL, respectively, compared with 190 and 500 mg/dL in the control group.

Of the 18 patients in the study group, 13 were determined as deficient (<200 pg/ml), and five as severely deficient (<160 pg/ml).

Anxiety disorder was present in 12 (16%) cases in the headache group and 8 (66.6%) of these were determined with vitamin $B_{12}$ deficiency.

## Discussion

Although several different neurological disorders have been reported in children with vitamin $B_{12}$ deficiency, to the best of our knowledge, there has been no study in the literature related to whether or not there is a relationship between vitamin $B_{12}$ deficiency and patients with tension-type headache [187–191].

The hypothesis of the current study was that tension-type headache in children may be associated with vitamin $B_{12}$ deficiency.

In a study of 16 children and adolescents with tension-type headache, 60% were found to have concomitant psychiatric diagnoses, with anxiety and depressive disorders being the most common [192].

The rate of patients with anxiety disorder together with tension-type headache was 16% (12 children).

The current study also found a high incidence of vitamin $B_{12}$ deficiency in those with headache and anxiety disorder.

These results showed that the anxiety and depression caused by vitamin $B_{12}$ deficiency could be a cause of tension-type headache.

## Conclusions

The findings of the present study showed a significant relationship between tension-type headache and serum vitamin $B_{12}$ level.

It is noticeable from this study that children with vitamin $B_{12}$ deficiency could present with different neurological findings.

These results have shown that apart from neuropsychiatric evaluation, routine measurement of vitamin $B_{12}$ levels could be useful in children with tension-type headache.

## Acknowledgement

*A machine generated summary based on the work of Calik, Mustafa; Aktas, Mehmet Salih; Cecen, Emre; Piskin, Ibrahim Etem; Ayaydın, Hamza; Ornek, Zuhal; Karaca, Meryem; Solmaz, Abdullah; Ay, Halil. 2018 in Neurological Sciences.*

# *The Role of the Autonomic Nervous System in Headache: Biomarkers and Treatment*

DOI: https://doi.org/10.1007/s11916-022-01079-x

## Abstract-Summary

A pathophysiological model for tension-type headache is proposed that is compatible with most physiological and behavioral literature.

For migraine, incorporating autonomic factors into the pathophysiology offers rationales for behavioral interventions that have been shown to be useful in migraine treatment and a biofeedback protocol is proposed.

Extended:

Future research should focus on understanding the mechanisms that seem to produce favorable results so as to improve interventions.

## Tension-Type Headache

"Tension-type headache (TTH) is the most common primary headache disorder with a prevalence of up to 78% in the general population and huge expenses in terms of health service.

Despite its high incidence and impact on life's quality, the knowledge on the pathophysiology and efficacious treatment of TTH was still limited" (p. 793) [193, 194].

Although TTH does not present the level of burden that has been found in migraine, it is far more common and thus represents a significant health challenge.

A recent review [195] concludes: "Despite being the most prevalent headache disorder, TTH pathophysiology remains poorly understood.

Patients with TTH tend to have muscles that are harder and tender to palpation, and may have more frequent trigger points of tenderness than patients without headache.

## Tension-Type Headache and Autonomic Indicators

Hedges' $g_s$ for both TTH and migraine indicated moderate effect sizes ($-0.63$) for both HA types, but more work needs to be done on TTH.

The studies that did look at that HA type did find similar effect sizes.

## Tension-Type Headache Pathophysiology

While most reviews conclude that the pathophysiology of TTH is unknown, and debate has continued on the role of peripheral versus central mechanisms of chronic TTH [19], our group has attempted to understand the pathophysiology from the perspective of peripheral pain sources that might have ANS mediation.

In a recent comprehensive review, Ashina and others [19] concluded: "Although the biological underpinnings remain unresolved, it seems likely that peripheral mechanisms are responsible for the genesis of pain in TTH, whereas central sensitization may be involved in transformation from episodic to chronic TTH" (p1, italics mine).

Evidence for sensitized pain pressure thresholds is a bit more solid: "This first meta-analysis addressing pressure pain thresholds differences in symptomatic and distant pain free areas between patients with tension-type headache and controls found low to moderate evidence supporting the presence of pressure pain hypersensitivity in the trigeminal and neck areas in tension-type headache in comparison with headache-free controls.

Sensitivity to pressure pain was widespread only in chronic, not episodic, tension-type headache (moderate evidence) [196] (p. 256)."

### The Sympathetically Mediated Trigger Point Spindle Model
Psychological stress activates alpha sympathetic fibers to TPs (here hypothesized a muscle spindles).

To test this hypothesis, my colleagues David Hubbard and Greg Berkoff used two needle EMG recordings, one inserted into an active trapezius TP and the second in nearby non-tender muscle [197].

We then published a number of studies that showed that various psychological stressors would dramatically increase activity in the TP, while the adjacent muscle remained quiet [198, 199].

In the McNulty and others study, patients were asked to do a stressful mental arithmetic task while EMG was monitored with one probe in or near the TP and the other nearby in non-tender muscle.

In all of this series of studies, the TP EMG activity proved very sensitive to stressful stimuli and in one study [200] reduced to the level of the adjacent site during a passive relaxation induction (autogenic training).

### The Role of the Parasympathetic System
Vagal 'tone' predominates over sympathetic tone at rest.

Under normal physiological conditions, abrupt parasympathetic stimulation will inhibit tonic sympathetic activation and its effects at rest and during exercise.

From Uijtdehaage and Thayer [201], "Sympathetic heart rate effects were substantially smaller with high levels of vagal tone than with low vagal background activity.

Vagal effects became progressively stronger with increasing sympathetic background activity, demonstrating the predominance of parasympathetic control of human heart rate" (p. 107).

By enhancing parasympathetic tone through either various biofeedback modalities or psychological/meditative procedures, we postulated that much longer pain and pressure relief would result, presumably based on the "Accentuated Antagonism" principles cited above.

### Heart Rate Variability Biofeedback
Results indicated that groups of non-drug therapy in comparison with only pharmacotherapy groups had statistically more pronounced decrease in the intensity of headache, a decrease in reactive anxiety and depression level, and an improvement of the quality of life.

The HRVB protocol produced an increase in indices of healthier ANS function.

ANS dysfunction (usually prolonged vagal withdrawal) and physical overstretch stimuli create sympathetic input to the TP.

In a parallel model [202], we found that children with functional abdominal pain had longer periods of vagal withdrawal than asymptomatic children and when HRVB was introduced, their vagal tone improved while symptoms reduced (r = 0.63).

## Current Clinical Model

In our current model, we propose combining HRVB (perhaps accompanied by an empirically based talk therapy) with one of the TP release procedures.

After mastery is demonstrated with physiological monitoring, the patient is instructed to use the breathing technique before, during, and after the TP release.

We are currently investigating this specific protocol against a credible comparison procedure measuring the length of pain and pressure relief.

## Migraine

Recent efforts have focused on the central nervous system mechanisms and acute and preventive treatments for migraine [203].

While this line of research has greatly improved our knowledge of the neurological nature of the migraine, less progress has been made on behavioral aspects of prevention.

## Migraine and Dysautonomia

Peroutka [204] postulated that the ANS played a significant role in migraine.

Through an improved understanding the role of autonomic changes in pathogenesis of migraine, it may be possible to develop even more effective treatments for migraine sufferers" (p. 153).

In a meta-analysis, de Coo and others [205] reported acute relief of cluster HA using vagal nerve stimulation (VNS).

One study [206] also reported acute relief in migraine.

The intervention described above, HRVB, has been shown to affect resting level autonomic flexibility and thus may be a candidate for migraine prevention.

Consistent with the idea that interventions that target ANS flexibility may be useful, in a recent meta-analysis [207], Wu and others concluded that despite limitations in methodology, "Yoga therapy may benefit to reduce the headache frequency of migraine patients" (p. 147).

## Biofeedback

Biofeedback has been used for migraine treatment for many years.

In a meta-analysis of this literature, Kisan and others [208] found that biofeedback modalities either alone or in combination with other therapies produced treatment advantages over controls (medium effect size).

Nestoriuc and Martin [209], in an excellent review, summarized the literature similarly: Various forms of biofeedback are effective for migraine and tension-type headache.

Although not reviewed here, the outcome effects from biofeedback seem to endure for extended periods, whether booster treatments are provided or not.

One recent random controlled trial [210] found that "…an App-based HRV biofeedback was feasible and acceptable on a time-limited basis for people with migraine.

Changes in the primary clinical outcome did not differ between biofeedback and control; however, high users of the app reported more benefit than low user" (p. 41).

## Conclusions

There has emerged a general consensus that non-pharmacological interventions can add treatment gains to traditional and the newer medical treatments for headache including migraine.

I have tried to emphasize the role that the ANS plays in migraine as a way of explaining the findings that a wide variety of interventions (including sham procedures and placebos) are effective in reducing HA frequency and, in a few studies, pain intensity.

HRVB has been shown to improve ANS flexibility in other applications and therefore may be a promising addition to the non-pharmacological armamentarium.

## [Section 12]

The role that the autonomic nervous system (ANS) plays in headache has historically been under-valued.

I review the scientific literature on the role of the ANS in migraine and tension-type headache.

This has allowed advances in understanding of the pathophysiology of both headache types and has led to some promising interventions.

## Acknowledgement

*A machine generated summary based on the work of Gevirtz, Richard. 2022 in Current Pain and Headache Reports.*

## *Diagnosis*

Machine generated keywords: tth, migraine tth, hormone, function, secondary headache, association, common trigger, sleep, ichd, headache clinic, reference, trigger, disturbance, diagnosis, threshold.

## Reference Programme: Diagnosis and Treatment of Headache Disorders and Facial Pain. Danish Headache Society, 3rd Edition, 2020

DOI: https://doi.org/10.1186/s10194-021-01228-4

**Abstract-Summary**

Headache and facial pain are among the most common, disabling and costly diseases in Europe, which demands for high quality health care on all levels within the health system.

The role of the Danish Headache Society is to educate and advocate for the needs of patients with headache and facial pain.

The Danish Headache Society has launched a third version of the guideline for the diagnosis, organization and treatment of the most common types of headaches and facial pain in Denmark.

The recommendations for the primary headaches and facial pain are largely in accordance with the European guidelines produced by the European Academy of Neurology.

The guideline should be used a practical tool for use in daily clinical practice for primary care physicians, neurologists with a common interest in headache, as well as other health-care professionals treating headache patients.

The guideline first describes how to examine and diagnose the headache patient and how headache treatment is organized in Denmark.

**Introduction**

The vast majority of Danes suffering from headache are treated in the primary sector and should for the most part continue to be treated there in the future, but there is an increasing need for clear guidelines for examining and organizing specialist treatment of severe and rare headache conditions.

There are international guidelines and general recommendations for the treatment of migraines and other primary headache diseases.

The Danish Headache Society created a working committee to update the Danish reference program for headache diseases and facial pain from 2010.

The objective is to create common guidelines for diagnosing, organizing and treating the most common primary headache diseases such as migraines, tension-type headache and cluster headache as well as trigeminal neuralgia in Denmark, as well as describe important warning signs of serious life-threatening and other secondary headache conditions.

**Diagnosis and Organization**

Warning signals, in the medical history or the physical examination, which warrant further examination, are (see also Section 7 "Secondary Forms of Headache"): New onset headache Thunderclap headache (sudden onset of severe headache) Sudden headache occurring during strenuous physical or sexual activity Headache with atypical aura (lasts over 1 h or includes motor outcomes) Headache with aura developed while using birth control pills New onset of headache in a patient with cancer or HIV infection Headache accompanied by fever Headache accompanied by neurological outcomes phrased migraine aura Progressive headache over weeks New onset headache in patients under 10 years of age or over 40 years of age Headache, which is position-dependent Physical and neurological examination is performed to rule out or confirm secondary headaches.

CT / MRI scan is most often not indicated in a patient with a long history of headache, but should be performed if the history or physical examination is unclear or indicates that the headache is due to secondary condition.

## Migraine with and Without Aura

Non-pharmacological interventions are an important part of the treatment for some headache patients, although there is generally only sparse evidence for the effect of this type of intervention.

Information about the causes of migraine and the possibilities for treatment, thorough physical examination, as well as simply taking the patient seriously, can have a beneficial effect in some patients.

A combination of triptan and NSAIDs may be more effective in some patients than each drug alone [211].

Approximately 20–50% of patients experience recurrence of migraine within 48 h. An additional dose of triptan is usually effective in these cases.

Botulinum type A toxin (Botox) is in Denmark so far only approved for the preventive treatment of chronic migraine (headache $\geq$15 days per month, of which at least 8 days with migraine) in patients who have shown insufficient response or intolerance to other migraine preventive drugs.

## Tension-Type Headache

In patients with frequent episodic and chronic tension-type headaches, the central nervous system has been shown to be hypersensitive to pain stimuli.

There is a well-documented effect of weak analgesics in the individual episodes of tension-type headaches, while the effect is often limited in chronic tension-type headache [212].

Preventive treatment may be indicated in patients with chronic tension-type headache, if there is insufficient effect of non-pharmacological treatment and when medication overuse headache is excluded [213].

Several placebo-controlled studies have shown an effect of the tricyclic antidepressant amitriptyline [212], which is first choice for preventive treatment of chronic tension-type headache.

In episodic tension-type headache, reported pain from pericranial musculoskeletal tissues as well as stress are likely to play an important role, while altered central pain modulation is involved in the chronic form.

In patients with chronic tension-type headache, analgesics rarely have an effect, so preventive treatment with amitriptyline, mirtazapine or venlafaxine may be indicated.

**Cluster Headache**

Cluster headache is divided into two types: An episodic type seen in 80–90% of patients, where the attacks occur in bouts lasting 4–12 weeks separated by attack-free periods of varying length (weeks-years); and a chronic type seen in 10–20% of patients, with bouts lasting longer than 9 months per year.

In chronic cluster headache, in patients with an atypical presentation, onset after 40 years of age or in treatment refractory cluster headache, a cerebral MR scan should be performed to exclude tumours, midline malformations, pathology in the cavernous sinus, pituitary gland and hypothalamus [214].

Non-pharmacological treatment has not been shown to have an effect in cluster headache [214].

The dosage of the preventive treatment should be gradually reduced if patients are attack-free for 14 days (please be aware that patients may experience milder attacks and/or autonomic symptoms indicating that the bout is still active) or when patients sense that the bout has ended.

**Medication Overuse Headache**

Medication overuse headache (MOH) is a chronic headache occurring at least 15 days a month in patients with pre-existing headache.

MOH is treated by withdrawal therapy (stop of the overuse of short-term medication) [215], either by a complete stop of all short-term medication for a 2 months period, or by a reduced intake of short-term medication to maximum 2 days a week in average.

Danish guidelines have recommended to postpone start of preventive headache medication to the end of 2 months withdrawal therapy for two reasons: 1) The headache pattern becomes clearer during withdrawal, and a correct diagnosis would help find the best treatment option for preventive medication; 2) It seemed that some patients did not need preventives after withdrawal.

MOH should be prevented via information to patient with pre-existing headache and a restrictive approach to prescription of short-term medication.

**Secondary Types of Headache**

Most common in obese people Papilledema is the most prominent feature The headache may worsen in the supine position and be worst in the morning In addition to headaches, there may be neck pain/back pain, visual field defects, transient visual obscurations, abduction paresis and pulsating tinnitus Suspected cases require acute hospitalization (important differential diagnosis: sinus vein thrombosis) and neuro-radiological examination, possibly measurement of the cerebrospinal pressure, which will be elevated more than 25 cm $H_2O$ Untreated intracranial hypertension can lead to permanent visual impairment or blindness Investigation and treatment: see national neurological treatment guide.

Link: http://neuro.dk/wordpress/nnbv/primaer-hjernetumor-lavgradsgliom/. Typical headache accompanied by fever and neck stiffness May present with cognitive impairment, photophobia or petechiae May present with seizures Investigation and treatment: see national neurological treatment guide.

## Trigeminal Neuralgia

In approximately 15% of TN patients, there is an underlying symptomatic cause of pain (not including a neurovascular contact).

It is not possible to accurately identify all patients with symptomatic TN based on pain characteristics, clinical examination or treatment response.

As TN usually has an unpredictable pattern of pain frequency and intensity, dose(s) of medical treatment should be titrated and tapered according to pain level.

At complete pain freedom lasting more than 1 month, it is advised to taper off medication by reducing, e.g. carbamazepine by 100 mg or gabapentin by 300 mg every 7th–14th day (or comparable doses of other TN drugs) [216].

Titrate 100 mg every third day until pain freedom or unacceptable side effects Typical maintenance dose is 100–600 mg BID Daily doses of 1800 mg or more may be necessary [2].

Approximately 30% of all TN patients do not have sufficient effect from medical treatment or have unacceptable medical side effects.

## Hormones and Migraines

Women with migraines with aura should be informed that they have a slightly increased risk of an ischemic stroke in the brain, but that the risk is very small if there are no other risk factors and if they refrain from smoking and taking oestrogen-containing birth control pills.

If contraception is needed in women with migraine with aura, birth control pills with the lowest possible oestrogen content are preferred, and the patient must be informed of the increased risk of ischemic stroke.

In case of need for contraception, where a worsening of migraine without aura is experienced at the same time, the following can be tried: Use of oestrogen-containing contraceptive pills, where there is no contraceptive pill break through several cycles, e.g. by taking birth control pills continuously for 9 weeks (instead of the usual 3 weeks) followed by a 7 day pill-free period.

## Children and Headaches

Generally inadequate evidence in relation to both acute and preventive treatment of headache diseases in children and adolescents and there is a great need for further randomized placebo-controlled trials (RCTs).

Triptan-related side effects in children/adolescents are comparable to side effects observed in adults.

Treatment with beta-blockers (propranolol or metoprolol) and flunarizine has a comparable preventive effect in children and adolescents [217, 218].

With the recent development of calcitonin gene-related peptide (CGRP) antagonist treatment, which appears to have an effect and good safety profile in adults, it can be hoped that these new types of preventive treatment also play a role in the preventive treatment of migraines in children.

Prevention with amitriptyline may have an effect on chronic tension-type headaches in children, but there are no placebo-controlled studies.

**Acknowledgement**

*A machine generated summary based on the work of Schytz, Henrik W.; Amin, Faisal M.; Jensen, Rigmor H.; Carlsen, Louise; Maarbjerg, Stine; Lund, Nunu; Aegidius, Karen; Thomsen, Lise L.; Bach, Flemming W.; Beier, Dagmar; Johansen, Hanne; Hansen, Jakob M.; Kasch, Helge; Munksgaard, Signe B.; Poulsen, Lars; Sørensen, Per Schmidt; Schmidt-Hansen, Peter T.; Cvetkovic, Vlasta V.; Ashina, Messoud; Bendtsen, Lars. 2021 in The Journal of Headache and Pain.*

## *Validation of an Algorithm for Automated Classification of Migraine and Tension-Type Headache Attacks in an Electronic Headache Diary*

DOI: https://doi.org/10.1186/s10194-020-01139-w

**Abstract-Summary**

This study evaluates the accuracy of an automated classification tool of single attacks of the two major primary headache disorders migraine and tension-type headache used in an electronic headache diary.

One hundred two randomly selected reported headache attacks from an electronic headache-diary of patients using the medical app M-sense were classified by both a neurologist with specialisation in headache medicine and an algorithm, constructed based on the ICHD-3 criteria for migraine and tension-type headache.

The level of agreement between the headache specialist and the algorithm was compared by using a kappa statistic.

The neurologist and the algorithm classified migraines with aura (MA), migraines without aura (MO), tension-type headaches (TTH) and non-migraine or non-TTH events.

Of the 102 headache reports, 86 cases were fully agreed on, and 16 cases not, making the level of agreement unweighted kappa 0.74 and representing a substantial level of agreement.

The substantial level of agreement indicates that the classification tool is a valuable instrument for automated evaluation of electronic headache diaries, which can thereby support the diagnostic and therapeutic clinical processes.

Extended:

The level of agreement between the neurologist and the algorithm's classification of 102 single headache events resulted in 86 cases of agreement and 16 cases of disagreement.

The findings from this validity assessment in the below section of results.

Future research can use this classification algorithm for large scale database analysis for epidemiological studies, for example to investigate whether migraine and tension-type headache are diagnostic types or points on a severity continuum [219].

## Background

Regarding treatments, patients with high severity of migraine and headache-related disability should receive acute and, if necessary, preventive migraine-specific therapy [220].

To resolve this need, in this paper, we present an algorithm that applies the ICHD-3 criteria to single headache events recorded in a migraine management app's database.

Our goal is to provide an efficient means to classify patient headache events as migraine or tension-type headache.

The aim being to investigate how accurately an algorithm classifies patient headache events as migraine or tension-type headache in electronic health diaries using ICHD criteria.

As validation, both a neurologist specialised in headache medicine and the algorithm classified the headache-diary data from a medical apps' database.

Patients use this medical app for documenting headaches as well as potential trigger factors, all of which get summarized in reports for doctors.

## Methods

We developed an algorithm to classify primary headache disorders according to ICHD-3 criteria for both definite and probable Migraine without Aura, Migraine with Aura, and TTH as for usage in the M-sense app.

In the first phase, a computer-based algorithm based on ICHD-3 criteria was run and classified the 102 single headache events taken from the M-sense database.

Of the validation study, the headache specialist classified the same 102 headache events also according to the criteria of ICHD-3 with information about an existing diagnosis of migraine and tension-type headache.

Based on the evaluation using the headache sheet, the neurologist assigned the classification of migraine without aura (MO), migraine with aura (MA), TTH, or non-migraine or non-TTH (non-classifiable).

We calculated the kappa statistic to compare the algorithm's classification results to each of the neurologist's classifications based on the single-entry headache sheets.

## Results

The level of agreement between the neurologist and the algorithm's classification of 102 single headache events resulted in 86 cases of agreement and 16 cases of disagreement.

From the neurologist's answers to the short questionnaire, we deduced that the algorithm correctly applied the ICHD-3 criteria in the 11 cases of category 1–4.

For subcategory five, in which the neurologist had categorized four cases as non-classifiable in contrast to the algorithm's identification as MO or TTH, three of four of these cases had a short headache duration <30 min in common.

For the other case, the neurologist corrected his classification.

For subcategory six, wherein the neurologist identified a case to be migraine without aura and the algorithm non-classifiable, we found that the algorithm was not coded to interpret the relevant ICHD criteria correctly.

**Discussion**

Results from the current study demonstrate that the investigated algorithm for identifying headaches is a valid instrument for automated evaluation of electronic headache diaries.

This result is not surprising, given that the evaluation of a whole headache diary by classifying large numbers of individual attacks is a tedious task that requires high levels of concentration and does not reflect common clinical practice in headache diagnosis.

One study identified that agreement between neurologists asked to assign a headache diagnosis based on the review of videotaped patient interviews, ranged in a kappa from 0.55 to 0.81 [221].

Since migraine and TTH themselves are phenomenological diagnoses, other possible diagnoses, such as secondary headaches, must be excluded via differential diagnosis which is reflected by the criterion E in ICHD-3.

Criterion A in ICHD-3 defines the number of attacks or headache days that are necessary before a diagnosis can be made [222].

**Conclusion**

The results of this study confirm the accuracy of an algorithm for automated classification of MA, MO, and TTH, with a substantial level of agreement to a neurologist specialized in headache medicine.

Study's results, additional diagnostic functionalities of headache management apps can be implemented.

Future research can use this classification algorithm for large scale database analysis for epidemiological studies, for example to investigate whether migraine and tension-type headache are diagnostic types or points on a severity continuum [219].

**Acknowledgement**

*A machine generated summary based on the work of Roesch, Aaron; Dahlem, Markus A; Neeb, Lars; Kurth, Tobias. 2020 in The Journal of Headache and Pain.*

## *Machine Learning-Based Automated Classification of Headache Disorders Using Patient-Reported Questionnaires*

DOI: https://doi.org/10.1038/s41598-020-70992-1

**Abstract-Summary**

Classification of headache disorders is dependent on a subjective self-report from patients and its interpretation by physicians.

We aimed to apply objective data-driven machine learning approaches to analyze patient-reported symptoms and test the feasibility of the automated classification of headache disorders.

The self-report data of 2162 patients were analyzed.

The first layer classified between migraine and others, the second layer classified between tension-type headache (TTH) and others, and the third layer classified between trigeminal autonomic cephalalgia (TAC) and others, and the fourth layer classified between epicranial and thunderclap headaches.

In the test cohort, our stacked classifier obtained accuracy of 81%, sensitivity of 88%, 69%, 65%, 53%, and 51%, and specificity of 95%, 55%, 46%, 48%, and 51% for migraine, TTH, TAC, epicranial headache, and thunderclap headaches, respectively.

We showed that a machine-learning based approach is applicable in analyzing patient-reported questionnaires.

Extended:

The first layer classified the most dominant subtype (i.e., migraine) and the rest (i.e., non-migraine).

## Introduction

The diagnosis of headache disorders is highly dependent on self-report from patients and the interpretation of the self-report by clinicians.

The International Classification of Headache Disorder (ICHD) was published to aid a standardized diagnosis of headache disorders [223].

There have been efforts to aid the diagnosis of primary headache disorders using neurophysiological tests [224], neuroimaging [225, 226], and blood-based biomarkers [227, 228]; however, these have not replaced clinical interviews.

Previous studies have mainly focused on migraine with little focus on the differential diagnosis of other headache disorders [229, 230].

The clinical diagnosis of headache disorders should, however, be based on a holistic approach since a single characteristic cannot replace the proper diagnosis.

We aimed to analyze self-reported symptoms of patients to classify four headache disorders including migraine, by using machine learning approaches.

## Methods

We applied the least absolute shrinkage and selection operator (LASSO) [231] in choosing a few important features for each stacked classifier layer.

These features were chosen as the set of stable features and the threshold of three was chosen to maximize the classifier performance on average in the left-out fold in the training cohort within the tenfold cross-validation.

The selected stable features were used to train the stacked XGBoost classifier.

To ensure the methods used in our study are well-suited in classifying headache subtypes, we compared our feature selection method (LASSO) with support vector machine recursive feature elimination (SVM-RFE) [232] and minimum-redundancy maximum-relevancy (mRMR) [233] approaches.

The numbers of the selected features using mRMR and SVM-RFE for each classifier layer were fixed as those of LASSO.

We also compared XGBoost with other binary classifiers such as k-nearest neighbor (k-NN), support vector machine (SVM), and random forest in each of the stacked layers with features selected by LASSO.

**Results**

The top three prominent features in the fourth layer (epicranial headache vs. thunderclap headache) were location: retroauricular, nature of pain: electric shock-like, and nature of pain: jabbing, assuming epicranial headache as the positive subtype in the specific headache syndromes classifier.

The stacked XGBoost classifier using the selected features attained an accuracy of 82%, sensitivity of 87%, 66%, 85%, 65%, and 64% for the five subtypes, and specificity of 94%, 54%, 58%, 63%, and 57% for the five subtypes in the training cohort.

The stacked XGBoost classifier using the selected features led to an accuracy of 81%, sensitivity of 88%, 69%, 65%, 53%, and 51% for the five subtypes, and specificity of 95%, 55%, 46%, 48%, and 51% for the five subtypes in the test cohort.

We compared XGBoost with k-NN, SVM, and random forest classifiers in each of the stacked layers in terms of overall accuracy, minimum sensitivity, and minimum specificity.

**Discussion**

We applied a machine learning approach to classify major headache disorders using questionnaires completed by patients in a real-world setting.

The performance of the machine learning approach in the classification of migraine was excellent however, its accuracy in classifying headache disorders other than migraine was inferior to that in classifying migraine.

Our study is one of the first studies to apply machine learning in the analysis of patient-reported questionnaires to classify primary headache disorders [229].

Existing studies on the classification of headache disorders with machine learning have focused on a few selected headache disorders such as migraine and tension-type headache due to challenges with sample size [229, 230].

This important feature should be always considered in the differential diagnosis of secondary and primary headaches, but it has not been listed in the ICHD-3 criteria for migraine, TTH, and epicranial headaches [223].

**Acknowledgement**

*A machine generated summary based on the work of Kwon, Junmo; Lee, Hyebin; Cho, Soohyun; Chung, Chin-Sang; Lee, Mi Ji; Park, Hyunjin. 2020 in Scientific Reports.*

## *Primary Headaches During Lifespan*

DOI: https://doi.org/10.1186/s10194-019-0985-0

**Abstract-Summary**

Primary headaches, especially migraine, are cyclic disorders with a complex sequence of symptoms within every headache attack.

The clinical presentation of migraine shows an age-dependent change with a significantly shorter duration of the attacks and occurrence of different paroxysmal symptoms, such as vomiting, abdominal pain or vertigo, in childhood and, in contrast, largely an absence of autonomic signs and a more often bilateral headache in the elderly.

The differences in the clinical presentation are in agreement with the idea that the connectivity of hypothalamic areas with different brainstem areas, especially the central parasympathetic areas, is important for the clinical manifestation of migraine, as well as, the change during lifespan.

**Introduction**

Pain perception changes with age and is different in very young and very old patients.

In a systematic review of 12 studies, Tumi and others [234] found that in the elderly subjects (mean age: 62 years) the pressure pain thresholds were lower than in the younger subjects (mean age: 22 years).

The heat pain thresholds did not differ.

Another systematic review reports that the pain thresholds increase with age.

Concerning gender differences in children, Boerner and others [235] stated that in the majority of studies there were no differences in the pain thresholds between girls and boys if the children were younger than 12 years.

Experimental data concerning pain perception in the trigeminal area in very young children are missing.

**Background**

In the same study, the 6-month prevalence in the 65–75-year-old group was about 3.5% for migraine and about 12.5% for tension-type headache, with females affected 2–1.5 times more often [236], and in a study from northern Italy the prevalence of migraine after the 75th year was 2.7% for males and 7.6% for females [237].

Concerning the severity of the primary headache patients over 70 years old with migraine, about 41% report on headache on 10–14 days per month [238, 239] and the average age of patients with chronic migraine is higher than that of patients with episodic migraine [240].

Aura symptoms with or without accompanying headache seem to occur more often in the elderly; in the group of 18–29-year-olds about 15.2% have auras compared to 41% of the patients aged 70 years and older [238, 241, 242].

The self-reported prevalence of tension-type headache in a Danish twin study was 86% (females slightly higher than males) and after the age of 39 years the prevalence declined for both sexes [243, 244].

**Discussion**

One general feature, especially in migraine and less also in cluster headache, seems to be a decrease in autonomic symptoms during aging.

Such a study would help to answer the question of whether the change in the reactivity of the autonomic system during life could be a reason for the decline in the prevalence of the autonomic symptoms during ageing and also why migraine symptoms in very young children are not as typical as in adolescents.

It is unclear if this immature control of the cortical control of autonomic functions is somewhat related to the time of migraine onset as well as clinical symptoms in children.

The episodic syndromes in infancy, which often are precursor symptoms of a later migraine, would be best explained by a temporarily disturbed descending inhibition, especially, reduced inhibition of the vestibular system (benign paroxysmal vertigo), of the descending axial motor system (benign paroxysmal torticollis, spinal vestibular pathways), and of the area postrema (cyclic vomiting) or the vagal control of the intestinal tract (abdominal migraine).

**Conclusions**

Headache symptoms change during lifespan, especially, in migraine.

In the elderly autonomic symptoms are less prominent and the headache becomes more featureless.

**Acknowledgement**

*A machine generated summary based on the work of Straube, Andreas; Andreou, Anna. 2019 in The Journal of Headache and Pain.*

# Co-occurrence of Pain Syndromes

DOI: https://doi.org/10.1007/s00702-019-02107-8

**Abstract-Summary**

Two concurrent visceral pains from internal organs sharing at least part of their central sensory projection can give rise to viscero-visceral hyperalgesia, i.e., enhancement of typical pain symptoms from both districts.

Visceral pain, headache and musculoskeletal pains (myofascial pain from trigger points, joint pain) can enhance pain and hyperalgesia from fibromyalgia.

Myofascial pain from trigger points can perpetuate pain symptoms from visceral pain conditions and trigger migraine attacks when located in the referred pain area from an internal organ or in cervico-facial areas, respectively.

A strong message in these pain syndrome co-occurrence is that effective treatment of one of the conditions can also improve symptoms from the other, thus suggesting a systematic and thorough evaluation of the pain patient for a global effective management of his/her suffering.

**Introduction**

Fibromyalgia has a very high degree of co-occurrence with a number of visceral, myofascial and craniofacial pain conditions [245–247].

The reasons behind co-occurrence of a number of pain conditions in the same patient, probably complex and multifactorial, are still the subject of active investigation.

Independently of the possible underlying mechanisms, however, the co-existence of several pain conditions in the same patient may involve significant interactions of symptoms leading to enhancement of pain manifestations, which can be very difficult to manage, to changes in the pain pattern, which may complicate diagnosis.

In this narrative review we describe some of the most frequent pain associations in patients, namely visceral pain, myofascial pain, fibromyalgia and headache, addressing their clinical presentation, possible underlying mechanisms and profiles of their interaction with consequent implications for management, by reporting the results of the most relevant studies in the field.

## Co-occurrence of Visceral Pain Syndromes

Cardiac revascularization performed in a subgroup of the comorbid patients produced resolution of cardiac symptoms and also a significant decrease in pain symptoms from the gallbladder, i.e., of number and intensity of biliary colics over a period of 1 month subsequent to surgery as compared to a 1-month period prior to surgery and of referred muscle hyperalgesia in the upper right abdominal quadrant at the cystic point as revealed by increased electrical pain thresholds at this level.

At both a retrospective and prospective 1-year study, comorbid women presented significantly higher urinary pain symptoms (number and intensity of renal colics, referred muscle hyperalgesia in the lumbar region documented as a decreased electrical pain threshold) than women with urinary calculosis only and significantly higher menstrual pain symptoms (number of painful menstrual cycles and referred abdominal muscle hyperalgesia/lowered electrical pain thresholds in rectus abdominis) than women with dysmenorrhea only.

## Pain Co-occurrence in Myofascial Pain Syndromes from Trigger Points

As originally described by Simons [248], myofascial pain syndromes (MPS) are a "complex of sensory, motor and autonomic symptoms that are caused by myofascial trigger points", whereby trigger points (TrPs) are "spots of exquisite tenderness and hyperirritability in muscles or their fascia, localized in taut, palpable bands of muscle fibers which mediate a local twitch response (LTR) of muscle fibers under a specific type of palpation—called snapping—and, if sufficiently hyperirritable, give rise to pain, tenderness and autonomic phenomena as well as dysfunction in areas usually remote from their site, called targets."

Trigger point formation can also be secondary to visceral painful events, in this case TrPs occur in muscle structures located in the referred pain area from a specific viscus as a consequence of the "parietalization" process of visceral pain, especially when the visceral algogenic process has been particularly prolonged or intense or repetitive (e.g., as in the case of colics) [249].

## Pain Co-occurrence in Fibromyalgia

In basal conditions in fibromyalgia plus symptomatic calculosis there was a significant direct linear correlation between the amount of visceral pain experienced by the patients (in terms of number of previously biliary colics) and FMS symptoms, i.e., the spontaneous diffuse musculoskeletal pain, and a significant inverse linear correlation between the number of colics and the muscle pain thresholds ($p < 0.0001$).

Affaitati and others [250], for instance, found that local anesthetic injection of TrPs (two infiltrations on day 1 and day 4), vs placebo-like injection, of trigger points in the trapezius or infraspinatus muscle in comorbid fibromyalgia patients not only reduced the regional pain and tenderness due to the myofascial related pain syndrome, but also had a significant impact onto FMS specific pain, in terms of reduction of fibromyalgia diffuse spontaneous pain, tenderness at tender point level and hyperalgesia in skin, subcutis and muscle in nonpainful areas as evaluated through measurement of pain thresholds to pressure and electrical stimulation.

**Pain Co-occurrence in Headache**
The majority of IBS patients display a generalized increase in pain sensitivity, testifying central sensitization, similarly to patients with migraine and tension-type headache at a high frequency of attacks/chronic [251–253].

Comorbidity in endometriosis is high: it is estimated that about 20% of women with endometriosis present other pain conditions, namely IBS, PBS, vulvodynia, fibromyalgia and particularly headache, mostly migraine, with data in some studies showing that the frequency of chronic headache is significantly higher in patients with migraine plus endometriosis than in those with migraine only [254–257].

The finding of a general hypersensitivity being a function of the number of migraine attacks (thresholds being lower in chronic than high frequency episodic migraine in both migraine-only patients and migraine patients plus fibromyalgia) confirm and extend the results by de Tommaso and others [258] who demonstrated that pain at tender points significantly correlated with headache frequency in comorbid patients.

**Conclusions**
Co-occurrence of pain conditions is common in patients.

The mechanisms behind the mutual influences of symptoms in co-existing pain conditions are also probably multiple, one contributing factor could be represented by modulation of phenomena of hyperexcitability in the central nervous system by the noxious peripheral inputs from one or the other condition.

Independently of mechanisms, however, clinical studies clearly indicate that in comorbid patients treatment of one condition appears crucial not only to treat that condition per se but also to reduce symptoms from one or more other pain comorbidities, probably by reducing the noxious overload onto the central nervous system.

The strong clinical message in co-occurrence of pain conditions is thus to always carry out a thorough patient evaluation and undertake a treatment which is not limited to the most evident and clinically manifest disease but also extended to even mild concurrent conditions, to obtain a better overall pain control.

**Acknowledgement**
*A machine generated summary based on the work of Affaitati, Giannapia; Costantini, Raffaele; Tana, Claudio; Cipollone, Francesco; Giamberardino, Maria Adele. 2019 in Journal of Neural Transmission.*

# *Characteristics of Headache Disorders, According to ICHD-III in an Outpatient Headache Clinic in Sohag Governorate, Egypt*

DOI: https://doi.org/10.1186/s41983-021-00271-x

## Abstract-Summary

The primary headache disorders are more common that of secondary headache.

The 3rd edition of the International Classification of Headache Disorders (ICHD-III) is considered as a helpful tool for classification and diagnosis of different headache disorders.

Primary headache disorders were found in 89% (most of them is episodic in nature 76.2%), secondary headache disorders in about 10%, and painful cranial neuropathy was present in 0.8%.

Primary headache associated with sexual activity was present in 1% of the total number of headache patients, and episodic cluster headache was found in 0.8%.

Male to female ratio was 1:3, 3:5, and 1:1 in primary headache, secondary headache, and painful cranial neuropathy respectively.

This study estimates the frequency and characterizes different headache disorders, according to ICHD-III in an outpatient headache clinic at Sohag Governorate, Egypt.

## Introduction

The headache can be classified to primary headache disorders which include migraine, tension-type headache (TTH), and cluster headache, and less common secondary type of headache which may be due to intracranial neoplasms, epileptic seizures, or intracranial infections [57, 259].

In Egypt, a population-based study conducted in Fayoum Governorate revealed that the 1-year headache prevalence was 51.4%, and the most common primary headache subtype was episodic tension type headache (24.5%), followed by episodic migraine (17.3%) [260].

A study conducted in Saudi Arabia revealed that tension headache was also the commonest primary headache with a prevalence of 9.5% then migraine with prevalence 5.0% [261].

The aim of this hospital-based cross-sectional study is to investigate the frequency and characteristics of different types of headache in the light of recent headache classification namely ICHD-III.

## Methods

Each patient was subjected to full medical and neurological evaluation including history of precipitating factors for each headache attack, comorbid medical conditions, and educational level based on the International Standard Classification of Education (ISCED) [262].

Patients with unclassified headache disorders were excluded from the study to accurately estimate the percentage of primary and secondary headache disorders.

Patients who reported headaches at a frequency of more than 15 days/month over a period of 3 months were classified as chronic headache which include chronic migraine (CM), chronic tension-type headache (CTTH), medication overuse headache (MOH), new daily persistent headache (NDPH), chronic paroxysmal hemicrania, SUNA, or hemicrania continua (HC).

## Results

The participants' age ranged from 11 to 78 years with a mean age of 34.8 ± 13 years.

The percent of chronic headache in males was 30.5% while in females was 21.4% with p value 0.03.

## Discussion

Although some previous studies reported that TTH is the most common type of primary headache all over the world [2], migraine was the most common presentation in our series, and this may be explained by the under-recognition of TTH by patients and health practitioners for its less disability than migraine.

We found that episodic migraine was found in 40.6% of the total number of headache patients, chronic migraine in 10%, episodic TTH in 29.2% of the total number of headache participants, chronic TTH in 4.4%, and episodic cluster headache in 0.8% of the total number of headache participants, and this in agreement with previous study which reported that episodic migraine was present in 35.3%, chronic migraine in 3.9%, episodic TTH in 45.3%, chronic TTH in 5.6%, and cluster headache in 3.4% [260].

## Acknowledgement

*A machine generated summary based on the work of Mohamed, Al-Amir Bassiouny. 2021 in The Egyptian Journal of Neurology, Psychiatry and Neurosurgery.*

# *The Applicability Research of the Diagnostic Criteria for 6.7.2 Angiography Headache in the International Classification of Headache Disorders, 3rd Edition*

DOI: https://doi.org/10.1186/s10194-021-01373-w

## Abstract-Summary

Angiography headache (AH) is common but not negligible, and the criteria for AH have been based on only a few studies.

Two hundred and seventy-nine patients completed this prospective, non-randomized study, including 107 patients who underwent cerebral angiography, 101 patients who underwent coronary intervention and 71 patients who underwent extremities arterial intervention.

The incidence of headache was 22.4% (24/107) in cerebral angiography group, 23.8% (24/101) in coronary intervention group, and 16.9% (12/71) in extremities arterial intervention group.

Two types of headache were observed in cerebral angiography group and coronary intervention group, one during and one after the procedure, while only postoperative headache was observed in extremities arterial intervention group.

Previous headache history was a risk factor for headache in the three groups (p = 0.003 in cerebral angiography group, p = 0.006 in coronary intervention group, and p = 0.016 in extremities arterial intervention group).

The diagnostic criteria for 6.7.2 angiography headache in ICHD-3 may miss a number of cerebral AH with onset later than 24 h after the procedure.

The incidence of headache was high during and after angiography and interventional procedure.

It was suggested that the definition of headache due to coronary intervention and headache due to extremities arterial intervention should be added in ICHD.

Extended:

The incidence of headache was 7.5% (8/107) during, 6.5% (7/107) within 24 h and 12.1% (13/107) within 2–14 days respectively after the procedure in cerebral angiography group.

The incidence of headache was 6.9% (7/101) during, 6.9% (7/101) within 24 h and 14.9% (15/101) within 2–14 days respectively after the procedure in coronary intervention group.

The incidence of headache was 8.5% (6/71) within 24 h and 11.3% (8/71) within 2–14 days respectively after the procedure in extremities arterial intervention group.

The incidence of headache during the procedure was 7.5% (8/107) in cerebral angiography group and 6.9% (7/101) in coronary intervention group.

The incidence of headache in the cerebral angiography and coronary intervention group was similar, slightly higher than that in extremities arterial intervention group, and there was no statistical significance in the incidence of headache in the three groups.

## Background

Previous studies have reported that the incidence of headache in cerebral angiography ranges from 6.9% to 55.6% [263–268].

The criteria defined the onset of cerebral AH to no more than 24 h after cerebral angiography and headache resolved within 72 h after the angiography.

In clinical practice we found that headache duration was less than 24 h in many patients with cerebral AH.

Nearly half of patients still had headaches after 24 h of cerebral angiography, and about a third of patients have more than one headache after cerebral angiography.

## Methods

Demographic information and related medical history such as: age, gender, body mass index (BMI), education level ≥high school or not, history of tobacco and alcohol, allergy history, history of intervention, history of hypertension, diabetes, hyperlipidemia, cerebral infarction and information of previous headache history were collected before procedure after informed consent was obtained from patients and their family members.

In the immediate postoperative investigation, all of the patients were informed about the possibility of "flushing" after the injection of contrast media and were instructed to differentiate this phenomenon from a headache.

If a patient with a previous headache reported a headache attack, the characteristics of headache were retrospectively analyzed by two independent neurologists to determine whether the headache type was similar or different from the previous headache.

**Results**

Twenty-four of 101 (23.8%) patients in coronary intervention group developed headache within 2 weeks.

Coronary intervention group—Among the 101 patients in coronary intervention group, 11.9% (12/101) patients had a history of headache, including 7 migraine, 4 TTH and 1 other type headache.

Extremities arterial intervention group—Of the 71 patients in extremities arterial intervention group, 11.3% (8/71) had a history of headache (2 migraine, 3 TTH and 3 other types of headache).

In coronary intervention group, after adjusting for sex, education level, history of headache, history of hypertension, hyperlipidemia, interventional pathway and X-ray exposure time in Logistic regression model, patients with history of headache had an increased risk of coronary intervention-related headache compared with those without history of headache (OR = 5.929; 95% CI, 1.676–20.977; p = 0.006).

**Discussion**

In the cerebral angiography group and coronary intervention group of our study, the intraoperative headache occurred within 1 h after the beginning of the procedure, the duration time was less than 1 h. Most of the patients had mild to moderate throbbing headache, and the headache characteristics were similar to 8.1.1.1 immediate NO donor-induced headache in ICHD-3 [107, 269, 270].

Throbbing pain was more common in all groups no matter intraoperative or postoperative headache. There were both 41.7% (10/24) patients of cerebral angiography group and coronary intervention group, and 25.0% (3/12) patients of extremities arterial intervention group had more than one headache occurred during the 2 weeks' follow up. Analysis of potential risk factors that may lead to headache showed that previous headache history was a common risk factor among the three groups, and female was a risk factor in cerebral angiography group.

**Conclusion**

The incidence of headache was 22.4% in cerebral angiography group, 23.8% in coronary intervention group, and 16.9% in extremities arterial intervention group.

Female and history of headache were risk factors in cerebral angiography group, and history of headache was a risk factor in coronary intervention group and extremities arterial intervention group.

There were no differences in headache onset time, duration and VAS of intraoperative headache between cerebral angiography group and coronary intervention group.

The headache onset time, duration and VAS of postoperative headache were similar in three groups.

**Acknowledgement**

*A machine generated summary based on the work of Lu, Chenglong; Zhang, Leyi; Wang, Jun; Cao, Xiangyu; Jia, Xin; Ma, Xiaohui; Zhang, Ran; Wang, Lin; Yang, Ying; Meng, Fanchao; Yu, Shengyuan; Liu, Ruozhuo. 2022 in The Journal of Headache and Pain.*

## *Tension-Type Headache in the Emergency Department Diagnosis and Misdiagnosis: The TEDDi Study*

DOI: https://doi.org/10.1038/s41598-020-59171-4

### Abstract-Summary

We evaluated the use of the International Classification of Headache Disorders (ICHD) criteria for TTH in the ED.

We performed a cross-sectional study including all ED patients with a definite TTH diagnosis in their discharge report for 2.5 years.

We evaluated whether the ICHD criteria for TTH were referenced and met.

We analysed discrepancies concerning anamnesis or prior history and reclassified patients.

A total of 211 out of 2132 patients fulfilled the criteria (9.9%).

Criteria A-D were referenced in 60–84% of patients and met in 16–74% of these patients.

After re-reclassification, 21 patients fulfilled the criteria for TTH (5) or probable TTH (16).

Only a minority of patients fulfilled the ICHD criteria.

### Introduction

Tension-type headache (TTH) is the most common primary headache disorder [118, 271].

Given the mild nature of the disorder, few patients seek assistance, and in headache unit-based series, it is not a frequent diagnosis, accounting for 16% of all diagnoses [272].

It seems remarkable that in some ED-based series, TTH diagnosis accounts for up to 25–33% of all headache visits [273, 274]; particularly when other series are performed by neurologists or using ICHD criteria diagnosis, TTH represents only 1–6% of total headache patients [275–279].

We hypothesize that TTH is probably overdiagnosed in the ED setting, which might represent a risk for patients with nondetected secondary headaches.

The first objective was to analyse the percentage of patients who fulfilled the ICHD [280] criteria for tension-type headache and the percentage of patients presenting each of the different criteria.

The third objective was to analyse whether patients could be re-classified as having other headache disorders by using the ICHD-3 criteria.

## Patients and Methods

Our study population included patients who visited the emergency department due to headache.

The inclusion criteria were as follows: 1) patients visiting the ED because of headache and 2) patients with a definite diagnosis of "tension-type headache" in the ED discharge report.

We excluded patients with 1) some degree of uncertainty in the diagnosis, such as "possible" or "probable"; 2) another headache diagnosed at the same time; and 3) no available information in the patient chart.

We screened all the patients who visited the ED during the study period because of headache by using the ED database, which codifies patients by initial reason for consultation.

For the third objective, two headache specialists (NGG, DGA) independently reviewed each case and analysed the information present in the discharge reports.

We did not anticipate any sample size a priori but included all possible patients during the study period.

## Results

Period, 2132 patients visited the ED because of headache.

Only five patients fulfilled all ICHD criteria for TTH (2.4% of the included patients).

Regarding prior medical history, 44 patients (20.85%) had some condition able to produce headache.

After reviewing all the discharge reports, only 21 patients (9.9% of the included sample, 0.98% of the total sample) fulfilled the ICHD-3 criteria for tension-type headache (5) or probable tension-type headache (16).

The diagnosis was more often appropriate in patients who underwent fundoscopy ($\chi^2$ test, 1 df, p = 0.004).

Regarding complementary exams, laboratory exams were performed in 32.6% of patients.

Laboratory exams including erythrocyte sedimentation rate (ESR) or C-reactive protein (CRP) were performed in 48.6% of patients older than 65 years old.

At discharge, 21.3% of patients were referred for a neurological examination.

## Discussion

We systematically analysed a series of patients with definite TTH diagnosis according to whether the diagnostic criteria were mentioned and fulfilled in the discharge report.

The main findings of our study were that only a minority of patients, only 2.4% of the whole sample, fulfilled the ICHD criteria for TTH.

Other series included patients who were diagnosed with TTH who had pulsating (23.8%) and hemicranial headaches (20.1%) [281].

The typical TTH phenotype is probably the most unspecific, and many conditions might have similar features, such as migraine, hemicrania continua, primary cough headache, primary exercise headache, primary headache associated with sexual activity, external-pressure headache, hypnic headache, new daily persistent headache and the vast majority of secondary headache disorders [280, 282].

Misdiagnosis might be related to the classification of patients based on pain phenotype; however, headache diagnosis should be performed by integrating prior medical history, headache anamnesis, presence of other symptoms and neurological examination, not solely by headache phenotype [282, 283].

## Conclusion

In our sample, TTH was overdiagnosed in an emergency department, as only 2.4% of the patients fulfilled all ICHD criteria for TTH.

Inconsistencies in prior medical history or anamnesis were present in the discharge reports in one-fifth and four-fifths of patients, respectively.

Our analysis of medical records allowed us to reclassify these patients as having other primary or secondary headaches.

## Acknowledgement

*A machine generated summary based on the work of García-Azorín, D.; Farid-Zahran, M.; Gutiérrez-Sánchez, M.; González-García, M. N.; Guerrero, A. L.; Porta-Etessam, J. 2020 in Scientific Reports.*

# *Sleep and Tension-Type Headache*

DOI: https://doi.org/10.1007/s11910-019-0953-8

## Abstract-Summary

This review discusses recent evidence for the association between TTH and sleep disturbances.

Further, the close association of TTH with sleep disturbances is more robust in subjects with chronic TTH than in those with episodic TTH.

Growing evidence highlights the association of TTH with psychiatric comorbidity, which is closely associated with sleep disturbances.

Recent advances in our understanding of the association between sleep and TTH will help in improved diagnosis and treatment of TTH and sleep disturbances.

## Introduction

Tension-type headache (TTH) is a prevalent neurological disorder and was estimated to affect 1.89 billion people globally in 2016 [1, 177].

The majority of individuals with TTH on 15 days or less per month are classified as having episodic tension-type headache (ETTH).

TTH is the most common headache disorder that is often associated with sleep disturbances [284–286].

Sleep-related headache disorders included migraine, cluster headache, chronic paroxysmal hemicrania, hypnic headache, and secondary headaches.

The most common sleep-related headache, TTH, was not listed [287].

ICHD-3 described the association of migraine, cluster headache, hypnic headache, primacy cough headache, sleep apnea headache, headache attributed to fasting, and high-altitude headache with sleep but did not include the association between sleep and TTH [107].

**Methods**

The search included full papers and abstracts published in English published until 2018.

Search strings were entered into PubMed as free text with no limits to minimize the possibility of omitting relevant records.

The search retrieved 224 records from the PubMed search.

Additional searches were performed with fewer or more terms to ensure that all potentially relevant studies were identified.

**Results**

Sleep disturbances were the second most common trigger of TTH in a clinic-based study including 334 patients with TTH [288].

An actigraphic study reported that excessive sleep was associated with more severe headache intensity in TTH participants [289].

In a Korean general population-based study, the prevalence of insomnia (Insomnia Severity Index [ISI] total score $\geq$10) among participants with TTH was significantly higher than that among participants without headache (13.2% vs. 5.8%, p < 0.001).

The prevalence of RLS was significantly higher in individuals with TTH than in non-headache individuals (8.0% vs. 3.6%, p = 0.018) in a general population-based study.

The association of TTH with sleep disturbances and mood disorders has been reported in cross-sectional and longitudinal studies [290].

If a TTH patient reports insomnia, sleep-prone prophylactic treatment medication may improve both TTH and insomnia.

**Conclusions**

TTH is the most common primary headache type which shows a significant association with sleep in its onset, change in prevalence, and clinical presentations.

TTH-like headaches can occur in association with sleep, sleep-apnea headaches, and hypnic headaches.

TTH is significantly associated with sleep apnea, insomnia, insufficient sleep, poor sleep quality, RLS, EDS, and bruxism in occurrence and symptom exacerbation, especially in CTTH.

More attention should be paid to the evaluation and treatment of these sleep disturbances during the treatment of TTH.

**Acknowledgement**

*A machine generated summary based on the work of Cho, Soo-Jin; Song, Tae-Jin; Chu, Min Kyung. 2019 in Current Neurology and Neuroscience Reports.*

# Migraine and Tension Headache Comorbidity with Hypothyroidism in Egypt

DOI: https://doi.org/10.1186/s41983-020-00208-w

## Abstract-Summary

Subclinical and overt hypothyroidism were significantly higher in patients with migraine and TTH (p = 0.001) than control subjects.

Patients with migraine and TTH showed significantly more abnormal thyroid gland morphology than healthy control (p = 0.027).

Patients having migraine and TTH more prone to develop hypothyroidism when compared with control group.

Patients with chronic TTH are susceptible to develop hypothyroidism (either subclinical or overt) when compared with patients having frequent or infrequent TTH.

Extended:

Subclinical and overt hypothyroidism were significantly higher in our patients more than control (p = 0.001).

Patients with migraine headache were diagnosed according to the International Classification of Headache Disorders (ICHD)-III beta criteria [291].

Patients with migraine or TTH had 3.73 times higher odds to exhibit hypothyroidism (BLR = 1.316, 95% CI = 1.82–7.64, p = 0.001).

## Introduction

Migraine and tension type headache (TTH) disorders are among the top six most prevalent disorders and the third cause of disability worldwide in individuals under the age of 50 with a major impact on activities of daily living and quality of life [7, 292].

Tension-type headache (TTH) is defined as a mild to moderate band-like pressure headache associated with some somatic and emotional symptoms.

Hypothyroidism represents one of non-neurological comorbidities of migraine.

Many studies defined a bidirectional relationship between migraine, TH, and hypothyroidism including underlying pathophysiological aspects.

The purpose of this study was to investigate the potential association between hypothyroidism in patients with migraine and tension headache.

## Subjects and Methods

Patients with migraine headache were diagnosed according to the International Classification of Headache Disorders (ICHD)-III beta criteria [291].

Patients with tension type headache was diagnosed according to the International Classification of Headache Disorders (ICHD)-III beta criteria [107].

Completely normal laboratory tests (complete blood count, creatinine, liver function tests) Exclusion criteria included patients that were beyond the range of 18–55 years, showed abnormal neurological examination, and or had chronic illness known to affect thyroid dysfunction (chronic kidney disease, psychiatric disorders) were excluded from the study.

To compare quantitative data for two groups, independent-samples t test was used for normally distributed data in both groups with no significant outliers otherwise the alternative non-parametric test (Mann-Whitney U test) was used.

To compare quantitative data for >2 groups, one-way ANOVA test was used for normally distributed data in all groups with no significant outliers otherwise the alternative non-parametric test (Kruskal-Wallis H test) was used.

## Results

Subclinical and overt hypothyroidism were significantly higher in our patients more than control (p = 0.001).

Binary logistic regression (BLR) analysis was run to assess the influence of having migraine or TTH versus no headache on the likelihood that participants will exhibit hypothyroidism (subclinical or overt).

Logistic regression analysis was also run to assess the influence of having chronic tension headache vs other types (frequent and infrequent) on the likelihood that participants will exhibit hypothyroidism (subclinical or overt).

Migraine patients were significantly younger than tension type headache patients (p = 0.001).

Using intragroup comparative statistics, hypothyroidism is significantly expressed in chronic TTH more than TTH with infrequent or even frequent attacks (p = 0.009).

## Discussion

The female preponderance in our study was consistent with Khan and his colleagues which found higher prevalence of both migraine and TTH in patients with hypothyroidism [293].

We have found in our study of 212 patients (migraine and tension headache) that there was significantly higher proportion with subclinical (23.3%) and overt hypothyroidism (6%), as compared to the control subjects of 9% and 1%.

The subclinical and overt hypothyroidism prevalence in our patients with migraine and tension headache were also higher than that reported in the general population.

Regarding sub analysis of migraine patients, there were no significant differences between migraine with aura, migraine without aura, or chronic migraine as regards thyroid function or morphology (p = 0.137 and p = 0.468 respectively) and this is consistent with a recent Russian study who reported negative results regarding comorbidities of migraine and hypothyroidism with abnormal levels of TSH in only 5% of their migraine patients.

## Conclusion

The limited number of patients and control (small sample size) beside we did not recruit other cases of primary headache disorder may be a limitation of our study.

Study the response of patients suffering from migraine or tension headache using conventional measures and having hypothyroidism when controlling thyroid function.

Sufficient number of patients with migraine, tension headache and control subjects for detection the accurate relationship.

Study the relationship between other types of primary headache disorders and hypothyroidism.

Study if there is relationship between primary headache disorders and thyroid dysfunction whether hypo or hyperthyroidism.

**Acknowledgement**

*A machine generated summary based on the work of Abou Elmaaty, Ali A.; Flifel, Mohamed E.; Belal, Tamer; Zarad, Carmen A. 2020 in The Egyptian Journal of Neurology, Psychiatry and Neurosurgery.*

## *Quantitative Analysis of the Retinal Nerve Fiber Layer, Ganglion Cell Layer and Optic Disc Parameters by the Swept Source Optical Coherence Tomography in Patients with Migraine and Patients with Tension-Type Headache*

DOI: https://doi.org/10.1007/s13760-018-1041-6

**Abstract-Summary**

The aim of the study was to measure the thicknesses of the inner retinal segments and optic nerve head (ONH) parameters in migraineurs and patients with tension-type headache (TTH) in headache-free period using swept source optical coherence tomography (SS-OCT) and to compare the outcomes with each other and those of healthy subjects.

Macular ganglion cell inner plexiform layer (mGCIPL), macular ganglion cell complex (mGCC), circumpapillary retinal nerve fiber layer (cpRNFL), and ONH parameters were evaluated using SS-OCT, and the areas under the receiver-operating characteristic (ROC) curves were calculated to determine the ability of these parameters to distinguish between the patient and normal eyes.

There were not statistically significant differences between the measurements acquired from migraineurs, TTH patients, and the controls.

SS-OCT presented reproducible and reliable measurements of posterior segment layers of the eyes, especially in sectoral configuration, and the parameters did not show significant difference between the groups.

Extended:

The aim of this study was to determine whether a similarity is present between the migraineurs and TTH patients regarding retinal structures, because we have previously demonstrated that the TTH patients had similar visual field defects in the attack period like the patients with migraines [294].

## Introduction

Although vasoconstriction of cerebral and retinal blood vessels is a transient phenomenon, the chronic nature of the migraine might cause permanent changes in the structure of the brain and retina [295].

In a study, it was reported that there could be visual field defect also in TTH patients and a continuum between the migraine headache and the TTH headache [294].

Many investigators measured the thicknesses of posterior pole retinal layers and choroid with optical coherence tomography (OCT), given the influence of migraine headache on the posterior segment of the eye.

The purpose of the current study was to measure the thicknesses of retinal layers and optic nerve head (ONH) parameters in migraineurs and patients with TTH using the SS-OCT and also to review whether there are similar characteristics in TTH patients by comparing the results with those of migraine patients and healthy subjects.

## Methods

Both normal individuals and patients with headaches who were eligible for the study underwent a complete ophthalmologic examination that comprised refraction and detection of visual acuity level, measurement of intraocular pressure, and biomicroscopy of anterior segment and posterior segment.

If all the participants had a best-corrected visual acuity of 20/20, refractive error of between $-3.00$ D and $+2.00$ D in sphere, intraocular pressure of 21 mmHg or less, normal looking ONH, and retina on ophthalmoscopy, their eyes were evaluated in the present study.

Distributed average and sectoral values of mGCIPL thickness, mGCC thickness, cpRNFL thickness, and ONH parameters were compared between normal and patient eyes using the independent sample t test.

The diagnostic accuracy of each retinal layer thickness and ONH parameters to differentiate between normal and patient eyes was determined by calculating the areas under the receiver-operating characteristic (ROC) curves.

## Results

The great majority of all groups consisted of the females.

The number of the females with migraine and with TTH were 20 (87%), and 18 (82%) respectively, against the proportion of 88% (22/25) of the control group.

When the influence of disease duration and the attack frequency for both groups of headache patients on retinal structures were evaluated, no relationship was defined between them.

## Discussion

We assessed the ability of mGCIPL, mGCC, cpRNFL, and ONH parameters; rim area, disc area, HCDR, VCDR, and cup volume to distinguish the migraineous eyes from the TTH and healthy eyes using SS-OCT image acquisition modality.

Through the analysis of cpRNFL, macula, and choroid with OCT, several authors have studied whether the posterior segments are involved in migraine patients.

Although a different equipment was employed to measure the retinal parameters in the present study, we obtained similar results to Tan and others In general, thinning in RNFL has been detected in patients.

Most of the retinal parameters in migraine and TTH patients in the current study were detected as slightly thicker than those in controls.

**Acknowledgement**

*A machine generated summary based on the work of Yener, Arif Ülkü; Korucu, Osman. 2018 in Acta Neurologica Belgica.*

# Sensory Function in Headache: A Comparative Study Among Patients with Cluster Headache, Migraine, Tension-Type Headache, and Asymptomatic Subjects

DOI: https://doi.org/10.1007/s10072-020-04384-8

**Abstract-Summary**

The purpose of the present study was to evaluate and compare sensory function in the trigeminocervical region in patients with CH, MH, and TH and healthy controls (HC).

TH presented significantly lower PPT values compared with CH ($p < 0.015$), MH ($p < 0.048$), and HC ($p < 0.009$), while MH demonstrated significantly lower values than HC ($p = 0.001$–$0.023$).

When analyzing TDT, CH in the symptomatic side presented significantly higher values in V1 compared with MH ($p = 0.001$), TH ($p < 0.001$), and HC ($p < 0.001$) and in V2 compared with TH ($p = 0.035$).

With regard to 2PDT, CH-s presented significantly higher values in V1 with respect to HC ($p = 0.016$) but lower values in V2 compared with MH ($p < 0.001$) and TH ($p = 0.003$).

The results of the present study indicate specific and different altered mechanical sensory thresholds in CH, MH, and TH patients compared with HC subjects.

Extended:

With regard to the TDT, post hoc comparisons using Bonferroni test evidenced that CH-s presented significantly higher values in V1 compared with MH ($p = 0.001$), TH ($p < 0.001$), and HC ($p < 0.001$) and in V2 compared with TH ($p = 0.035$).

The results of the present study indicated that CH patients demonstrated hypoaesthesia in V1 area of the symptomatic side.

Future studies should consider these limitations, as well as research with other sensory modalities.

Future studies are warranted to further elucidate this data.

## Introduction

Baseline deficits of mechanical sensory function have demonstrated to be predictive of poor prognosis and higher risk for the development of chronic pain in different clinical subgroups including headaches [296, 297].

Somatosensory disturbances including mechanical, thermal, and electrical sensory function have been consistently shown to be a feature of patients with primary headaches.

Most of these studies have focused on migraine, while evidence of sensory function in other primary headaches is underrepresented.

Our study had a double purpose: first, to estimate and compare sensory function in the trigeminocervical region in patients with CH, MH, and TH and healthy controls (HC), and second, to determine if sensory function correlates with any clinical variable.

We hypothesized that CM, MH, and TH would evidence alterations in sensory function compared with HC and these disturbances would be specific for each type of headache based on its different pathophysiological basis.

## Materials and Methods

CH patients (n = 16) were 9 males (56.2%) and 7 females (43.8%) with an average age of 41.9 (SD = 6.8) years.

TH patients (n = 71) were 12 males (16.9%) and 59 females (83.1%) with an average age of 38.3 (SD = 13.7) years.

TDT and PDT were measured with a set of 20 calibrated Semmes-Weinstein monofilaments (Saehan, marking number 1.65–6.65; force 0.005–447 g) delivering a precise amount of pressure [298, 299].

To determine TDT and PDT, the method of limits was used, following a standardized protocol of five ascending and descending series [300].

In the descending series, monofilaments were applied in decreasing order of strength until the patient no longer detected the stimulus.

For PDT, the patient was instructed to indicate when the tactile sensation of the monofilament changed to sensation of prick.

## Results

An initial comparative analysis showed no significant difference (p > 0.05) in any of the QST variables with regard to the examined side in MH, TH, and HC groups.

Regarding PPT, TH presented significantly lower PPT values in V1, V2, cranium, upper trapezius muscle, C2-C3 facet joint, suboccipital muscles, and thenar eminence compared with CH-s (p < 0.015), CH-a (p < 0.001), MH (p < 0.048), and HC (p < 0.009).

MH showed significantly higher TDT in V1, V2, and V3 compared with TH (p < 0.037) and in the thenar eminence compared with CH patients (p = 0.003).

When analyzing 2PDT, CH-s presented significantly higher values in V1 with respect to HC (p = 0.016) but lower values in V2 compared with MH (p < 0.001) and TH (p = 0.003).

## Discussion

The results of the present study evidence specific and different altered mechanical sensory thresholds in CH, MH, and TH patients compared with HC subjects.

MH patient showed statistically significant lower PPT values compared with HC in V2, upper trapezius muscle, C2–C3 facet joint, and suboccipital muscles.

MH patient showed statistically significant lower PPT values compared with HC in V2, upper trapezius muscle, C2–C3 facet joint, and suboccipital muscles but no differences in TDT.

MH patients exhibited significantly higher TDT values in V1, V2, and V3 compared with TH but significantly lower TDT in V1 compared with CH-s. Although differences with the control group were not found for TDT, MH sensory profile could be intermediate with respect to CH and TH.

TH patients consistently showed statistically significant lower PPT values in V1, V2, upper trapezius muscle, C2–C3 facet joint, suboccipital muscles, and thenar eminence compared with CH, MH, and HC.

## Conclusions

This study is the first attempt to investigate mechanical sensory function in the three types of primary headache and asymptomatic subjects throughout the entire craniofacial region: in the three divisions of the trigeminal nerve (V1, V2, and V3), neck (superficial cervical plexus), and ear (trigeminal and facial nerves), including a control region (hand).

The results of the present study evidence specific and different altered mechanical sensory thresholds in CH, MH, and TH patients compared with HC subjects.

QST variables also evidenced some negligible correlations with BMI, headache intensity, and time elapsed since the first headache.

## Acknowledgement

*A machine generated summary based on the work of Malo-Urriés, Miguel; Estébanez-de-Miguel, Elena; Bueno-Gracia, Elena; Tricás-Moreno, José Miguel; Santos-Lasaosa, Sonia; Hidalgo-García, César. 2020 in Neurological Sciences.*

# *Cognitive Performance in Patients with Chronic Tension-Type Headache and Its Relation to Neuroendocrine Hormones*

DOI: https://doi.org/10.1186/s41983-020-0150-3

## Abstract-Summary

Depression is highly prevalent in chronic tension-type headache (CTTH) patients attending the clinical settings.

Cognitive impairment and neuroendocrine dysregulation had been reported in patients with depression and patients with CTTH.

To assess the cognitive performance and investigate its possible relations to neuroendocrine levels in patients with CTTH.

Patients with CTTH, depression, and control subjects were recruited.

Both patients with CTTH and depression had impaired cognitive performance.

The hormonal levels significantly correlated with cognitive function in patient groups, especially patients with CTTH.

Patients with CTTH had cognitive dysfunction which could be related to neuro-endocrine hormonal dysregulation.

Extended:

Patients with CTTH often suffer from memory impairment, sleep disturbance, and other psychiatric disorders especially anxiety and depression [301].

Patients with CTTH were in active episodes of headache when the blood samples were obtained.

Patients with CTTH usually suffering from poor cognitive performance.

Patients with CTTH had cognitive dysfunction and prominent hormonal changes.

## Introduction

Several studies reported impaired cognitive performance in patients with migraine [302, 303].

Studies that evaluate the cognitive function of patients with CTTH are rare, the previous study reported cognitive impairment and neuroendocrine dysregulation in those patients [304].

Many neuroendocrine hormones dysregulation, including hormones of the hypothalamus-pituitary-adrenal (HPA) axis, hypothalamus-pituitary-thyroid (HPT) axis, and hypothalamus-pituitary-gonadal (HPG) axis were associated and correlated with impaired cognitive performance in different medical disorders [305–315].

The cognitive impairment reported in CTTH could be the result of neuroendocrine hormones alteration or the effect of associated depression.

We aimed to (1) assess the cognitive performance and measure the serum concentration of neuroendocrine hormones [corticotropin-releasing hormone (CRH), adrenocorticotropic hormone (ACTH), cortisol, thyroid-stimulating hormone (TSH), free triiodothyronine (FT3), and free thyroxine (FT4)] in patients with CTTH. (2) Investigate the possible relations between cognitive performance and neuroendocrine hormones.

## Subjects and Methods

In a cross-sectional case-control study, we investigated 100 patients with CTTH, 97 patients with depression, and 105 control subjects without headache or depression for cognitive performance and serum levels of neuroendocrine hormones.

Depression was diagnosed in accordance with the Diagnostic and Statistical Manual of Mental Disorders, 5th edition [316].

Patients with CTTH were in active episodes of headache when the blood samples were obtained.

Blood samples were immediately centrifuged at 3000 rpm for 5 min and sera were separated and kept in labeled sterile microtubes at −80 °C until the hormones were assayed.

An enzyme-linked immunosorbent assay was performed to detect the basal serum concentrations of neuroendocrine hormones including CRH, ACTH, CORTISOL, TSH, FT3, and FT4.

The statistical analysis was performed with non-parametric $\chi^2$ between gender, and pain severity in the studied groups.

Regression analysis was performed to identify the effect of different hormones on cognitive function.

## Results

In patients with CTTH, the serum levels of CRH, ACTH, cortisol, and TSH had significant negative effects on MoCA scores (r − .314, p = .001; r − .378, p = .000; r− .222, p .027; r − .388, p = .000, respectively) while the serum level of FT4 had positive effect on the MoCA score (r .372, p = .000).

The serum levels of CRH, ACTH, TSH were positively (r .202, p = .044; r .285, p = .004; r .416, p = .000, respectively) and serum level of FT4 was negatively (r − .388, p = .000) correlated with BDI score among patients with CTTH.

In patients with depression, the serum levels of CRH, ACTH, cortisol, and TSH were positive (r .403, p = .000; r .288, p = .004; r 0427, p = .000; r .834, p = .000, respectively) and serum levels of FT3 and FT4 were negative (r − .357, p = .000 and r − .523, p = .000) correlated with BDI score.

## Discussion

Both patients with CTTH and patients with depression had cognitive impairment without significant differences between them.

Ping and others [304] reported an impairment in cognitive function, especially memory, in patients with CTTH.

The correlation between serum levels of neuroendocrine hormones and cognitive functions showed significant negative effects of CRH, ACTH, cortisol, and TSH and positive effects of FT4 on cognitive function in patients with CTTH, and ACTH, and TSH appeared to be the independent hormones related to cognitive function.

In patients with depression, the only significant negative correlation was reported with TSH which might suggest that the cognitive impairment in patients with CTTH may be related to alterations in functions of HPA and PT axes and not due to the presence of comorbid depression, specially, patients with depression had more prominent hormonal dysregulation than patients with CTTH.

## Conclusion

Patients with CTTH had cognitive dysfunction and prominent hormonal changes.

The hormonal changes may be the cause of the cognitive decline in patients with CTTH.

## Acknowledgement

*A machine generated summary based on the work of Kotb, Mamdouh Ali; Kamal, Ahmed M.; Al-Malki, Daifallah; Abd El Fatah, Aliaa S.; Ahmed, Yassmin M. 2020 in The Egyptian Journal of Neurology, Psychiatry and Neurosurgery.*

## *Geographical Differences in Trigger Factors of Tension-Type Headaches and Migraines*

DOI: https://doi.org/10.1007/s11916-019-0760-6

**Abstract-Summary**

We discussed the types and frequencies of trigger factors of primary headache [migraine and tension-type headache (TTH)] among adult patients.

We assessed the influence of geographical location, ethnicity and gender on the various trigger factors of a migraine and a TTH.

We also evaluated the trigger factors among the multi-ethnic Southeast Asian adult patients.

Stress is one of the most common trigger factors for patients with migraines and TTHs worldwide.

These patients have much difficulty in adapting to the high level of sensitivity, and the sensitized brain is therefore more vulnerable to trigger factors.

The geographical location factor has an influence on the trigger factors of headaches.

Change in weather and sunlight are important commonly identified trigger factors for headaches.

Gender differences in some trigger factors are present among the patients with headaches, especially sunlight and sleep deprivation.

This will enable proper identification of trigger factors, leading to a decrease in the number of headache episodes and an improvement in quality of life for patients.

Extended:

Gender differences in some trigger factors were present among patients with headaches.

**Introduction**

In a community study conducted in Malaysia, the most common trigger factors for migraines and TTHs were sunlight, sleep deprivation and stress [317].

The most common trigger factors for both TTHs and migraines in previous studies were sleep deprivation, stress, change of weather and sunlight [288, 318–326].

Sunlight was the most common trigger factor in the primary headache patients (47%) in one community study conducted in Malaysia [317].

In a study conducted on the patients with migraines in a general population of Mexican-Americans in San Diego County, USA, change of weather was the second most frequently reported trigger factor in the female migraineurs (54.4%) [327].

In a clinic-based study conducted in Holland, sleep deprivation was the third most common trigger factor among patients with headaches [325].

In a previous community study also conducted in Malaysia, menstruation was a triggering factor in 31 and 18.2% of the patients with migraines and TTHs, respectively [317].

**Acknowledgement**

*A machine generated summary based on the work of Tai, Mei-Ling Sharon; Yet, Sharon Xue Er; Lim, Ting Chung; Pow, Zhen Yuan; Goh, Cheng Beh. 2019 in Current Pain and Headache Reports.*

## Drug-Naïve Egyptian Females with Migraine Are More Prone to Sexual Dysfunction Than Those with Tension-Type Headache: A Cross-Sectional Comparative Study

DOI: https://doi.org/10.1007/s13760-020-01504-1

**Abstract-Summary**

All the participants were evaluated by the Arabic version of the female sexual function index (ArFSFI: 19 items), the abridged 5-item version of the international index of erectile function (IIEF-5), hospital anxiety and depression scale (HADS: 14 items), visual analog scale (VAS) score, and the headache impact test questionnaire (HIT-6TM: 6 items).

A significant correlation was noticed between scores of total ArFSFI in women with TTH and their partners' IIEF-5 scores ($r = 0.773$, $p < 0.001$).

Significant negative correlations were also found between scores of total ArFSFI in women with migraine ($r -0.327$, $p\ 0.011$), HADS-A scores ($r -0.504$, $p < 0.001$), HADS-D scores ($r -0.579$, $p < 0.001$), HITS scores ($r -0.413$, $p\ 0.001$), VAS scores ($r\ 0.737$, $p < 0.001$), and their partners' IIEF-5 scores ($r -0.839$, $p < 0.001$).

Our study had shown a bidirectional relation between SD, anxiety, and depression subscales of HADS in females with migraine only ($28.49 \pm 9.46$, $13.54 \pm 4.44$, $15.17 \pm 7.73$ respectively, $p\ 0.009$), while females with migraine and SD reported statistical higher scores of anxiety and depression ($25.21 \pm 11.70$, $12.71 \pm 4.20$, $17.95 \pm 8.05$, respectively, $p\ 0.006$).

**Introduction**

Migraine and tension-type headache (TTH) are the most prevalent types of primary headache (PH) [328, 329].

It is postulated that PH is commonly associated with SD and comorbid psychiatric disorders, such as anxiety and depression [330].

We aimed in this observational case-control study to determine the rate of SD in drug naïve women with migraine and TTH as the primary objective for the study.

We aimed to determine whether migraine or TTH is associated with more devastating impact on sexual function as a secondary objective for the study.

**Methods and Materials**

Male partners of patients and control were evaluated against the abridged 5-item version of the international index of erectile function (IIEF-5) to determine their sexual functions; each item is scored on a five-point ordinal scale where lower values represent poorer sexual function.

It is worth mentioning that all affected females were asked to fill out the headache impact test questionnaire (HIT-6TM: 6 items) to determine the impact of headache on the patient's daily activities; it is a brief instrument covering a broad content of headache-related quality of life across the following domains: pain, social functioning, role functioning, vitality, cognitive functioning, and psychological distress.

Patients with migraine were also evaluated by The Migraine-Specific Quality of Life Questionnaire; a 14-item questionnaire designed to measure how migraines affect and/or limit daily functioning across three domains: 7 items assessing how migraines limit one's daily social and work-related activities, 4 items assessing how migraines prevent these activities and 3 items assessing the emotions associated with migraines.

**Discussion**

The current study had revealed that circumcised females with TTH were significantly depressed than uncircumcised females, while circumcised females with migraine revealed significantly lower total FSFI scores together with significant impairment of their partners' erectile function than uncircumcised females.

Our study had shown that migraine had a more devastating impact than TTH on sexual functions of the affected females and their partners which could be seen in consistence with the findings demonstrated by Secuteri and others (1976) [331]. The prevalence of SD among migraine and/or TTH patients is still contradictory.

Nappi and others (2012) who studied sexual functions in females with TTH accompanied by migraine using FSFI and female sexual distress scale found that FSFI scores were lower in the patients group [330].

Our study is one of the few studies that evaluated the sexual functions of females suffering from migraine and TTH together with the presence of controls that strengthen the findings of our study.

**Acknowledgement**
*A machine generated summary based on the work of Ahmed, Hossam El Din Hosni; GamalEl Din, Sameh Fayek; Oraby, Mohammed Ibrahim; Elhameed, Heba Mohammad Abd; Ahmed, Ahmed Ragab. 2020 in Acta Neurologica Belgica.*

## *Treatment*

Machine generated keywords: tth, manual, care, therapy, efficacy, medication, physical, effectiveness, episodic tth, neck, tensiontype headache, tensiontype, adolescent, usual, nsaid.

# *Aids to Management of Headache Disorders in Primary Care (2nd Edition)*

DOI: https://doi.org/10.1186/s10194-018-0899-2

## Abstract-Summary

The Aids to Management are a product of the Global Campaign against Headache, a worldwide programme of action conducted in official relations with the World Health Organization.

The common headache disorders (migraine, tension-type headache and medication-overuse headache) are major causes of ill health.

These Aids to Management, with the European principles of management of headache disorders in primary care as the core of their content, combine educational materials with practical management aids.

The Aids to Management may be individually downloaded and, as is the case for all products of the Global Campaign against Headache, are available without restriction for non-commercial use.

## Preface

Medical management of headache disorders does not, for the vast majority of people affected by them, require specialist skills or investigations.

Aids to management of headache disorders in primary care (2nd edition) updates the 1st edition, published 11 years ago [332].

It has undergone review by a wider consultation group of headache experts, including representatives of the member national societies of EHF, primary-care physicians from eight countries of Europe, and lay advocates from member organisations of the European Headache Alliance.

The European principles of management of headache disorders in primary care, laid out in 14 sections, are the core of the content.

Any of seven information leaflets may be offered to patients to improve their understanding of their headache disorders and their management.

LTB and EHF offer these aids for use without restriction for non-commercial purposes, as is the case for all products of the Global Campaign against Headache [333].

## European Principles of Management of Headache Disorders in Primary Care

Key points of information are: ■ migraine is a common disorder which, while it may be disabling, is benign; ■ it is often familial, and probably genetically inherited; ■ it cannot be cured but can be successfully treated; ■ trigger or predisposing factors are common in migraine, and should be identified and avoided or modified when possible, but not all can be; ■ a headache calendar helps good management by recording over time: ■ the symptoms and pattern of attacks (eg, menstrual relationship); ■ medication use (thus identifying overuse); ■ regular activity (eg, sport or exercise 2–3 times per week) may reduce intensity and frequency of migraine attacks.

**Instruments and Other Materials to Aid Diagnosis and Management of Headache Disorders in Primary Care**

Diagnostic criteria: A. Headache (migraine-like or tension-type-like) on ≥15 days/month for >3 months, and fulfilling criteria B and C B. Occurring in a patient who has had at least five attacks fulfilling criteria B–D for 1.1 Migraine without aura and/or criteria B and C for 1.2 Migraine with aura C. On ≥8 days/month for >3 months, fulfilling any of the following.

Diagnostic criteria: A. At least 10 episodes of headache occurring on 1–14 days/month on average for >3 months (≥12 and <180 days/year) and fulfilling criteria B–D B. Lasting from 30 min to 7 days C. At least two of the following four characteristics: [1].

Diagnostic criteria: A. Headache occurring on ≥15 days/month in a patient with a pre-existing headache disorder B. Regular overuse for >3 months of one or more drugs that can be taken for acute and/or symptomatic treatment of headache[1,2] C. Not better accounted for by another ICHD-3 diagnosis.

**Patient Information Leaflets to Aid Headache Management in Primary Care (2nd Edition)**

Headache management is greatly facilitated when the patient understands his or her headache disorder and the treatment being proposed for it.

Good treatment of patients with any headache disorder therefore begins with explanations of their disorder and the purpose and means of management.

■ Explanation is a crucial element of preventative management in patients with frequent migraine or tension-type headache, who are at particular risk of escalating medication consumption.

The general principles of headache management place education and reassurance of patients first.

To assist, Lifting The Burden (LTB) has produced a series of Patient Information Leaflets (PILs).

**Translation, and the Preservation of Original Meaning, of Materials Developed to Improve Headache Management**

Coordination of the translation A translation coordinator, who oversees but does not carry out the translation, is selected according to the following criteria: ■ a headache expert; ■ bilingual in English and the target language (ideally a native speaker and a resident of the country of the target language); ■ has ability to mediate between different translators and to understand the points of view of lay and professional translators.

Coordination of the translation A translation coordinator, who oversees but does not carry out the translation, is selected according to the following criteria: ■ has technical knowledge (ie, understands the concepts underlying the questions or instrument being translated); ■ bilingual in English and the target language (ideally a native speaker and a resident of the country of the target language); ■ has ability to mediate between different translators and to understand the points of view of lay and professional translators.

**Acknowledgement**

*A machine generated summary based on the work of Steiner, T. J.; Jensen, R.; Katsarava, Z.; Linde, M.; MacGregor, E. A.; Osipova, V.; Paemeleire, K.; Olesen, J.; Peters, M.; Martelletti, P. 2019 in The Journal of Headache and Pain.*

# Variables Associated with Use of Symptomatic Medication During a Headache Attack in Individuals with Tension-Type Headache: A European Study

DOI: https://doi.org/10.1186/s12883-020-1624-8

**Abstract-Summary**

Pharmacological treatment of patients with tension-type headache (TTH) includes symptomatic (acute) and prophylactic (preventive) medication.

No previous study has investigated variables associated to symptomatic medication intake in TTH.

Differences between patients using or not using symptomatic medication, depending on self-perceived effectiveness, and time (early during an attack, i.e., the first 5 min, or when headache attack is intense) when the symptomatic medication was taken were calculated.

One hundred and thirty-six (n = 136, 80%) reported symptomatic medication intake for headache (73% NSAIDs).

Patients taking symptomatic medication in general showed lower headache frequency and lower depressive levels than those patients not taking medication.

Symptomatic medication was more effective in patients with lower headache history, frequency, and duration, and lower emotional burden.

No differences in pressure pain sensitivity were found depending on the self-perceived effectiveness of medication.

Patients taking 'late symptomatic' medication exhibited more widespread pressure pain sensitivity than those taking 'early medication'.

This study found that the effectiveness of symptomatic medication was associated with better headache parameters (history, frequency, or duration) and lower emotional burden.

Further, consuming early symptomatic medication at the beginning of a headache attack (the first 5 min) could limit widespread pressure pain sensitivity.

Extended:

One hundred and sixty-eight (n = 168, 99%) were finally included in the analysis as they returned the headache diary with medication intake data.

One hundred and sixty (n = 160, 95%) were diagnosed with TTH associated to pericranial tenderness whereas the remaining 8 (5%) were not associated to pericranial tenderness.

One hundred and thirty-six (81%) reported taking symptomatic medication for their headache: 62 (45.5%) took simple analgesics (paracetamol) whereas the remaining 74 (54.5%) took NSAID (ibuprofen: n = 57, 42%; ketoprofen: n = 7, 5%; naproxen: n = 10, 7.5%).

Symptomatic medication was more effective in those patients with lower frequency and shorter duration of headaches, shorter history of pain, and lower emotional burden of headache.

This study found that the use of symptomatic acute medication for TTH was associated with a lower headache frequency and lower depressive symptoms, but not to other clinical/psychological outcomes.

## Background

Pharmacological treatment of patients with TTH includes symptomatic (acute) and prophylactic medication.

A recent study observed that NSAIDs consumption in people with TTH almost reached 90% and that patient's preferences on medication intake was slightly different from clinical guideline recommendations [334].

No study has previously investigated the association of these variables to symptomatic medication intake in TTH patients.

Considering the impact [335] and personal burden [336] associated to this headache disorder, better understanding of the variables associated with symptomatic medication intake may help to better identify some critical areas for future research on symptomatic medication treatment of individuals with TTH.

The aim of this longitudinal observational study was to investigate potential associations of clinical, psychological and sensitivity outcomes with use of symptomatic medication in individuals suffering from TTH.

## Methods

This previous analysis found that patients with TTH taking prophylactic medication (i.e., amitriptyline) had higher frequency and burden of headaches, worse sleep quality and higher depressive levels than those TTH patients not taking prophylactic medication [337].

In this diary, they registered if the symptomatic medication drug used for headache (when taken); the time when they take the medication: 'early symptomatic' (at the beginning of the attack, in the first 5 min) or 'late symptomatic' (when the headache was intense, defined as >7 on a NPRS); and the self-perceived effectiveness of the medication (i.e., absent, moderate or total pain relief at 2 h without the use of other medication) [338].

Differences between grouped patients in clinical features, burden of headache (HDI-E, HDI-P), depression (HADS-D), anxiety (HADS-A, STAI-T, STAI-S) and sleep quality (PSQI) were compared using one-way analysis of variance (ANOVA).

## Results

One hundred and thirty-six (81%) reported taking symptomatic medication for their headache: 62 (45.5%) took simple analgesics (paracetamol) whereas the remaining 74 (54.5%) took NSAID (ibuprofen: n = 57, 42%; ketoprofen: n = 7, 5%; naproxen: n = 10, 7.5%).

Patients reported that they took symptomatic medication in 70% of the headache attacks (mean 8.8 ± 1 headache per month), not in all.

Significant differences in the distribution of individuals with frequent episodic (FETTH) and chronic (CTTH) tension-type headache (p = 0.021), headache frequency (p = 0.015) and depression (HADS-D, p = 0.021) were observed between patients taking or not taking symptomatic medication.

Fifty-eight (43%) reported taking 'early symptomatic' medication, whereas the remaining 78 (57%) took 'late symptomatic' medication.

## Discussion

This is the first study investigating variables associated with the use of symptomatic medication intake in patients with TTH and when the medication is taken (early or late during the headache attack).

81% of our sample of patients with TTH reported taking medication for their headache attacks, data similar to a recent study conducted in Italy where 90% of individuals with TTH were symptomatic medication users [334].

It seems that higher frequency of headache [134] and emotional factors [339] can lead to hyperalgesic response to the central nervous system; therefore, symptomatic medication may be more effective in patients with lower central sensitization.

An important finding of this study was that patients taking symptomatic medication at the beginning of the headache attack ('early symptomatic medication') showed lower widespread pressure pain sensitivity than those subjects taking the medication when the headache was intense ('late symptomatic medication').

## Conclusions

This study found that the use of symptomatic acute medication for TTH was associated with a lower headache frequency and lower depressive symptoms, but not to other clinical/psychological outcomes.

Higher effectiveness of symptomatic medication was associated with lower frequency and shorter duration of the headaches, shorter headache history, and lower emotional headache burden.

## Acknowledgement

*A machine generated summary based on the work of Fernández-de-las-Peñas, César; Palacios-Ceña, Maria; Castaldo, Matteo; Wang, Kelun; Guerrero-Peral, Ángel; Catena, Antonella; Arendt-Nielsen, Lars. 2020 in BMC Neurology.*

# Treatment of Tension-Type Headaches in Adolescents (14–15 Years Old): The Efficacy of Aminophenylbutyric Acid Hydrochloride

DOI: https://doi.org/10.1007/s12668-018-0507-6

## Abstract-Summary

The research covered 64 adolescents aged 14–15 with tension-type headaches: 33 boys and 42 girls (11 boys and 20 girls with frequent episodic tension-type headache (ETTH) and 12 boys and 21 girls with chronic tension-type headache (CTTH)).

The reduction of tension-type headache intensity was assessed by 3-grade scale: "no change," "significantly reduced," and "completely stopped": 0—no, 1—very seldom, 2—often, and 3—permanently.

ETTH/CTTH associated symptoms are as follows: (1) difficulty of falling asleep and restless sleep ($0.91 \pm 0.83/1.54 + 1.26$), (2) difficulty of concentrating during the day ($0.61 + 0.92/2.04 + 1.21$), (3) morning sickness ($0.32 + 0.87/1.81 + 1.29$), (4) feeling ill in the morning with improvement in the second half of the day ($0.17 + 0.57/1\ 95 + 0.95$), (5) meteosensitivity ($0.58 + 1.01/1.59 + 1.22$), and (6) decrease in physical capability ($0.20 + 0.64/1.72 + 0.82$).

After 3 weeks, the pain in ETTH subgroup completely stopped in 27 children (79%) and significantly reduced in 7 (21%).

Associated symptoms of ETTH/CTTH are as follows: (1) difficulty of falling asleep and restless sleep ($0.26 + 0.44$, $p = 0.000093/0.45 + 0.80$, $p = 0.000224$), (2) difficulty of concentrating during the day ($0.17 + 0.38$, $p = 0.003707/0.54 + 0.85$; $p = 0.000007$), (3) morning sickness ($0.08 + 0.28$, $p = 0$.

Aminophenylbutyric acid hydrochloride (GABA receptor agonist) reduces the intensity of tension-type headache and has a positive effect on associated symptoms.

Extended:

Aminophenylbutyric acid hydrochloride has a positive effect on symptoms which were reasons for the complaint; however, it does not eliminate them at all.

## Introduction

At the age of 3, headache occurs in 3–8% children [340], at the age of 5—in 19.5%, and at the age of 7—in 37–51.5% of children and adolescents.

Tension-type headache (TTH) is one of the most common types of headache.

Episodic headache is the pain that occurs several times per month.

Non-frequent episodic TTH occurs not less than 1 day per month (<12 days per year); frequent episodic TTH is registered 1–15 days per month (<12 and >180 days per year).

Chronic TTH occurs several times per week, at least 15 times per month within 3 months (>180 days per year) [47].

The purpose of the study is to investigate efficacy of the synthetic analogue of GABA-beta-phenyl-gamma-aminobutyric acid hydrochloride in the treatment of TTH in adolescents ages 14–15.

## Materials and Methods

The inclusion criteria were as follows: the presence of a headache for at least 1 year, the correspondence to the criteria for a tension headache according to The International Classification of Headache Disorders, 3rd edition (beta version) [47].

The research covered 64 adolescents aged 14–15 with tension-type headaches: 33 boys and 42 girls (11 boys and 20 girls with frequent episodic tension-type headache (ETTH) and 12 boys and 21 girls with chronic tension-type headache (CTTH)).

TTH was diagnosed in accordance with International Headache Society [47].

After pre-assessment, all adolescents were prescribed aminophenylbutyric acid hydrochloride 250 mg three times a day for 3 weeks.

The reduction of tension-type headache intensity 3 weeks later was assessed by 3-grade scale: "no change," "significantly reduced," and "completely stopped": 0—no, 1—very seldom, 2—often, and 3—permanently.

## Results

In patients with CTTH, the most significant symptom associated with headache was lack of concentration during the day; meanwhile, other symptoms were presented equally.

After the second course of treatment, patients suffering from ETTH did not show any significant dynamic; however, adolescents with CTTH reported serious changes (AUHC rate decrease).

AUHC analysis shows that beta-phenyl-gamma-aminobutyric acid hydrochloride effects in patients suffering from ETTH develop faster comparing with those suffering from CTTH where positive effects appear later.

All adolescents suffering from either ETTH or CTTH have MTZ of pericranial and cervical muscles.

MTZs of pericranial muscles are revealed in 26% of individuals and MTZ of cervical muscle—in 17% of adolescents suffering from ETTH.

After treatment, active MTZs were not revealed in patients of both groups; meanwhile, latent MTZs were preserved in 50% of patients with CTTH and in 6% of adolescents (two individuals) with ETTH.

## Discussion

In response to complaints of headache, some parents carry hyperprotection; as a result, they subconsciously encourage passive coping strategy and simultaneously let their children avoid potentially stressful school environment [341].

One of the pathways of TTH is a lack of GABA transmission that causes biologically negative stress (dystress) as a reaction on homeostasis dysbalance (external and internal stressors rather than biologically positive stress (eustress)).

Our hypothesis is supported by efficacy of GABA-ergic agent—aminophenylbutyric acid hydrochloride, which has a positive effect on pain intensity and associated symptoms such as insomnia, meteosensitivity, and lack of concentration.

Treatment efficacy which was estimated by AUHC occurs later in patients suffering from CTTH comparing with patients suffering from ETTH that indicates on more profound dysfunction of stress-limiting system in case of chronic TTH.

Elimination of MTZ resulting from postural overloads and stress is a crucial point in patients suffering from TTH.

## Conclusions

TTH in children and adolescent that becomes increasingly an actual issue is related to lifestyle changing and stress-factors increasing.

GABA receptor agonists as beta-phenyl-gamma-aminobutyric acid hydrochloride (aminophenylbutyric acid hydrochloride) have a pathogenic effect activating stress-limiting factors and can be used as a treatment of stress-induced TTH.

**Acknowledgement**
*A machine generated summary based on the work of Esin, Oleg Radievich. 2018 in BioNanoScience.*

## *Efficacy and Feasibility of Behavioral Treatments for Migraine, Headache, and Pain in the Acute Care Setting*

DOI: https://doi.org/10.1007/s11916-020-00899-z

### Abstract-Summary

This narrative review examines the use of behavioral interventions for acute treatment of headache and pain in the emergency department (ED)/urgent care (UC) and inpatient settings.

Behavioral interventions demonstrate reductions of pain and associated disability in headache, migraine, and other conditions in the outpatient setting.

Behavioral treatments may be a useful addition for patients presenting with acute pain to hospitals and emergency departments.

There are few high-quality studies on behavioral treatments in the inpatient and emergency department settings.

### Introduction

Acute pain, headache, and migraine are common reasons for presentations to emergency departments and for admissions to the hospital [342].

Behavioral interventions are not a standard part of inpatient or emergency department (ED)/urgent care (UC) for migraine, headache, or pain treatment [343].

The safety and efficacy of many behavioral treatments for pain and headache has been demonstrated convincingly in the outpatient setting [344].

This review discusses the application of behavioral treatments for treating acute inpatient pain.

Given these physiologic differences, there may be different levels of effectiveness of behavioral interventions for acute pain compared with chronic pain.

We will review the evidence base of these interventions for acute pain, migraine, and headache.

### Evidence Base in the Outpatient Setting

Relaxation training, biofeedback, and cognitive behavioral therapy have strong evidence of effectiveness for migraine and tension-type headache management [345].

Haddock and others [346] analyzed 20 trials of home-based behavioral treatments (including home-based relaxation treatments, biofeedback, and minimal therapist contact CBT) and found them equally effective, or superior to, clinic-based interventions.

Holroyd and others [347] performed a trial of 203 adults with chronic tension-type headache randomly assigned amitriptyline or nortriptyline vs. placebo vs.

stress management therapy (relaxation and cognitive coping strategies taught over 3 face-to-face sessions and 2 telephone contacts) and found that pharmacotherapy was equally effective compared with behavioral therapy.

To the above well-established behavioral therapies for migraine, acceptance and commitment therapy (ACT), mindfulness-based interventions (MBCT and MBSR), and sleep interventions are emerging as potentially effective migraine treatments, but more data is needed before these can be definitively recommended [348].

### Evidence Base for Behavioral Treatments for Pain and Primary Headache in the Experimental and Acute Settings

Petter [349] randomized 198 adolescents to a mindful attention manipulation or control group prior to an experimental pain task (the cold pressor task, in which the subject places their hand in cold water and time submerged is measured).

The authors found no effect on pain, but interestingly, regular meditators in the mindful attention group reported lower pain intensity than mediators in the control condition (mean pain score on a 10-point scale were 5 and 6.5, p < 0.5).

Garland [350] and others ran a randomized-controlled trial of mindfulness for inpatient pain comparing mindfulness training vs. hypnotic suggestion vs. psycho-education for acute pain relief in the hospital setting.

The authors found that the single brief mindfulness or hypnotic suggestion intervention reduced pain more than the psychoeducation group.

The authors found significantly reduced pain intensity in the hypnosis group compared with the massage group while the patients were hospitalized (p = 0.008).

### Discussion

Despite the evidence base for many behavioral treatments delivered or taught in the outpatient setting, more robust studies in the inpatient setting are needed before they become a routine part of inpatient pain treatment.

Control groups can be no treatment (e.g., a waiting list control), minimal treatment (e.g., a very brief intervention), a non-specific active control (a condition in which no clear rationale for the treatment is provided), or a specific active controls (a condition where a clear rationale for the treatment is provided to the patient).

Ernst and others [351] classified barriers to behavioral treatment for migraine into patient and provider-related.

These treatments require patient buy-in and will not work for patients uninterested in these treatments [345] or patients in too much pain to focus on the interventions.

It may be possible to take a patient into a less stimulating treatment room of the ED to teach a behavioral intervention.

### Conclusion

There have been numerous studies on behavioral treatments for acute experimentally induced pain, with evidence for mindfulness-based therapies, relaxation, and hypnosis treatments.

There is a much smaller body of literature for the application of behavioral treatments to the management of headache, migraine, and pain in acute inpatient or emergency department or urgent care settings.

Some research supports the acute use of relaxation therapies, mindfulness-based therapies, hypnosis, and virtual reality-based delivery systems in these settings.

**Acknowledgement**
*A machine generated summary based on the work of Vekhter, Daniel; Robbins, Matthew S.; Minen, Mia; Buse, Dawn C. 2020 in Current Pain and Headache Reports.*

## Manual Therapy and Quality of Life in People with Headache: Systematic Review and Meta-analysis of Randomized Controlled Trials

DOI: https://doi.org/10.1007/s11916-019-0815-8

**Abstract-Summary**
People with headache usually experienced significantly lower health-related quality of life (HRQoL) than the healthy subjects.

The goal of this systematic review was to evaluate the effectiveness of manual therapy on HRQoL in patients with tension-type headache (TTH), migraine (MH) or cervicogenic headache (CGH).

Treatment was manual therapy compared to usual care or placebo.

The outcome was the HRQoL that could be measured by Headache Impact Test (HIT-6), Headache Disability Inventory (HDI), Migraine Disability Assessment Questionnaire (MIDAS) and Short Form Health Survey 12/36 (SF-12/36).

For HIT-6 scale, meta-analysis showed statistically significant differences in favour to manual therapy both after treatment (mean difference (MD) $-3.67$; 95% CI from $-5.71$ to $-1.63$) and at follow-up (MD $-2.47$; 95% CI from $-3.27$ to $-1.68$).

For HDI scale, meta-analysis showed statistically significant differences in favour to manual therapy both after treatment (MD $-4.01$; 95% CI from $-5.82$ to $-2.20$) and at follow-up (MD $-5.62$; 95% CI from $-10.69$ to $-0.54$).

Manual therapy should be considered as an effective approach in improving the quality of life in patients with TTH and MH, while in patients with CGH, the results were inconsistent.

Extended:

To increase the level of evidence, researchers should in future design primary studies that provide appropriate control groups and follow-up periods, using valid and reliable disease-specific outcome measures.

## Introduction

All recent literature reviews focused on the effectiveness of manual treatment in reducing the frequency, intensity and duration of attacks in headaches, especially on migraine (MH), tension-type headache (TTH) and cervicogenic headache (CGH) [131, 352–357]; however, none of the aforementioned reviews performed a quantitative analysis of the results of manual treatments on patients' quality of life.

Considering the multifactorial nature of headache, it would be more correct to adopt a broader approach, evaluating the effects of treatments also on other factors such as pharmacological consumption, stress, patient satisfaction or expectations, disability and impact on the quality of life [358, 359].

The aim of this systematic review was to research and summarize in a meta-analysis the results obtained on the quality of life in patients with headache when treated with manual therapy techniques compared to the pharmacological usual care or placebo.

## Methods

Measured results in the studies at the baseline and different follow-up were extracted; if necessary, the authors of the studies included were contacted [360–362].

The internal validity of the studies was independently assessed by two authors (FML, RM) using the Cochrane risk of bias (RoB) assessment tool [363].

The RoB for each study was assessed considering the following domains: selection bias (generation of random sequences and concealment of assignments), performance bias (blindness of participants and personnel), detection bias (blindness of evaluators), attrition bias (incomplete outcome data), reporting bias (selective reporting) and other sources of bias (sample size calculated on a different or unspecified outcome) [363].

Studies that did not provide usable results for the quantitative assessment of outcomes were included in the review but excluded from the meta-analysis; the results of these studies have been treated in a descriptive way.

## Results

At the post-treatment, the meta-analysis included five studies for a total of 413 patients; two studies had high risk of bias on TTH [159, 361], two studies had low risk of bias on TTH [364, 365] and one had low-risk of bias on MH [366].

In the MH subgroup (N = 105), the results showed a significant difference in favour of the treatment (MD −7.48; 95% CI from −0.57 to −4.39; p < 0.001; $I^2 = 0\%$); despite the absence of heterogeneity, the level of evidence remains low due to the presence of a single study.

At the follow-up, the meta-analysis included four studies, two had high risk of bias [159, 361] and two had low risk of bias [364, 365] for a total of 308 patients with TTH; the study on MH [366] did not show follow-up.

At the post-treatment, the meta-analysis included four studies, two had high risk of bias [159, 361] and two had low risk of bias [367, 368] for a total of 287 patients with TTH.

The study conducted on 39 subjects with TTH by Berggren and others [360] reported no significant difference between post-treatment and follow-up groups for any of the items on the scale, but the values were not reported in the study.

**Discussion**

Except for a few exceptions, manual therapy obtained more positive effect on quality of life compared to usual care or placebo when measured by the HIT-6 and HDI disease-specific scales in patients with TTH or MH [364, 366]; however, only the HIT-6 scale results reached the minimal clinical important difference [369–371].

These positive results are consistent with those obtained in a previous narrative review that investigated the general effects of manual therapy on patients with TTH [372].

The results obtained on CGH are to be taken with reserve: in fact, his type of disorder was included only in one study [373] where groups were composed by patients with different types of headache (MH, TTH, CGH and mixed).

The results obtained by the MIDAS and SF-36 scales have been tendentially positive compared to the baseline values for most of the groups; also in this case, manual therapy techniques seem to have a certain influence on different aspects of quality of life in people with TTH, especially in functional aspects.

**Conclusions**

Manual therapy has shown better effects compared to usual care and placebo in terms of quality of life patients with TTH and MH, but the results should be taken with caution due to the very low level of evidence and high risk of bias of the most influential studies.

In patients with CGH, the results are inconsistent, and there is a need to make new specific studies for this type of headache.

In the face of significant improvements compared to baseline and the absence of adverse effects, manual therapy should, therefore, be considered as a valid approach, being able to positively affect the quality of life of patients with headache.

**Acknowledgement**

*A machine generated summary based on the work of Falsiroli Maistrello, Luca; Rafanelli, Marco; Turolla, Andrea. 2019 in Current Pain and Headache Reports.*

## *Manual Joint Mobilisation Techniques, Supervised Physical Activity, Psychological Treatment, Acupuncture and Patient Education for Patients with Tension-Type Headache. A Systematic Review and Meta-analysis*

DOI: https://doi.org/10.1186/s10194-021-01298-4

**Abstract-Summary**

The evidence for their effects are limited.

The aim of this study was to review the evidence for manual joint mobilisation techniques, supervised physical activity, psychological treatment, acupuncture and patient education as treatments for TTH on the effect of headache frequency and quality of life.

The primary outcomes measured were days with headache and quality of life at the end of treatment along with a number of secondary outcomes.

The overall certainty of evidence was evaluated using the Grading of Recommendations, Assessment, Development, and Evaluation approach (GRADE).

Acupuncture might have positive effects on both primary outcomes.

Supervised physical activity might have a positive effect on pain intensity at the end of treatment and headache frequency at follow-up.

Manual joint mobilisation techniques might have a positive effect on headache frequency and quality of life at follow-up.

Psychological treatment might have a positive effect on stress symptoms at the end of treatment.

The overall certainty of evidence was downgraded to low and very low.

Based on identified benefits, certainty of evidence, and patient preferences, manual joint mobilisation techniques, supervised physical activity, psychological treatment, acupuncture, and patient education can be considered as non-pharmacological treatment approaches for TTH.

Some positive effects were shown on headache frequency, quality of life, pain intensity and stress symptoms.

Extended:

The overall certainty of evidence for each clinical question was based on the lowest rating of the primary outcome.

The overall certainty of evidence for the included studies assessed by using GRADE was low to very low owing to insufficient blinding of staff, participants and outcome assessors.

Supervised physical activity was defined as planned, repeated and structured physical activity [374].

Manual joint mobilisation techniques were defined as all manual techniques, mobilisation or manipulation within the normal range of motion of the joint, aimed at affecting the joints, muscles and connective tissues of the neck, chest and lower back.

## Background

A European expert panel recommended non-pharmacological treatment for TTH such as psychological approaches that included EMG biofeedback, cognitive-behavioural therapy and relaxation as well as physical therapy and acupuncture [213].

Non-pharmacological treatment may also be considered if TTH-patients suffer from unpleasant side effects and/or perceive the medical treatment as not effective.

No previous systematic review has evaluated the literature for the evidence of physical activity for TTH such as strength training and aerobic exercises.

Previous systematic reviews have evaluated the effect of psychological treatment on headache disorders [375–378].

The aim of the current study was to conduct a systematic review with meta-analyses and summarise the evidence for the following five separate treatment approaches for TTH: manual joint mobilisation techniques, supervised physical activity, psychological treatment, acupuncture, and patient education compared to other than the respective investigated modality on the effect of headache frequency and quality of life.

## Methods

The current review and NCG were based on the Population, Intervention, Comparison and Outcome (PICO) framework, with the methodology following the Grading of Recommendation, Assessment, Development, and Evaluation (GRADE) approach.

The Danish Knowledge Centre on Headache Disorders invited a multidisciplinary expert group with the purpose of developing a NCG for non-pharmacological treatment for patients with TTH as an aid to assist healthcare professionals and patients with TTH to identify and seek the most relevant non-pharmacological treatment strategies.

If studies of cervicogenic headache also included patients with TTH, there had to be a clear distinction between these two classifications based on ICHD 2–3 for both headache disorders and/or the classification proposed by Sjaastad and others for cervicogenic headache [379].

The investigated interventions included: 1) manual joint mobilisation techniques 2) supervised physical activity 3) psychological treatment 4) acupuncture and 5) patient education.

Data including population demographics, intervention and control details, outcome and time measurement were independently extracted, by two review authors, from relevant RCTs.

## Results

A weak recommendation is made for manual joint mobilisation techniques which can be considered as a supplement to medical treatment for patients with TTH.

A weak recommendation is made for supervised physical activity which can be considered as a supplement to medical treatment for patients with TTH.

A weak recommendation is made for psychological treatment which can be considered as a supplement to medical treatment for patients with TTH.

A weak recommendation is made for acupuncture which can be considered as a supplement to medical treatment for patients with TTH.

Based on consensus, it is recommended to consider using patient education as a supplement to medical treatment for patients with TTH.

## Discussion

The current study presented a systematic review of the evidence for manual joint mobilisation techniques, supervised physical activity, psychological treatment, acupuncture, and patient education as non-pharmacological treatment strategies for TTH regarding headache related outcomes, quality of life and disability.

In line with the current review, the NICE CG150 [380] reviewed the evidence for manual therapies, exercise, psychological therapies, acupuncture, and patient education and self-management also applying the GRADE approach.

In line with the NICE CG150, that found low to very low certainty of evidence for psychological treatment but were not able to form a recommendation.

Based on clinical experience, the multidisciplinary expert group of this review recommended patient education for patients with frequent and chronic TTH as they often seek knowledge about their disorder and tools to manage their life with chronic illness.

## Conclusion

Based on the identified benefits, the certainty of evidence, and patient preferences, the multidisciplinary expert group of this review concluded that manual joint mobilisation techniques, supervised physical activity, psychological treatment, acupuncture, and patient education can be considered as treatment approaches for TTH.

No serious adverse events were identified for any of the included studies.

This NCG can be used by healthcare professionals as an aid in identifying and directing the patient with TTH to the appropriate treatment strategy targeting the patient's needs and resources based on evidence.

## Acknowledgement

*A machine generated summary based on the work of Krøll, Lotte Skytte; Callesen, Henriette Edemann; Carlsen, Louise Ninett; Birkefoss, Kirsten; Beier, Dagmar; Christensen, Henrik Wulff; Jensen, Mette; Tómasdóttir, Hanna; Würtzen, Hanne; Høst, Christel Vesth; Hansen, Jakob Møller. 2021 in The Journal of Headache and Pain.*

## *A Short Review of the Treatment of Headaches Using Osteopathic Manipulative Treatment*

DOI: https://doi.org/10.1007/s11916-018-0736-y

## Abstract-Summary

This review highlights the importance of osteopathic manipulative treatment (OMT) in headache sufferers.

Patients with headaches that are refractory to other treatment options may also be candidates for OMT.

Multiple headache etiologies are amenable to this non-invasive treatment option and they will be reviewed here.

Many headache sufferers are unable to find relief through conventional treatment options.

OMT is a useful non-invasive treatment option with little to no side effects.

OMT is a non-invasive treatment option for individuals suffering from various types of headaches.

This treatment option is tailored to the individual needs of the patient and is delivered by licensed and experienced osteopathic physicians.

## Introduction

While ergots can relieve headache symptoms, these medications may also have severe cardiovascular contraindications [381].

Botulinum toxin injections have been FDA approved since 2010 as a treatment option for headaches, especially for patients who have more than 15 headaches per months, also known as chronic headaches [382]. In the PREEMPT 2 trial the results showed a significant decrease in migraines as well as a decrease in headache-related disability [383]. However, the drawbacks to utilizing this medication include cost (not always covered by commercial insurance companies), and it can be a painful treatment (approximately 30 injections per treatment).

Osteopathic manipulative treatment of the cranium and drainage of the glymphatic system not only has the ability to help individuals with headaches, it has also been theorized to help individuals with Alzheimer's disease [384].

OMT has been shown to decrease the symptoms of individuals with headaches caused by sinusitis [385].

OMT was seen to relieve the symptoms in individuals with a persistent headache after the removal of a tooth [386, 387].

## Review Article Methods

Article, an effort was made to look for articles explaining how osteopathic manipulative treatment can be used to treat headaches of varying etiologies.

This review demonstrates the broad range of effects that osteopathic manipulative treatment could have for headache sufferers.

Each article was analyzed for their use of osteopathic manipulative treatment and their connection to the change in symptoms seen in the patient.

Articles that used other methods along with osteopathic manipulative treatment were not excluded.

## Results

Osteopathic manipulative treatment was used in all seven of these studies and was used for different headache etiologies.

In all of the studies, osteopathic manipulative treatment was found to improve the symptoms of the patients.

Some of the articles have evidence of other treatments that were used with osteopathic manipulative treatment, they were not excluded.

## Discussion

Osteopathic manipulative treatment is capable of improving headache symptoms in patients that are unable or unwilling to tolerate other forms of treatment.

Consistently, individuals who were suffering from a headache and who received OMT had a reduction of symptoms.

More data is needed to determine if OMT increases the efficacy of other conventional headache treatments.

The data is sparse and the methods of reducing the symptoms of headaches are not completely comparable between studies, evidence has been shown of its effectiveness.

The limited number of articles made it challenging to fully assess the impact of OMT for headaches.

A standardization of OMT treatments needs to be created so that the results of different journal articles can be compared in a uniform fashion.

More studies should be completed containing OMT as the only treatment, instead of studies that have both OMT and conventional treatments.

## Conclusion

Headaches are a major debilitating condition for Americans and many of these individuals only use pharmacological agents to treat their symptoms.

Through treatment of the somatic dysfunctions that often cause headaches, relief can be found for those individuals.

With further research, headaches and migraines will be analyzed and treated differently.

With a different treatment and approach, the individuals suffering from these conditions will be able to gain back these lost work days and money currently being lost to this condition.

## Acknowledgement

*A machine generated summary based on the work of Whalen, John; Yao, Sheldon; Leder, Adena. 2018 in Current Pain and Headache Reports.*

# *Effectiveness of Mulligan Manual Therapy over Exercise on Headache Frequency, Intensity and Disability for Patients with Migraine, Tension-Type Headache and Cervicogenic Headache: A Protocol of a Pragmatic Randomized Controlled Trial*

DOI: https://doi.org/10.1186/s12891-021-04105-y

## Abstract-Summary

Non-pharmacological management of migraine, tension-type headache (TTH), and cervicogenic headache (CGH) may include spinal manual therapy and exercise.

Mulligan Manual Therapy (MMT) utilizes a protocol of headache elimination procedures to manage headache parameters and associated disability, but has only been evaluated in CGH.

This study aims to determine the effectiveness of MMT and exercise over exercise and placebo in the management of migraine, TTH, and CGH.

Two hundred ninety-seven participants with a diagnosis of migraine, TTH or CGH based on published headache classification guidelines will be included.

An assessor blind to group allocation will measure outcomes pre-and post-intervention as well as 3 and 6 months after commencement of treatment.

Participants will be allocated to one of the three groups: MMT and exercise; placebo and exercise; and exercise alone.

The primary outcome measure is headache frequency.

Secondary outcome measures are headache duration and intensity, medication intake, pressure pain threshold (PPT), range of motion recorded with the flexion rotation test, and headache disability recorded with Headache Activities of Daily Living Index (HADLI).

This pragmatic study will provide evidence for the effectiveness of MMT when compared with a placebo intervention and exercise on headache frequency, intensity, and disability.

Limitations are that baseline evaluation of headache parameters may be affected by recall bias.

The HADLI is not yet extensively evaluated for its psychometric properties and association between PPT and headache parameters is lacking.

Extended:

Participants will be included if they fulfil the following inclusion criteria: age more than 18 years and less than 60 years, pain intensity >6 on a 10 cm visual analogue scale at the time of presentation (to balance headache severity across different headache groups), a minimum 1-year history of headache with a minimum mean frequency of 1 per week.

Participants will be excluded if their headache diagnosis is other than, migraine, TTH or CGH.

Participants will be provided with an information sheet outlining the study protocol including duration of commitment, intervention, benefits and harms of the treatment, voluntary participation, right to withdraw, as well as confidentiality of data.

Participants will be advised to undertake similar exercise at home, unsupervised, once a day.

Participants will be asked to maintain an exercise diary to monitor compliance.

**Background**

Headache reproduction and resolution following manual palpation of the upper cervical spine in patients with primary headache [388, 389] indicates that manual therapy has the capacity to modulate the sensitivity of this nucleus.

The effects of such an approach on other headache forms have been reported in a case study [390] of a patient with features of migraine, but not in TTH and not in a formal RCT.

This paper aims to report the study protocol which will be used to investigate the short and mid-term effectiveness of MMT and exercise on headache frequency, intensity, disability, and duration as well as medication intake, upper cervical rotation range of motion, PPT and patient satisfaction compared with placebo and exercise and exercise alone in the management of migraine, TTH, and CGH.

**Methods/Design**

Participants will be included if they fulfil the following inclusion criteria: age more than 18 years and less than 60 years, pain intensity >6 on a 10 cm visual analogue scale at the time of presentation (to balance headache severity across different headache groups), a minimum 1-year history of headache with a minimum mean frequency of 1 per week.

Participants will then be randomly and equally allocated to one of three groups: MMT plus exercise; placebo plus exercise; or exercise alone by stratified randomization based on the type of headache.

MMT will be delivered at the discretion of the therapist, based on the initial and progressive assessment of the participant's cervical joint dysfunction and headache presentation.

To assess whether the participants were blind to intervention or not, after each treatment session the participants in the MMT and the placebo group will complete a questionnaire on whether they believed MMT treatment was received, partly received or not.

**Discussion**

A pragmatic effectiveness study design will enable a greater understanding of the true effect of MMT when compared with a placebo intervention and a control group in reducing various parameters of headache over a 6 months period.

This study will help us to understand the true net effect of MMT over placebo.

Recruitment will be a challenge due to the strict inclusion criteria but that could be strength of our study to involve a homogeneous population of headache sufferers with features of upper cervical articular dysfunction who might respond to MMT.

Previous studies using MMT targeting the upper cervical spine for headache management have not reported adverse events associated with its application.

The study will contribute to the evidence base for manual therapy management of headache and will lead to improved clinical decision making in the field of non-pharmacological management of headache.

**Acknowledgement**

*A machine generated summary based on the work of Satpute, Kiran; Bedekar, Nilima; Hall, Toby. 2021 in BMC Musculoskeletal Disorders.*

## Tension-Type Headache, Its Relation to Stress, and How to Relieve It by Cryotherapy Among Academic Students

DOI: https://doi.org/10.1186/s43045-020-00030-3

**Abstract-Summary**

Tension-type headache and stress are common students' problems suffering.

Alternative and complementary medicine, as cryotherapy, is effective for relieving physical and psychological pain; using ice compresses by placing it at the back of the neck, leads to relief of tension and anxiety, and gives feeling of relaxation and full of energy for doing daily life activities.

This study aimed to assess tension-type headache, its relation to stress, and how to relieve it by cryotherapy, among academic students.

After applying cryotherapy (ice compresses) in relieving TTH, students feel analgesia, relaxation, increased effort, and alertness, added to that decreased mental tension and recurrence of headache to a minimum level.

Extended:

Alternative and complementary medicine, like cryotherapy, is effective for relieving physical and psychological pain.

This study aimed to assess the relation between stress and TTH among academic students, as well as the role of cryotherapy.

The interpretation of the findings using two different research approaches offered a breadth and depth of understanding about the status of TTH after proceeding cryotherapy (ice compresses).

## Background

Growing evidence now supports that central factors are of greater significance, especially sensitization of neurons at spinal and supraspinal levels as well as decreased inhibition of nociceptive signals leading to an increased sensitivity to pain and thereby causing headaches [47, 391].

Topical cold treatment decreases the temperature of the skin and underlying tissues to a depth of 2–4 cm, decreasing the activation threshold of tissue nociceptors and the conduction velocity of pain nerve signals.

The significance of using it comes from the fact that this experience needs no money, no effort, little time, and effective safe alternative therapy for mental tension and TTH for academic students and other people who are suffering from mental tension and tension headache.

This study aimed to assess the relation between stress and TTH among academic students, as well as the role of cryotherapy.

## Methods

The technical design includes the research design, study setting, sample, and tools of data collection.

Three tools were used to collect data for this study.

This phase deals with the preparation of the study design; data collection tool was adapted by the researcher.

Reviewing literature studies and other available resources related to TTH, stress, among academic students, and role of cryotherapy to relieve tension-type headache, for the preparations of data collection tools.

Stage II: Instructional guidelines about cryotherapy (ice compression) were introduced for a group of six students as follows: The subjects of the study were informed about the therapeutic use of locally applied coolants at the back of the neck and its effect in reducing TTH.

## Results

Disturbed appetite, disturbed sleep, and doing daily living activity with little effort. Anxiety symptoms Feeling like loaded with a lot of things, and need to do many things at the same time. Level of performance of daily activities We are not satisfied about our achievements regarding daily activities. Mood changes From time to time, between nervousness and calmness Sleep quality Getting up with difficulty, disturbed sleep, between many and little hours Appetite Disturbed appetite, and sometimes we have no time to eat. What is the effect of ice compresses on TTH? Do ice compresses relieve TTH?

No mental tension or hard tidiness around head like before. The recurrence of headache decreased to a large extent. The intensity of headache low intensity to very little degree, and some of them advised their family to use ice compresses to relieve their TTH. Mental tension after ice compresses Decreased tidiness, tension, and anxiety to a minimum level. Stress feeling It is a good method of stress management. Did you observe any physical problems after using ice compresses?

## Discussion

Regarding physical symptoms of stress, in this study, it was found that slightly less than two-thirds (63.5) of the students felt neck pain to a large degree.

This result matches with Kjaergaard [391], who found that stress leads to an increased sensitivity to pain and thereby causes headaches.

This is comparable to a study one by Ahmad and Qaisy [392] who reported that students can potentially experience different types of stress that can affect their mental and social health and their academic achievement.

As in a studies by [213, 393, 394] about associations with exposure to stressors in adolescents which have been reported with TTH and is cryotherapy (ice compresses) in relieving TTH, students feel analgesia, relaxation, increased effort, and alertness, added to that decreased mental tension and recurrence of headache to a minimum level.

## Conclusion

After applying cryotherapy (ice compresses) in relieving TTH, students feel analgesia, relaxation, increased effort, and alertness, added to that decreased mental tension and recurrence of headache to a minimum level.

1. Cryotherapy (ice compresses) is a non-pharmacological therapy for TTH relief.
2. Ice compresses can be added as a new method of stress management.
3. Ice compression is a rapid and effective method for TTH management.
4. More research is needed about the role of ice compression in the relief of physical and psychological pain.
5. More research is needed about the role of ice compression in the relief of multiple sclerosis.

## Acknowledgement

*A machine generated summary based on the work of Hassan, Mona; Asaad, Tarek. 2020 in Middle East Current Psychiatry.*

## *Safety and Efficacy of Melatonin in Chronic Tension-Type Headache: A Post-Marketing Real-World Surveillance Program*

DOI: https://doi.org/10.1007/s40122-020-00207-y

### Abstract-Summary

About 2–3% of patients with TTH progress to chronic TTH with daily or near-daily headache, warranting preventive treatment.

The treatment of chronic TTH is complex and very often associated with significant tolerability issues.

The aim of this surveillance program was to evaluate the efficacy of melatonin (Melaxen®) in patients with TTH and disruption of circadian rhythms in real-world practice.

Sixty-one patients with chronic TTH were enrolled.

A significant decrease in the number of headache days per month, VAS pain intensity, HAM-A, HAM-D and HIT-6 scores, and an improvement in sleep quality were observed throughout the study.

Melatonin is an effective and safe alternative for the treatment of chronic TTH.

### Digital Features

This article is published with digital features, including a summary slide, to facilitate understanding of the article.

To view digital features for this article go to https://doi.org/10.6084/m9.figshare.13055717.

### Introduction

In about 2–3% of patients, TTH progresses to chronic TTH with daily or near-daily headache.

Chronic TTH is the second most prevalent chronic headache after chronic migraine [395].

The treatment of chronic TTH is complex.

To high levels of anxiety and depression, chronic TTH is frequently associated with disruption of circadian rhythms and sleep [284].

The authors concluded that sleep problems increase the risk of chronic pain in pain-free individuals, worsen the long-term prognosis of existing headache and chronic musculoskeletal pain, and influence daily fluctuations in clinical pain.

In the recent consensus article published in 2019 by the European Headache Federation, it is clearly stated that in the absence of registered prophylactic drugs for chronic TTH, a broad range of drugs can be attempted resting on individual clinical responsibility [396].

### Methods

Eligible subjects were aged 18–65 and diagnosed with chronic TTH, according to the International Classification of Headache Disorders, version 3 [107].

To confirm headache frequency, all subjects completed a headache diary during the 30-day baseline period.

VAS pain intensity assessments, Hamilton Anxiety Rating Scale (HAM-A), Hamilton Depression Rating Scale (HAM-D), HIT-6 and Levin sleep quality scores were obtained at the baseline visit, at month 1 and month 2.

The primary endpoint was the change in the monthly number of headache days at month 1 (treatment phase) and month 2 (follow-up) compared to the baseline headache frequency.

Secondary endpoints included the change in headache intensity, levels of depression, anxiety and HIT-6 disability, and sleep quality at day 30 and day 60 compared to the corresponding baseline values.

Change in the analgesic intake during month 1 and month 2 of the study compared to the baseline period was also included into the preplanned analysis.

## Results

A median decrease in headache frequency over 33% was observed in 93.4% of patients.

In 6.6% of patients, no change in headache frequency was observed.

At 30 days after the end of the study (on day 60), a significant decrease in headache frequency was still observed in 29/61 (47.5%) patients.

This decrease was observed in 56/61 (92%) patients and was stable during the 30-day follow-up period.

Anxiety levels also decreased significantly during the treatment period, and remained significant at visit 3, despite the tendency to rise again during the follow-up period.

After 30 days of treatment, a significant increase in sleep quality was observed, with a median of 44.6%.

No further changes in analgesic intake were observed during the 30-day follow-up period.

All patients completed the study and the follow-up period.

## Discussion

The effect of melatonin was easily observable—the majority of patients reported an over 30% decrease in headache frequency.

Patients with temporomandibular disorder taking 5 mg of melatonin for 28 days experienced significant improvements in pain scores (−44%), pressure pain threshold (+39%), and sleep quality; the effect on pain was independent from that on sleep [397].

The anxiolytic effect of melatonin documented in a variety of studies may also be of special importance in the treatment of chronic pain [398, 399].

This is in line with the reports of other authors who studied the effect of melatonin in the treatment of various diseases and pain syndromes [400, 401], while in controlled studies melatonin has demonstrated a safety profile comparable with that of placebo [402].

To date, this is the largest study of melatonin efficacy in chronic TTH, which also evaluated the dynamics of depression and anxiety levels and headache impact on day-to-day activities.

**Acknowledgement**
*A machine generated summary based on the work of Danilov, Andrei B.; Danilov, Alexey B.; Kurushina, Olga V.; Shestel, Elena A.; Zhivolupov, Sergey A.; Latysheva, Nina V. 2020 in Pain and Therapy.*

## *The Best from East and West? Acupuncture and Medical Training Therapy as Monotherapies or in Combination for Adult Patients with Episodic and Chronic Tension-Type Headache: Study Protocol for a Randomized Controlled Trial*

DOI: https://doi.org/10.1186/s13063-019-3700-1

**Abstract-Summary**
This study aims to evaluate the feasibility and efficacy of a complex health intervention, based on the combination of conventional Western medicine and traditional Chinese medicine (TCM), in an outpatient department of a university hospital for patients with frequent episodic or chronic tension-type headaches.

This is a prospective randomized controlled pilot study with four balanced treatment arms (usual care, acupuncture, training, and training plus acupuncture).

After completion of the intervention, two follow-up evaluations will be performed 3 and 6 months after the start of treatment.

At predefined times, the various outcomes (pain intensity, health-related quality of life, pain duration, autonomic regulation, and heart rate variability) as well as the participants' acceptance of the complex treatment will be evaluated with valid assessment instruments (Migraine Disability Assessment, PHQ-D, GAD-7, and SF-12) and a headache diary.

The acupuncture treatment will be based on the rules of TCM, comprising a standardized combination of acupuncture points and additional points selected according to individual pain localization.

In supplementary analyses, the proportion of treatment responders (those with a 50% reduction in the frequency of pain episodes) will be determined for each treatment arm.

This trial may provide evidence for the additive effects of acupuncture and medical training therapy as a combination treatment and may scientifically support the implementation of this complex health intervention.

Extended:

The acupuncture treatment comprises a standardized combination of points plus additional individual points identified by location (meridian).

## Background

Despite the evidence in support of the effectiveness of acupuncture and MTT, we could not identify any studies evaluating the efficacy of a combination of acupuncture and MTT for tension-type headaches in comparison with the two treatment modalities alone or with usual care.

Acupuncture as a treatment modality in traditional Chinese medicine (TCM) is combined with MTT, a classical Western medical treatment.

To the classical outcomes of headache studies, which will be used to evaluate the efficacy of the two methods regarding pain, analgesic consumption, anxiety, and depression, this study will also address whether the two therapies affect individual psychological stress levels, as an association between increased stress levels and tension-type headaches has been reported.

TMD as a comorbidity has no impact on treatment outcomes for tension-type headaches in the study setting.

## Methods/Design

Those who fulfill any of the following criteria will be excluded: Those participating or having participated during the last 30 days prior to the initial screening examination in another clinical trial. Those who have been treated with acupuncture or MTT for tension-type headaches within the last 6 months prior to the initial examination. Those with a serious psychiatric disorder. Those with substance dependence or misuse. Those using headache medication for >10 days per month. Those with a severe neurological or severe medical disease. Pregnant women. Nursing women. Women planning to become pregnant during the study period. Those with migraine whose attacks occur more frequently than once per year. Those with unstable angina pectoris. Those with New York Heart Association functional classification III–IV heart failure. Those with uncontrollable or untreatable arterial hypertension. Those suffering from headaches due to other medical causes (e.g. pseudotumor cerebri, sleep apnea syndrome, or newly developed daily headaches). Subjects who refuse to undergo the assigned intervention and those who fail to complete the assessments will be excluded.

## Discussion

We expect to find positive treatment effects in all intervention groups for all outcomes in comparison with the usual care or control group.

We expect to demonstrate the additive effects of acupuncture and MTT as a combination treatment and to provide scientific evidence to support the implementation of this complex health intervention.

We believe that analyzing the correlations between the various outcome parameters with the applied treatment will provide information about the levels at which the effects occur.

Extracts from the results of the study will be made accessible to the public, after their publication in journals, on the homepage of the clinic and in newsletters, as well as the print and online media of the Hannover Medical School press office (for example MHH Info, research reports, and information for patients and doctors).

Such changes will also be recorded in diaries if possible, to enable a correction of the results where necessary. Unspecific treatment effects.

**Acknowledgement**

*A machine generated summary based on the work of Schiller, J.; Kellner, T.; Briest, J.; Hoepner, K.; Woyciechowski, A.; Ostermann, A.; Korallus, C.; Sturm, C.; Weiberlenn, T.; Jiang, L.; Egen, C.; Beissner, F.; Stiesch, M.; Karst, M.; Gutenbrunner, C.; Fink, M. G. 2019 in Trials.*

# References


1. Stovner LJ, Nichols E, Steiner TJ, et al. Global, regional, and national burden of migraine and tension-type headache, 1990-2016: a systematic analysis for the Global Burden of Disease Study 2016. Lancet Neurol. 2018;17:954–76.
2. Stovner LJ, Hagen K, Jensen R, Katsarava Z, Lipton R, Scher A, Steiner T, Zwart JA. The global burden of headache: a documentation of headache prevalence and disability worldwide. Cephalalgia. 2007;27:193–210.
3. Stovner LJ, Al Jumah M, Birbeck GL, Gururaj G, Jensen R, Katsarava Z, Queiroz LP, Scher AI, Tekle-Haimanot R, Wang SJ, Steiner TJ. The methodology of population surveys of headache prevalence, burden and cost: principles and recommendations from the global campaign against headache. J Headache Pain. 2014;15:5.
4. GBD 2019 Demographics Collaborators. Global age-sex-specific fertility, mortality, healthy life expectancy (HALE), and population estimates in 204 countries and territories, 1950–2019: a comprehensive demographic analysis for the Global Burden of Disease Study 2019. Lancet. 2020;396(10258):1160–203. https://doi.org/10.1016/S0140-6736(20)30977-6.
5. GBD 2016 Neurology Collaborators. Global, regional, and national burden of neurological disorders, 1990–2016: a systematic analysis for the Global Burden of Disease Study 2016. Lancet Neurol. 2019;18(5):459–80. https://doi.org/10.1016/S1474-4422(18)30499-X.
6. Fuensalida-Novo S, Parás-Bravo P, Jiménez-Antona C, Castaldo M, Wang K, Benito-González E, et al. Gender differences in clinical and psychological variables associated with the burden of headache in tension-type headache. Women Health. 2020;60(6):652–63.
7. GBD 2016 Disease and Injury Incidence and Prevalence Collaborators. Global, regional, and national incidence, prevalence, and years lived with disability for 328 diseases and injuries for 195 countries, 1990–2016: a systematic analysis for the Global Burden of Disease Study 2016. Lancet. 2017;390:1211–59. https://doi.org/10.1016/S0140-6736(17)32154-2.
8. Shahbeigi S, Fereshtehnejad S-M, Mohammadi N, et al. Epidemiology of headaches in Tehran urban area: a population-based cross-sectional study in district 8, year 2010. Neurol Sci. 2013;34(7):1157–66. https://doi.org/10.1007/s10072-012-1200-0.
9. Ayatollahi SMT, Moradi F, Ayatollahi SAR. Prevalences of migraine and tension-type headache in adolescent girls of shiraz (southern Iran). Headache. 2002;42(4):287–90. http://www.ncbi.nlm.nih.gov/pubmed/12010386. Accessed Nov 16, 2018.
10. Fallahzadeh H, Alihaydari M. Prevalence of migraine and tension-type headache among school children in Yazd, Iran. J Pediatr Neurosci. 2011;6(2):106–9. https://doi.org/10.4103/1817-1745.92818.
11. Herekar AA, Ahmad A, Uqaili UL, et al. Primary headache disorders in the adult general population of Pakistan—a cross sectional nationwide prevalence survey. J Headache Pain. 2017;18(1):28. https://doi.org/10.1186/s10194-017-0734-1.
12. Romdhane NA, Ben Hamida M, Mrabet A, et al. Prevalence study of neurologic disorders in Kelibia (Tunisia). Neuroepidemiology. 1993;12(5):285–99. https://doi.org/10.1159/000110330.
13. Bener A, Swadi H, Qassimi EM, Uduman S. Prevalence of headache and migraine in schoolchildren in the United Arab Emirates. Ann Saudi Med. 1998;18(6):522–4. http://www.ncbi.nlm.nih.gov/pubmed/17344729. Accessed 16 Nov 2018.

14. Bahrami P, Zebardast H, Zibaei M, Mohammadzadeh M, Zabandan N. Prevalence and characteristics of headache in Khoramabad, Iran. Pain Physician. 2012;15(4):327–32. http://www.ncbi.nlm.nih.gov/pubmed/22828686. Accessed 16 Nov 2018.

15. Bessisso MS, Bener A, Elsaid MF, Al-Khalaf FA, Huzaima KA. Pattern of headache in school children in the State of Qatar. Saudi Med J. 2005;26(4):566–70. http://www.ncbi.nlm.nih.gov/pubmed/15900361. Accessed 16 Nov 2018.

16. Free 2018 ICD-10-CM Codes. https://www.icd10data.com/ICD10CM/Codes. Accessed 4 Jun 2018.

17. Ashina M, et al. Migraine: epidemiology and systems of care. Lancet. 2021; https://doi.org/10.1016/S0140-6736(20)32160-7.

18. Institute for Health Metrics and Evaluation. GHDx. http://ghdx.healthdata.org/gbd-results-tool.

19. Ashina S, Mitsikostas DD, Lee MJ, Yamani N, Wang S-J, Messina R, et al. Tension-type headache. Nat Rev Dis Prim. 2021;7(1):24.

20. Eigenbrodt AK, et al. Diagnosis and management of migraine in ten steps. Nat Rev Neurol. 2021;17:501–14.

21. Sanderson JC, et al. Headache-related health resource utilisation in chronic and episodic migraine across six countries. J Neurol Neurosurg Psychiatry. 2013;84:1309–17.

22. Katsarava Z, Mania M, Lampl C, Herberhold J, Steiner TJ. Poor medical care for people with migraine in Europe—evidence from the Eurolight study. J Headache Pain. 2018;19:10.

23. The World Health Organization. Atlas of headache disorders and resources in the world 2011. Geneva: World Health Organization; 2011. p. 72. https://doi.org/10.1097/01.tp.0000399132.51747.71.

24. Steiner TJ, et al. Structured headache services as the solution to the ill-health burden of headache: 1. Rationale and description. J Headache Pain. 2021;22:78.

25. Amin FM, Aristeidou S, Baraldi C, et al. The association between migraine and physical exercise. J Headache Pain. 2018;19:83.

26. Houle TT, Butschek RA, Turner DP, et al. Stress and sleep duration predict headache severity in chronic headache sufferers. Pain. 2012;153:2432–40.

27. Varkey E, Hagen K, Zwart JA, et al. Physical activity and headache: results from the Nord-Trondelag Health Study (HUNT). Cephalalgia. 2008;28:1292–7.

28. Shaik MM, Hassan NB, Tan HL, et al. Quality of life and migraine disability among female migraine patients in a tertiary hospital in Malaysia. Biomed Res Int. 2015;2015:523717. https://doi.org/10.1155/2015/523717.

29. Kroll LS, Hammarlund CS, Westergaard ML, et al. Level of physical activity, well-being, stress and self-rated health in persons with migraine and co-existing tension-type headache and neck pain. J Headache Pain. 2017;18:46.

30. Iigaya M, Sakai F, Kolodner KB, et al. Reliability and validity of the Japanese Migraine Disability Assessment (MIDAS) Questionnaire. Headache. 2003;43:343–52.

31. Leonardi M, Raggi A, Bussone G, et al. Health-related quality of life, disability and severity of disease in patients with migraine attending to a specialty headache center. Headache. 2010;50:1576–86.

32. Michel P, Dartigues JF, Lindoulsi A, et al. Loss of productivity and quality of life in migraine sufferers among French workers: results from the GAZEL cohort. Headache. 1997;37:71–8.

33. Sharma K, Remanan R, Singh S. Quality of life and psychiatric comorbidity in Indian migraine patients: a headache clinic sample. Neurol India. 2013;61:355–9.

34. Abu-Arafeh I, Razak S, Sivaraman B, Graham C. Prevalence of headache and migraine in children and adolescents: a systematic review of population-based studies. Dev Med Child Neurol. 2010;52:1088–97.

35. Wöber-Bingöl C. Epidemiology of migraine and headache in children and adolescents. Curr Pain Headache Rep. 2013;17(6):341.

36. Heinrich M, Morris L, Kröner-Herwig B. Self-report of headache in children and adolescents in Germany: possibilities and confines of questionnaire data for headache classification. Cephalalgia. 2009;29(8):864–72.
37. Wober C, Wober-Bingol C, Uluduz D, Aslan TS, Uygunoglu U, Tufekci A, Alp SI, Duman T, Surgun F, Emir GK, Demir CF, Balgetir F, Ozdemir YB, Auer T, Siva A, Steiner TJ. Undifferentiated headache: broadening the approach to headache in children and adolescents, with supporting evidence from a nationwide school-based cross-sectional survey in Turkey. J Headache Pain. 2018;19:18.
38. Anttila P, Metsähonkala L, Aromaa M, Sourander A, Salminen J, Helenius H, et al. Determinants of tension-type headache in children. Cephalalgia. 2002;22(5):401–8.
39. Pothmann R, Frankenberg SV, Muller B, Sartory G, Hellmeier W. Epidemiology of headache in children and adolescents: evidence of high prevalence of migraine. Int J Behav Med. 1994;1(1):76–89.
40. Antonaci F, Voiticovschi-Iosob C, Di Stefano AL, Galli F, Ozge A, Balottin U. The evolution of headache from childhood to adulthood: a review of the literature. J Headache Pain. 2014;15:15.
41. Karwautz A, Wöber C, Lang T, Böck A, Wagner-Ennsgraber C, Vesely C, et al. Psychosocial factors in children and adolescents with migraine and tension-type headache: a controlled study and review of the literature. Cephalalgia. 1999;19(1):32–43.
42. Juang K-D, Wang S-J, Fuh J-L, Lu S-R, Chen Y-S. Association between adolescent chronic daily headache and childhood adversity: a community-based study. Cephalalgia. 2004;24(1):54–9.
43. Kröner-Herwig B, Heinrich M, Morris L. Headache in German children and adolescents: a population-based epidemiological study. Cephalalgia. 2007;27(6):519–27.
44. Bugdayci R, Ozge A, Sasmaz T, Kurt AO, Kaleagasi H, Karakelle A, et al. Prevalence and factors affecting headache in Turkish schoolchildren. Pediatr Int. 2005;47(3):316–22.
45. Đuranović V, Bošnjak-Mejaški V. Glavobolje u dječjoj dobi. In: Demarin V, editor. Znanstveni pristup dijagnostici i terapiji glavobolja. Zagreb: HAZU; 2005. p. 139–56.
46. Đuranović V, Mejaški-Bošnjak V, Lujić L, Krakar G. Glavobolje u djetinjstvu i adolescenciji. Medix. 2005;59:81–5.
47. Headache Classification Committee of the International Headache Society (IHS). The International Classification of Headache Disorders (beta version). Cephalalgia. 2013;33(9):629–808.
48. Tavasoli A, Aghamohammadpoor M, Taghibeigi M. Migraine and tension-type headache in children and adolescents presenting to neurology clinics. Iran J Pediatr. 2013;23:536–40.
49. Matar AK, Kerem NC, Srugo I, Genizi J. Primary headache in children and adolescents–diagnosis and treatment. Harefuah. 2015;154:795–8.
50. Sedlic M, Mahovic D, Kruzliak P. Epidemiology of primary headaches among 1,876 adolescents: a cross-sectional survey. Pain Med. 2016;17:353–9. https://doi.org/10.1093/pm/pnv033.
51. Vuković V, Plavec D, Pavelin S, Janculjak D, Ivanković M, Demarin V. Prevalence of migraine, probable migraine and tension-type headache in the Croatian population. Neuroepidemiology. 2010;35:59–65. https://doi.org/10.1159/000310940.
52. Vuković-Cvetković V, Plavec D, Lovrenčić-Huzjan A. Prevalence of chronic headache in Croatia. Biomed Res Int. 2013;2013:837613. https://doi.org/10.1155/2013/837613.
53. Rasmussen BK, Jensen R, Schroll M, Olesen J. Epidemiology of headache in a general population—a prevalence study. J Clin Epidemiol. 1991;44:1147–57.
54. Castillo J, Muñoz P, Guitera V, Pascual J. Epidemiology of chronic daily headache in the general population. Headache. 1999;39:190–6.
55. Sjaastad O, Pettersen H, Bakketeig LS. The Vågå study, epidemiology of headache. The prevalence of ultrashort paroxysms. Cephalalgia. 2001;21:207–15.

56. Lyngberg AC, Rasmussen BK, Jorgensen T, Jensen R. Has the prevalence of migraine and tension-type headache changed over a 12-year period? A Danish population survey. Eur J Epidemiol. 2005;20:243–9.

57. Grande RB, Aaseth K, Gulbrandsen P, Lundqvist C, Russell MB. Prevalence of primary chronic headache in a population-based sample of 30- to 44-year-old persons: the Akershus study of chronic headache. Neuroepidemiology. 2008;30(2):76–83. https://doi.org/10.1159/000116244.

58. Hagen K, Zwart JA, Aamodt AH, Nilsen KB, Brathen G, Helde G, Stjern M, Tronvik EA, Stovner LJ. A face-to-face interview of participants in HUNT 3: the impact of the screening question on headache prevalence. J Headache Pain. 2008;9:289–94.

59. Ferrante T, Castellini P, Abrignani G, Latte L, Russo M, Camarda C, Veronesi L, Pasquarella C, Manzoni GC, Torelli P. The PACE study: past-year prevalence of migraine in Parma's adult general population. Cephalalgia. 2012;32:358–65.

60. Ferrante T, Manzoni GC, Russo M, Taga A, Camarda C, Veronesi L, Pasquarella C, Sansebastiano G, Torelli P. The PACE study: past-year prevalence of tension-type headache and its subtypes in Parma's adult general population. Neurol Sci. 2015;36:35–42.

61. Kandil MR, Hamed SA, Fadel KA, Khalifa HE, Ghanem MK, Mohamed KO. Migraine in Assiut governorate, Egypt: epidemiology, risk factors, comorbid conditions and predictors of change from episodic to chronic migraine. Neurol Res. 2016;38:232–41.

62. Russell MB, Aaseth K, Grande RB, Gulbrandsen P, Lundqvist C. Which strategy should be applied? Design of a Norwegian epidemiological survey on chronic headache. Acta Neurol Scand. 2007;115(suppl. 187):59–63.

63. Hagen K, Zwart JA, Vatten L, Stovner LJ, Bovim G. Head-HUNT: validity and reliability of a headache questionnaire in a large population-based study in Norway. Cephalalgia. 2000;20:244–51.

64. Montazeri A, Vahdaninia M, Ebrahimi M, Jarvandi S. The Hospital Anxiety and Depression Scale (HADS): translation and validation study of the Iranian version. Health Qual Life Outcomes. 2003;2003(1):14. https://doi.org/10.1186/1477-7525-1-14.

65. Eysenck MW. Happiness facts and myths. London: Erlbaum; 1990.

66. Ellis A. Why rational emotive behavior therapy is the most comprehensive and effective form of behavior therapy? J Ration Emot Cogn Behav Ther. 2004;22:85–92. https://doi.org/10.1023/B:JORE.0000025439.78389.52.

67. Yu S, et al. The prevalence and burden of primary headaches in China: a population-based door-to-door survey. Headache. 2012;52:582–91.

68. Alzoubi KH, et al. Prevalence of migraine and tension-type headache among adults in Jordan. J Headache Pain. 2009;10:265–70.

69. Schwartz BS, Stewart WF, Simon D, Lipton RB. Epidemiology of tension-type headache. JAMA. 1998;279:381–3.

70. Stovner LJ, et al. The global burden of headache: a documentation of headache prevalence and disability worldwide. Cephalalgia. 2007;27:193–210.

71. Winkler A, et al. The prevalence of headache with emphasis on tension-type headache in rural Tanzania: a community-based study. Cephalalgia. 2009;29:1317–25.

72. Leonardi M, et al. Global burden of headache disorders in children and adolescents 2007-2017. Int J Environ Res Public Health. 2020;18:250.

73. Lyngberg AC, Rasmussen BK, Jorgensen T, Jensen R. Prognosis of migraine and tension-type headache: a population-based follow-up study. Neurology. 2005;65:580–5.

74. Fernandez-de-Las-Penas C. Myofascial head pain. Curr Pain Headache Rep. 2015;19:28.

75. Kocer A, Kocer E, Memisogullari R, Domac FM, Yuksel H. Interleukin-6 levels in tension headache patients. Clin J Pain. 2010;26:690–3.

76. Sarchielli P, Alberti A, Floridi A, Gallai V. L-Arginine/nitric oxide pathway in chronic tension-type headache: relation with serotonin content and secretion and glutamate content. J Neurol Sci. 2002;198:9–15.

77. Ashina S, et al. Increased pain sensitivity in migraine and tension-type headache coexistent with low back pain: a cross-sectional population study. Eur J Pain. 2018;22:904–14.
78. Ashina S, Bendtsen L, Ashina M. Pathophysiology of tension-type headache. Curr Pain Headache Rep. 2005;9:415–22.
79. Palacios-Cena M, et al. Trigger points are associated with widespread pressure pain sensitivity in people with tension-type headache. Cephalalgia. 2018;38:237–45.
80. Langemark M, Jensen K, Jensen TS, Olesen J. Pressure pain thresholds and thermal nociceptive thresholds in chronic tension-type headache. Pain. 1989;38:203–10.
81. Buchgreitz L, Lyngberg AC, Bendtsen L, Jensen R. Frequency of headache is related to sensitization: a population study. Pain. 2006;123:19–27.
82. Bendtsen L, Jensen R, Olesen J. Decreased pain detection and tolerance thresholds in chronic tension-type headache. Arch Neurol. 1996;53:373–6.
83. Ashina S, Bendtsen L, Ashina M, Magerl W, Jensen R. Generalized hyperalgesia in patients with chronic tension-type headache. Cephalalgia. 2006;26:940–8.
84. de Tommaso M, et al. Clinical features of headache patients with fibromyalgia comorbidity. J Headache Pain. 2011;12:629–38.
85. Schoenen J, Jensen R. In: Olesen J, et al., editors. The headaches. Philadelphia: Lippincott, Williams & Wilkins; 2005. p. 701–9.
86. Palacios-Ceña M, et al. Variables associated with the use of prophylactic amitriptyline treatment in patients with tension-type headache. Clin J Pain. 2019;35:315–20.
87. Diener HC, et al. Pathophysiology, prevention, and treatment of medication overuse headache. Lancet Neurol. 2019;18:891–902.
88. Diener HC, et al. European Academy of Neurology guideline on the management of medication-overuse headache. Eur J Neurol. 2020;27:1102–16. An important guideline on the management of MOH, a complication of primary headaches including migraine and TTH.
89. Grande RB, Aaseth K, Benth J, Lundqvist C, Russell MB. Reduction in medication-overuse headache after short information. The Akershus study of chronic headache. Eur J Neurol. 2011;18:129–37.
90. Gildir S, Tüzün EH, Eroğlu G, Eker L. A randomized trial of trigger point dry needling versus sham needling for chronic tension-type headache. Medicine. 2019;98:e14520.
91. Vázquez-Justes D, Yarzábal-Rodríguez R, Doménech-García V, Herrero P, Bellosta-López P. Effectiveness of dry needling for headache: a systematic review. Neurologia. 2020; https://doi.org/10.1016/j.nrl.2019.09.010.
92. Ashina S, et al. Health-related quality of life in tension-type headache: a population-based study. Scand J Pain. 2021; https://doi.org/10.1515/sjpain-2020-0166.
93. Wang SJ, Fuh JL, Lu SR, Juang KD. Quality of life differs among headache diagnoses: analysis of SF-36 survey in 901 headache patients. Pain. 2001;89:285–92.
94. Penacoba-Puente C, Fernandez-de-Las-Penas C, Gonzalez-Gutierrez JL, Miangolarra-Page JC, Pareja JA. Interaction between anxiety, depression, quality of life and clinical parameters in chronic tension-type headache. Eur J Pain. 2008;12:886–94.
95. Friedman AP. Migraine and other common headaches. World Wide Abstr Gen Med. 1959;2:10–20.
96. Kolb LC. Psychiatric and psychogenic factors in headache in headache: diagnosis and treatment. Philadelphia: F.A. Davis Co.; 1959. p. 259–98.
97. Langemark M, Olesen J. Pericranial tenderness in tension headache. A blind, controlled study. Cephalalgia. 1987;7(4):249–55.
98. Sahler K. Epidemiology and cultural differences in tension-type headache. Curr Pain Headache Rep. 2012;16(6):525–32.
99. Castillo J, et al. Kaplan Award 1998. Epidemiology of chronic daily headache in the general population. Headache. 1999;39(3):190–6.
100. Ulrich V, Gervil M, Olesen J. The relative influence of environment and genes in episodic tension-type headache. Neurology. 2004;62(11):2065–9.

101. Buchgreitz L, et al. Increased pain sensitivity is not a risk factor but a consequence of frequent headache: a population-based follow-up study. Pain. 2008;137(3):623–30. This was a longitudinal study following TTH patients for 12 years, demonstrating that increased pain sensitivity was a consequence and not merely a risk factor for development of chronic headache.
102. Langemark M, et al. Pressure pain thresholds and thermal nociceptive thresholds in chronic tension-type headache. Pain. 1989;38(2):203–10.
103. Fernandez-de-Las-Penas C, et al. Increased pericranial tenderness, decreased pressure pain threshold, and headache clinical parameters in chronic tension-type headache patients. Clin J Pain. 2007;23(4):346–52.
104. Schoenen J, et al. Cephalic and extracephalic pressure pain thresholds in chronic tension-type headache. Pain. 1991;47(2):145–9.
105. Sandrini G, et al. Abnormal modulatory influence of diffuse noxious inhibitory controls in migraine and chronic tension-type headache patients. Cephalalgia. 2006;26(7):782–9.
106. Terrin A, et al. A prospective study on osmophobia in migraine versus tension-type headache in a large series of attacks. Cephalalgia. 2020;40(4):337–46.
107. Headache Classification Committee of the International Headache Society (IHS). The International Classification of Headache Disorders, 3rd edition. Cephalalgia. 2018;38(1):1–211.
108. Banzi R, et al. Selective serotonin reuptake inhibitors (SSRIs) and serotonin-norepinephrine reuptake inhibitors (SNRIs) for the prevention of tension-type headache in adults. Cochrane Database Syst Rev. 2015;5:CD011681.
109. Bendtsen L, Jensen R. Mirtazapine is effective in the prophylactic treatment of chronic tension-type headache. Neurology. 2004;62(10):1706–11.
110. Nestoriuc Y, et al. Biofeedback treatment for headache disorders: a comprehensive efficacy review. Appl Psychophysiol Biofeedback. 2008;33(3):125–40.
111. Benito-González E, Palacios-Ceña M, Fernández-Muñoz JJ, Castaldo M, Wang K, Catena A, Arendt-Nielsen L, Fernández-de-las-Peñas C. Variables associated with sleep quality in chronic tension-type headache: a cross-sectional and longitudinal design. PLoS One. 2018;13:e0197381.
112. Palacios-Ceña M, Fernández-Muñoz JJ, Castaldo M, Wang K, Guerrero-Peral Á, Arendt-Nielsen L, Fernández-de-las-Peñas C. The association of headache frequency with pain interference and the burden of disease is mediated by depression and sleep quality, but not anxiety, in chronic tension type headache. J Headache Pain. 2017;18:19.
113. Valente TW. Network interventions. Science. 2012;337:49.
114. Gómez Penedo JM, Rubel JA, Blättler L, Schmidt SJ, Stewart J, Egloff N, Grosse Holtforth M. The complex interplay of pain, depression, and anxiety symptoms in patients with chronic pain: a network approach. Clin J Pain. 2020;36:249–59.
115. Åkerblom S, Cervin M, Perrin S, Rivano Fischer M, Gerdle B, McCracken LM. A network analysis of clinical variables in chronic pain: a Study from the Swedish Quality Registry for Pain Rehabilitation (SQRP). Pain Med. 2021;22:1591–602.
116. Costantini G, Epskamp S, Borsboom D, Perugini M, Mottus R, Waldorp LJ, Cramer AOJ. State of the aRt personality research: a tutorial on network analysis of personality data in R. J Res Pers. 2015;54:13–29.
117. Fernández-de-las-Peñas C, Florencio LL, Plaza-Manzano G, Arias-Buría JL. Clinical reasoning behind non-pharmacological interventions for the management of headaches: a narrative literature review. Int J Environ Res Public Health. 2020;17:4126.
118. Jensen RH. Tension-type headache—the normal and most prevalent headache. Headache. 2018;58(2):339–45.
119. Yu S, Han X. Update of chronic tension-type headache. Curr Pain Headache Rep. 2015;19(1):469. This intensive review summaries the update knowledge on CTTH regarding pathogenesis and therapeutic strategies.
120. Filatova E, Latysheva N, Kurenkov A. Evidence of persistent central sensitization in chronic headaches: a multi-method study. J Headache Pain. 2008;9(5):295–300.

121. de Tommaso M, et al. Photic driving response in primary headache: diagnostic value tested by discriminant analysis and artificial neural network classifiers. Ital J Neurol Sci. 1999;20(1):23–8.

122. Wang W, Wang GP, Ding XL, Wang YH. Personality and response to repeated visual stimulation in migraine and tension-type headaches. Cephalalgia. 1999;19(8):718–24; discussion 697–8.

123. Chen WT, Hsiao FJ, Ko YC, Liu HY, Wang PN, Fuh JL, et al. Comparison of somatosensory cortex excitability between migraine and "strict-criteria" tension-type headache: a magnetoencephalographic study. Pain. 2018;159(4):793–803.

124. Chen WT, Chou KH, Lee PL, Hsiao FJ, Niddam DM, Lai KL, et al. Comparison of gray matter volume between migraine and "strict-criteria" tension-type headache. J Headache Pain. 2018;19(1):4.

125. Andersen S, Petersen MW, Svendsen AS, Gazerani P. Pressure pain thresholds assessed over temporalis, masseter, and frontalis muscles in healthy individuals, patients with tension-type headache, and those with migraine-a systematic review. Pain. 2015;156(8):1409–23.

126. Avramidis T, Bougea A, Hadjigeorgiou G, Thomaides T, Papadimitriou A. Blink reflex habituation in migraine and chronic tension-type headache. Neurol Sci. 2017;38(6):993–8.

127. Valeriani M, de Tommaso M, Restuccia D, le Pera D, Guido M, Iannetti DG, et al. Reduced habituation to experimental pain in migraine patients: a CO(2) laser evoked potential study. Pain. 2003;105(1–2):57–64.

128. Vuralli D, et al. Somatosensory temporal discrimination remains intact in tension-type headache whereas it is disrupted in migraine attacks. Cephalalgia. 2016:333102416677050.

129. Bezov D, Ashina S, Jensen R, Bendtsen L. Pain perception studies in tension-type headache. Headache. 2011;51(2):262–71.

130. Chen Y. Advances in the pathophysiology of tension-type headache: from stress to central sensitization. Curr Pain Headache Rep. 2009;13(6):484–94.

131. Fernández-de-Las-Peñas C, Cuadrado ML. Physical therapy for headaches. Cephalalgia. 2016;36(12):1134–42.

132. Zito G, Jull G, Story I. Clinical tests of musculoskeletal dysfunction in the diagnosis of cervicogenic headache. Man Ther. 2006;11(2):118–29.

133. Lipchik GL, Holroyd KA, O'Donnell FJ, et al. Exteroceptive suppression periods and pericranial muscle tenderness in chronic tension-type headache: effects of psychopathology, chronicity and disability. Cephalalgia. 2000;20:638–46.

134. Buchgreitz L, Lyngberg AC, Bendtsen L, et al. Frequency of headache is related to sensitization: a population study. Pain. 2006;123:19–27.

135. Sakai F, Ebihara S, Akiyama M, et al. Pericranial muscle hardness in tension-type headache. A non-invasive measurement method and its clinical application. Brain. 1995;118(Pt 2):523–31.

136. Ashina M, et al. Muscle hardness in patients with chronic tension-type headache: relation to actual headache state. Pain. 1999;79(2–3):201–5.

137. Shah JP, Thaker N, Heimur J, et al. Myofascial trigger point then and now: a historical and scientific perspective. PM R J. 2015;7:746–61.

138. Simons D, Travell J. Travell & Simons' myofascial pain and dysfunction: the trigger point manual. Baltimore: Williams & Wilkins; 1999.

139. Olesen J. Clinical and pathophysiological observations in migraine and tension-type headache explained by integration of vascular, supraspinal and myofascial inputs. Pain. 1991;46:125–32.

140. Calandre EP, Hidalgo J, García-Leiva JM, et al. Trigger point evaluation in migraine patients: an indication of peripheral sensitization linked to migraine predisposition? Eur J Neurol. 2006;13:244–9.

141. Fernández-de-Las-Peñas C, Cuadrado ML, Pareja JA. Myofascial trigger points, neck mobility and forward head posture in unilateral migraine. Cephalalgia. 2006;26:1061–70.

142. Tali D, Menahem I, Vered E, et al. Upper cervical mobility, posture and myofascial trigger points in subjects with episodic migraine: case-control study. J Bodyw Mov Ther. 2014;18:569–75.
143. Fernandez-de-las-Penas C, et al. Trigger points in the suboccipital muscles and forward head posture in tension-type headache. Headache. 2006;46(3):454–60.
144. Sohn J, Choi H, Lee S-M, et al. Differences in cervical musculoskeletal impairment between episodic and chronic tension-type headache. Cephalalgia. 2010;30:1514–23.
145. Fernandez-de-Las-Penas C, et al. Myofascial trigger points and their relationship to headache clinical parameters in chronic tension-type headache. Headache. 2006;46(8):1264–72.
146. Fernandez-de-Las-Penas C, et al. Referred pain from trapezius muscle trigger points shares similar characteristics with chronic tension type headache. Eur J Pain. 2007;11(4):475–82.
147. Simons DG, Hong C-Z, Simons LS. Endplate potentials are common to midfiber myofacial trigger points. Am J Phys Med Rehabil. 2002;81:212–22.
148. Ge HY, Monterde S, Graven-Nielsen T, et al. Latent myofascial trigger points are associated with an increased intramuscular electromyographic activity during synergistic muscle activation. J Pain. 2014;15:181–7.
149. Yu SH, Kim HJ. Electrophysiological characteristics according to activity level of myofascial trigger points. J Phys Ther Sci. 2015;27:2841–3.
150. Wytrążek M, Huber J, Lipiec J, et al. Evaluation of palpation, pressure algometry, and electromyography for monitoring trigger points in young participants. J Manip Physiol Ther. 2015;38:232–43.
151. Ferracini GN, Florencio LL, Dach F, et al. Myofascial trigger points and migraine-related disability in women with episodic and chronic migraine. Clin J Pain. 2017;33:109–15.
152. Ferracini GN, Chaves TC, Dach F, et al. Relationship between active trigger points and head/neck posture in patients with migraine. Am J Phys Med Rehabil. 2016;95:831–9.
153. Florencio LL, Ferracini GN, Chaves TC, et al. Active trigger points in the cervical musculature determine the altered activation of superficial neck and extensor muscles in women with migraine. Clin J Pain. 2017;33:238–45.
154. Landgraf MN, Biebl JT, Langhagen T, et al. Children with migraine: provocation of headache via pressure to myofascial trigger points in the trapezius muscle? A prospective controlled observational study. Eur J Pain. 2018. Epub ahead of print 26 Sept 2017; https://doi.org/10.1002/ejp.1127.
155. Fernandez-de-Las-Penas C, et al. The local and referred pain from myofascial trigger points in the temporalis muscle contributes to pain profile in chronic tension-type headache. Clin J Pain. 2007;23(9):786–92.
156. Couppe C, et al. Myofascial trigger points are very prevalent in patients with chronic tension-type headache: a double-blinded controlled study. Clin J Pain. 2007;23(1):23–7.
157. Harden RN, et al. Botulinum toxin a in the treatment of chronic tension-type headache with cervical myofascial trigger points: a randomized, double-blind, placebo-controlled pilot study. Headache. 2009;49(5):732–43.
158. Karadas O, et al. Efficacy of local lidocaine application on anxiety and depression and its curative effect on patients with chronic tension-type headache. Eur Neurol. 2013;70(1–2):95–101.
159. Moraska AF, et al. Myofascial trigger point-focused head and neck massage for recurrent tension-type headache: a randomized, placebo-controlled clinical trial. Clin J Pain. 2015;31(2):159–68.
160. Karadas O, Gul HL, Inan LE. Lidocaine injection of pericranial myofascial trigger points in the treatment of frequent episodic tension-type headache. J Headache Pain. 2013;14:44.
161. Gandolfi M, Geroin C, Valè N, et al. Does myofascial and trigger point treatment reduce pain and analgesic intake in patients undergoing Onabotulinumtoxin A injection due to chronic intractable migraine? A pilot, single-blind randomized controlled trial. Eur J Phys Rehabil Med. 2018. Epub ahead of print 27 Jul 2017.; https://doi.org/10.23736/S1973-9087.17.04568-3.

162. Ghanbari A, Askarzadeh S, Petramfar P, et al. Migraine responds better to a combination of medical therapy and trigger point management than routine medical therapy alone. NeuroRehabilitation. 2015;37:157–63.
163. Giamberardino MA, Tafuri E, Savini A, et al. Contribution of myofascial trigger points to migraine symptoms. J Pain. 2007;8:869–78.
164. Ranoux D, Martiné G, Espagne-Dubreuilh G, et al. OnabotulinumtoxinA injections in chronic migraine, targeted to sites of pericranial myofascial pain: an observational, open label, real-life cohort study. J Headache Pain. 2017;18:75.
165. Sollmann N, Trepte-Freisleder F, Albers L, et al. Magnetic stimulation of the upper trapezius muscles in patients with migraine—a pilot study. Eur J Paediatr Neurol. 2016;20:888–97.
166. Lipton RB, Cady RK, Stewart WF, Wilks K, Hall C. Diagnostic lessons from the spectrum study. Neurology. 2002;58:S27–31.
167. Ashina M, et al. Plasma levels of calcitonin gene-related peptide in chronic tension-type headache. Neurology. 2000;55(9):1335–40.
168. Valeriani M, de Tommaso M, Restuccia D, Le Pera D, Guido M, Iannetti GD, Libro G, Truini A, Di Trapani G, Puca F, Tonali P, Cruccu G. Reduced habituation to experimental pain in migraine patients: a CO(2) laser evoked potential study. Pain. 2003;105:57–64.
169. Vuralli D, Boran HE, Cengiz B, Coskun O, Bolay H. Somatosensory temporal discrimination remains intact in tension-type headache whereas it is disrupted in migraine attacks. Cephalalgia. 2017;37:1241–7.
170. Borsook D, Maleki N, Becerra L, McEwen B. Understanding migraine through the lens of maladaptive stress responses: a model disease of allostatic load. Neuron. 2012;73:219–34.
171. Della Vedova C, Cathcart S, Dohnalek A, Lee V, Hutchinson MR, Immink MA, Hayball J. Peripheral interleukin-1β levels are elevated in chronic tension-type headache patients. Pain Res Manag. 2013;18:301–6.
172. Koçer A, Koçer E, Memişoğullari R, Domaç FM, Yüksel H. Interleukin-6 levels in tension headache patients. Clin J Pain. 2010;26:690–3.
173. Arruda MA, Guidetti V, Galli F, Albuquerque RC, Bigal ME. Primary headaches in childhood—a population-based study. Cephalalgia. 2010;30:1056–64.
174. Poyrazoğlu HG, Kumandas S, Canpolat M, Gümüs H, Elmali F, Kara A, Per H. The prevalence of migraine and tension-type headache among schoolchildren in Kayseri, Turkey: an evaluation of sensitivity and specificity using multivariate analysis. J Child Neurol. 2015;30:889–95.
175. Yılmaz Ü, Çeleğen M, Yılmaz TS, Gürçınar M, Ünalp A. Childhood headaches and brain magnetic resonance imaging findings. Eur J Paediatr Neurol. 2014;18:163–70.
176. Ozge A, Sasmaz T, Cakmak SE, Kaleagasi H, Siva A. Epidemiological-based childhood headache natural history study: after an interval of six years. Cephalalgia. 2010;30:703–12.
177. Fumal A, Schoenen J. Tension-type headache: current research and clinical management. Neurology. 2008;7:70–83. https://doi.org/10.1016/S1474-4422(07)70325-3.
178. Anttila P, Sourander A, Metsähonkala L, Aromaa M, Helenius H, Sillanpää M. Psychiatric symptoms in children with primary headache. J Am Acad Child Adolesc Psychiatry. 2004;43:412–9.
179. Balottin U, Fusar Poli P, Termine C, Molteni S, Galli F. Psychopathological symptoms in child and adolescent migraine and tension-type headache: a meta-analysis. Cephalalgia. 2013;33:112–22.
180. Bektaş Ö, Uğur C, Gençtürk ZB, Aysev A, Sireli Ö, Deda G. Relationship of childhood headaches with preferences in leisure time activities, depression, anxiety and eating habits: a population-based, cross-sectional study. Cephalalgia. 2015;35:527–37.
181. Amouroux R, Rousseau-Salvador C, Pillant M, Antonietti JP, Tourniaire B, Annequin D. Longitudinal study shows that depression in childhood is associated with a worse evolution of headaches in adolescence. Acta Paediatr. 2017;106:1961–5.
182. Martin VT, Vij B. Diet and headache: part 2. Headache. 2016;56:1553–62.

183. Lippi G, Mattiuzzi C, Meschi T, Cervellin G, Borghi L. Homocysteine and migraine. A narrative review. Clin Chim Acta. 2014;433:5–11.
184. Di Lorenzo C, Coppola G, Sirianni G, Di Lorenzo G, Bracaglia M, Di Lenola D, et al. Migraine improvement during short lasting ketogenesis: a proof-of-concept study. Eur J Neurol. 2015;22:170–7.
185. Bjørke-Monsen AL, Ueland PM. Cobalamin status in children. J Inherit Metab Dis. 2011;34:111–9.
186. De Benoist B. Conclusions of a WHO Technical Consultation on folate and vitamin B12 deficiencies. Food Nutr Bull. 2008;29(2 Suppl):238–44.
187. Koc A, Kocyigit A, Soran M, Demir N, Sevinc E, Erel O, Mil Z. High frequency of maternal vitamin B12 deficiency as an important cause of infantile vitamin B12 deficiency in Sanliurfa province of Turkey. Eur J Nutr. 2006;45:291–7.
188. Goraya JS, Kaur S, Mehra B. Neurology of nutritional vitamin B12 deficiency in infants: case series from India and literature review. J Child Neurol. 2015;30:1831–7.
189. Yilmaz S, Serdaroglu G, Tekgul H, Gokben S. Different neurologic aspects of nutritional B12 deficiency in infancy. J Child Neurol. 2016;31:565–8.
190. Erol I, Alehan F, Gümüs A. West syndrome in an infant with vitamin B12 deficiency in the absence of macrocytic anaemia. Dev Med Child Neurol. 2007;49:774–6.
191. Incecik F, Hergüner MO, Altunbaşak S, Leblebisatan G. Neurologic findings of nutritional vitamin B12 deficiency in children. Turk J Pediatr. 2010;52:17–21.
192. Sarioglu B, Erhan E, Serdaroglu G, Doering BG, Erermis S, Tutuncuoglu S. Tension-type headache in children: a clinical evaluation. Pediatr Int. 2003;45:186–9.
193. Bentivegna E, Luciani M, Paragliola V, Baldari F, Lamberti PA, Conforti G, et al. Recent advancements in tension-type headache: a narrative review. Expert Rev Neurother. 2021; https://doi.org/10.1080/14737175.2021.1943363.
194. Karikari TK, Charway-Felli A, Höglund K, Blennow K, Zetterberg H. Commentary: global, regional, and national burden of neurological disorders during 1990–2015: a systematic analysis for the Global Burden of Disease Study 2015. Front Neurol. 2018; https://doi.org/10.3389/fneur.2018.00201.
195. Steel SJ, Robertson CE, Whealy MA. Current understanding of the pathophysiology and approach to tension-type headache. Curr Neurol Neurosci Rep. 2021; https://doi.org/10.1007/s11910-021-01138-7.
196. Fernández-de-Las-Peñas C, Plaza-Manzano G, Navarro-Santana MJ, Olesen J, Jensen RH, Bendtsen L. Evidence of localized and widespread pressure pain hypersensitivity in patients with tension-type headache: a systematic review and meta-analysis. Cephalalgia. 2021; https://doi.org/10.1177/0333102420958384.
197. Hubbard DR, Berkoff GM. Myofascial trigger points show spontaneous needle EMG activity. Spine. 1993; https://doi.org/10.1097/00007632-199310000-00015.
198. McNulty WH, Gevirtz RN, Hubbard DR, Berkoff GM. Needle electromyographic evaluation of trigger point response to a psychological stressor. Psychophysiology. 1994; https://doi.org/10.1111/j.1469-8986.1994.tb02220.x.
199. Gevirtz R. The muscle spindle trigger point model of chronic pain. Biofeedback. 2006. https://search.proquest.com/openview/f4bc54e54c4365337df5a78da92f01e1/1?pq-origsite=gscholar&cbl=39806.
200. Banks SL, Jacobs DW, Gevirtz R, Hubbard DR. Effects of autogenic relaxation training on electromyographic activity in active myofascial trigger points. J Musculoskelet Pain. 1998; https://doi.org/10.1300/J094v06n04_03.
201. Uijtdehaage SH, Thayer JF. Accentuated antagonism in the control of human heart rate. Clin Auton Res. 2000; https://doi.org/10.1007/BF02278013.
202. Sowder E, Gevirtz R, Shapiro W, Ebert C. Restoration of vagal tone: a possible mechanism for functional abdominal pain. Appl Psychophysiol Biofeedback. 2010; https://doi.org/10.1007/s10484-010-9128-8.

203. Moran M. New migraine consensus statement on post-approval use of migraine therapies. Neurol Today. 2021;21(15):10.

204. Peroutka SJ. Migraine: a chronic sympathetic nervous system disorder. Headache. 2004; https://doi.org/10.1111/j.1526-4610.2004.04011.x.

205. de Coo IF, Marin JC, Silberstein SD, Friedman DI, Gaul C, McClure CK, et al. Differential efficacy of non-invasive vagus nerve stimulation for the acute treatment of episodic and chronic cluster headache: a meta-analysis. Cephalalgia. 2019; https://doi.org/10.1177/0333102419856607.

206. Goadsby PJ, de Coo IF, Silver N, Tyagi A, Ahmed F, Gaul C, et al. Non-invasive vagus nerve stimulation for the acute treatment of episodic and chronic cluster headache: a randomized, double-blind, sham-controlled ACT2 study. Cephalalgia. 2018; https://doi.org/10.1177/0333102417744362.

207. Wu Q, Liu P, Liao C, Tan L. Effectiveness of yoga therapy for migraine: a meta-analysis of randomized controlled studies. J Clin Neurosci. 2022; https://doi.org/10.1016/j.jocn.2022.01.018.

208. Kisan R, Sujan MU, Adoor M, Rao R, Nalini A, Kutty BM, et al. Effect of Yoga on migraine: a comprehensive study using clinical profile and cardiac autonomic functions. Int J Yoga. 2014; https://doi.org/10.4103/0973-6131.133891.

209. Nestoriuc Y, Martin A. Efficacy of biofeedback for migraine: a meta-analysis. Pain. 2007; https://doi.org/10.1016/j.pain.2006.09.007.

210. Minen MT, Corner S, Berk T, Levitan V, Friedman S, Adhikari S, et al. Heartrate variability biofeedback for migraine using a smartphone application and sensor: a randomized controlled trial. Gen Hosp Psychiatry. 2021; https://doi.org/10.1016/j.genhosppsych.2020.12.008. This is the first randomized controlled trial (n=52) of heart rate variability biofeedback for migraine. The authors concluded that the app-based HRV biofeedback was feasible and acceptable on a time-limited basis for people with migraine. Changes in the primary clinical outcome did not differ between biofeedback and control; however, high users of the app reported more benefit than low users.

211. Schytz HW, Bendtsen L. Sumatriptan plus naproxen for acute migraine attacks in adults. Ugeskr Laeger. 2014;176(32):V03140155.

212. Bendtsen L, Jensen R. Treating tension-type headache—an expert opinion. Expert Opin Pharmacother. 2011;12(7):1099–109. https://doi.org/10.1517/14656566.2011.548806.

213. Bendtsen L, et al. EFNS guideline on the treatment of tension-type headache—report of an EFNS task force. Eur J Neurol. 2010;17(11):1318–25. These are the most recent evidence-based guidelines for treatment of TTH.

214. May A, Leone M, Afra J, Linde M, Sándor PS, Evers S, Goadsby PJ, Task Force EFNS. EFNS guidelines on the treatment of cluster headache and other trigeminal-autonomic cephalalgias. Eur J Neurol. 2006;13(10):1066–77. https://doi.org/10.1111/j.1468-1331.2006.01566.x.

215. Diener HC, Antonaci F, Braschinsky M, Evers S, Jensen R, Lainez M, Kristoffersen ES, Tassorelli C, Ryliskiene K, Petersen JA. European academy of neurology guideline on the management of medication-overuse headache. Eur J Neurol. 2020;27(7):1102–16. https://doi.org/10.1111/ene.14268.

216. Bendtsen L, Zakrzewska JM, Heinskou TB, Hodaie M, Leal PRL, Nurmikko T, Obermann M, Cruccu G, Maarbjerg S. Advances in diagnosis, classification, pathophysiology, and management of trigeminal neuralgia. Lancet Neurol. 2020;19(9):784–96. https://doi.org/10.1016/S1474-4422(20)30233-7.

217. Bakhshandeh BM, Rahbarimanesh AA, Sadeghi M, et al. Comparison of propranolol and pregabalin for prophylaxis of childhood migraine: a randomised controlled trial. Acta Med Iran. 2015;53:276–80.

218. Stubberud A, Flaaen NM, McCrory DC, Pedersen SA, Linde M. Flunarizine as prophylaxis for episodic migraine: a systematic review with meta-analysis. Pain. 2019;160(4):762–72. https://doi.org/10.1097/j.pain.0000000000001456.

219. Turner DP, Smitherman TA, Black AK, Penzien DB, Porter JAH, Lofland KR, Houle TT. Are migraine and tension-type headache diagnostic types or points on a severity continuum? An exploration of the latent taxometric structure of headache. Pain. 2015;156:1200–7.
220. Charles A. Migraine. N Engl J Med. 2017;377(6):553–61.
221. Granella F, D'Alessandro R, Manzoni GC, Cerbo R, Colucci D'Amato C, Pini LA, et al. International Headache Society Classification: interobserver reliability in the diagnosis of primary headaches. Cephalalgia. 1994;14(1):16–20.
222. Olesen J. International Classification of Headache Disorders. Lancet Neurol. 2018;17(5):396–7.
223. Olesen J. Headache Classification Committee of the International Headache Society (IHS). The International Classification of Headache Disorders. Cephalalgia. 2018;38:1–211.
224. Zhu B, Coppola G, Shoaran M. Migraine classification using somatosensory evoked potentials. Cephalalgia. 2019;39:1143–55.
225. Lee MJ, et al. Dynamic functional connectivity of the migraine brain: a resting-state functional magnetic resonance imaging study. Pain. 2019;160:2776–86.
226. Chong CD, et al. Migraine classification using magnetic resonance imaging resting-state functional connectivity data. Cephalalgia. 2017;37:828–44.
227. Cernuda-Morollón E, et al. Interictal increase of CGRP levels in peripheral blood as a biomarker for chronic migraine. Neurology. 2013;81:1191–6.
228. Lee MJ, Lee SY, Cho S, Kang ES, Chung CS. Feasibility of serum CGRP measurement as a biomarker of chronic migraine: a critical reappraisal. J Headache Pain. 2018;19:53.
229. Krawczyk B, Simić D, Simić S, Woźniak M. Automatic diagnosis of primary headaches by machine learning methods. Cent Eur J Med. 2013;8:157–65.
230. Garcia-Chimeno Y, Garcia-Zapirain B, Gomez-Beldarrain M, Fernandez-Ruanova B, Garcia-Monco JC. Automatic migraine classification via feature selection committee and machine learning techniques over imaging and questionnaire data. BMC Med Inf Decis Making. 2017;17:38.
231. Tibshirani R. Regression shrinkage and selection via the lasso. J R Stat Soc Ser B. 1996;58:267–88.
232. Guyon I, Weston J, Barnhill S, Vapnik V. Gene selection for cancer classification using support vector machines. Mach Learn. 2002;46:389–422.
233. Peng H, Long F, Ding C. Feature selection based on mutual information: criteria of max-dependency, max-relevance, and min-redundancy. IEEE Trans Pattern Anal Mach Intell. 2005;27:1226–38.
234. El Tumi H, Johnson MI, Dantas PBF, Maynard MJ, Tashani OA. Age-related changes in pain sensitivity in healthy humans: a systematic review with meta-analysis. Eur J Pain. 2017;21(6):955–64.
235. Boerner KE, Birnie KA, Caes L, Schinkel M, Chambers CT. Sex differences in experimental pain among healthy children: a systematic review and meta-analysis. Pain. 2014;155(5):983–93.
236. Pfaffenrath V, Fendrich K, Vennemann M, Meisinger C, Ladwig KH, Evers S, Straube A, Hoffmann W, Berger K. Regional variations in the prevalence of migraine and tension-type headache applying the new IHS criteria: the German DMKG headache study. Cephalalgia. 2009;29(1):48–57.
237. Schwaiger J, Kiechl S, Seppi K, Sawires M, Stockner H, Erlacher T, Mairhofer ML, Niederkofler H, Rungger G, Gasperi A, Poewe W, Willeit J. Prevalence of primary headaches and cranial neuralgias in men and women aged 55-94 years (Bruneck Study). Cephalalgia. 2009;29(2):179–87.
238. Bigal ME, Libermann JN, Lipton RB. Age-dependent prevalence and clinical features of migraine. Neurology. 2006;67:246–51.
239. Mattsson P, Svärdsudd K, Lundberg PO, Westerberg CE. The prevalence of migraine in women aged 40-74 years: a population-based study. Cephalalgia. 2000;20(10):893–9.

240. Martins KM, Bordini CA, Bigal ME, Speciali JG. Migraine in the elderly: a comparison with migraine in young adults. Headache. 2006;46(2):312–6.
241. Wöber C, Brannath W, Schmidt K, Kapitan M, Rudel E, Wessely P, Wober-Bingol C. Prospective analysis of factors related to migraine attacks: the PAMINA study. Cephalagia. 2007;27:304–14.
242. Kelman L. Migraine changes with age: impact on migraine classification. Headache. 2006;46:1161–71.
243. Kaniecki RG. Tension-type headache in the elderly. Curr Pain Headache Rep. 2006;10(6):448–53.
244. Russell MB, Levi N, Saltyte-Benth J, Fenger K. Tension-type headache in adolescents and adults: a population based study of 33,764 twins. Eur J Epidemiol. 2006;21(2):153–60.
245. Duffield SJ, Ellis BM, Goodson N, Walker-Bone K, Conaghan PG, Margham T, Loftis T. The contribution of musculoskeletal disorders in multimorbidity: implications for practice and policy. Best Pract Res Clin Rheumatol. 2017;31(2):129–44.
246. Häuser W, Marschall U, Layer P, Grobe T. The prevalence, comorbidity, management and costs of irritable bowel syndrome. Dtsch Arztebl Int. 2019;116(27–28):463–70.
247. Lichtenstein A, Tiosano S, Amital H. The complexities of fibromyalgia and its comorbidities. Curr Opin Rheumatol. 2018;30(1):94–100.
248. Simons DG. Muscular pain syndromes. Adv Pain Res Ther. 1990;17:1–41.
249. Giamberardino MA, Affaitati G, Fabrizio A, Costantini R. Myofascial pain syndromes and their evaluation. Best Pract Res Clin Rheumatol. 2011b;25(2):185–98.
250. Affaitati G, Costantini R, Fabrizio A, Lapenna D, Tafuri E, Giamberardino MA. Effects of treatment of peripheral pain generators in fibromyalgia patients. Eur J Pain. 2011;15:61–9.
251. Caldarella MP, Giamberardino MA, Sacco F, Affaitati G, Milano A, Lerza R, Balatsinou C, Laterza F, Pierdomenico SD, Cuccurullo F, Neri M. Sensitivity disturbances in patients with irritable bowel syndrome and fibromyalgia. Am J Gastroenterol. 2006;101(12):2782–9.
252. Munakata J, Naliboff B, Harraf F, Kodner A, Lembo T, Chang L, Silverman DH, Mayer EA. Repetitive sigmoid stimulation induces rectal hyperalgesia in patients with irritable bowel syndrome. Gastroenterology. 1997;112(1):55–63.
253. Wilder-Smith CH, Robert-Yap J. Abnormal endogenous pain modulation and somatic and visceral hypersensitivity in female patients with irritable bowel syndrome. World J Gastroenterol. 2007;13(27):3699–704.
254. Chung MK, Chung RP, Gordon D. Interstitial cystitis and endometriosis in patients with chronic pelvic pain: the "Evil Twins" syndrome. JSLS. 2005;9(1):25–9.
255. Ferrero S, Pretta S, Bertoldi S, Anserini P, Remorgida V, Del Sette M, Gandolfo C, Ragni N. Increased frequency of migraine among women with endometriosis. Hum Reprod. 2004;19(12):2927–32.
256. Tervila L, Marttila P. Headache as a symptom of endometriosis externa. Ann Chir Gynaecol Fenn. 1975;64(4):239–41.
257. Tietjen GE, Bushnell CD, Herial NA, Utley C, White L, Hafeez F. Endometriosis is associated with prevalence of comorbid conditions in migraine. Headache. 2007;47(7):1069–78.
258. de Tommaso M, Sardaro M, Serpino C, Costantini F, Vecchio E, Prudenzano MP, Lamberti P, Livrea P. Fibromyalgia comorbidity in primary headaches. Cephalalgia. 2009;29:453–64.
259. Aaseth K, Grande RB, Kværner KJ, Gulbrandsen P, Lundqvist C, Russell MB. Prevalence of secondary chronic headaches in a population-based sample of 30-44-year-old persons. The Akershus study of chronic headache. Cephalalgia. 2008;28(7):705–13. https://doi.org/10.1111/j.1468-2982.2008.01577.x.
260. El-Sherbiny NA, Masoud M, Shalaby NM, Shehata HS. Prevalence of primary headache disorders in Fayoum Governorate, Egypt. J Headache Pain. 2015;16(1):85.
261. Rajeh SA, Awada A, Bademosi O, Ogunniyi A. The prevalence of migraine and tension headache in Saudi Arabia: a community-based study. Eur J Neurol. 1997;4(5):502–6.
262. Schneider SL. The international standard classification of education 2011. In: Class and stratification analysis. Emerald Group Publishing Ltd.; 2013. p. 365–79.

263. Gil-Gouveia RS, Sousa RF, Lopes L, et al. Post-angiography headaches. J Headache Pain. 2008;9:327–30. https://doi.org/10.1007/s10194-008-0057-3.
264. Ramadan NM, Gilkey SJ, Mitchell M, et al. Postangiography headache. Headache. 1995;35:21–4. https://doi.org/10.1111/j.1526-4610.1995.hed3501021.x.
265. Gündüz A, Göksan B, Koçer N, et al. Headache in carotid artery stenting and angiography. Headache. 2012;52:544–9. https://doi.org/10.1111/j.1526-4610.2012.02096.x.
266. Aktan Ç, Özgür Ö, Sindel T, et al. Characteristics of headache during and after digital substraction angiography: a critical re-appraisal of the ICHD-3 criteria. Cephalalgia. 2017;37:1074–81. https://doi.org/10.1177/0333102416665878.
267. Kwon M, Hong C, Joo J, et al. Headache after cerebral angiography: frequency, predisposing factors, and predictors of recovery. J Neuroimaging. 2016;26:89–94. https://doi.org/10.1111/jon.12290.
268. Qureshi AI, Naseem N, Saleem MA, et al. Migraine and non-migraine headaches following diagnostic catheter-based cerebral angiography. Headache. 2018;58:1219–24. https://doi.org/10.1111/head.13377.
269. Ashina M, et al. Nitric oxide-induced headache in patients with chronic tension-type headache. Brain. 2000;123(Pt 9):1830–7.
270. Thomsen L, Kruuse C, Iversen H, et al. A nitric oxide donor (nitroglycerin) triggers genuine migraine attacks. Eur J Neurol. 1994;1:73–80. https://doi.org/10.1111/j.1468-1331.1994.tb00053.x.
271. Bendtsen L, Jensen R. Tension-type headache: the most common, but also the most neglected, headache disorder. Curr Opin Neurol. 2006;19:305–9.
272. Guerrero ÁL, Rojo E, Herrero S, Neri MJ, Bautista L, Peñas ML, et al. Characteristics of the first 1000 headaches in an outpatient headache clinic registry. Headache. 2011;51(2):226–31.
273. Maizels M. Headache evaluation and treatment by primary care physicians in an emergency department in the era of triptans. Arch Intern Med. 2001;161:1969–73.
274. Dermitzakis EV, Georgiadis G, Rudolf J, Nikiforidou D, Kyriakidis P, Gravas I, et al. Headache patients in the emergency department of a Greek tertiary care hospital. J Headache Pain. 2010;11(2):123.
275. Sahai-Srivastava S, Desai P, Zheng L. Analysis of headache management in a busy emergency room in the United States. Headache. 2008;48:931–8.
276. Friedman BW, et al. Applying the International Classification of Headache Disorders to the Emergency Department: an assessment of reproducibility and the frequency with which unique diagnosis can be assigned to every acute headache presentation. Ann Emerg Med. 2007;49:409–19.
277. Relja G, Granato A, Capozzoli F, Maggiore C, Catalan M, Pizzolato G, et al. Nontraumatic headache in the emergency department: a survey in the province of Trieste. J Headache Pain. 2005;6(4):298–300.
278. Barton CW. Evaluation and treatment of headache patients in the emergency department: a survey. Headache. 1994;34:91–4.
279. Munoz-Ceron J, Marin-Careaga V, Peña L, Mutis J, Ortiz G. Headache at the emergency room: etiologies, diagnostic usefulness of ICHD-3 criteria, red and green flags. PLoS One. 2019;14(1):e0209728.
280. Headache Classification Committee of the International Headache Society (IHS). The International Classification of Headache Disorders, 3rd edition. Cephalalgia. 2018;38:1–211.
281. Li X, et al. Clinical characteristics of tension-type headache in the neurological clinic of university hospital in China. Neurol Sci. 2012;33:283–7.
282. Crystal SC, Robbins MS. Tension-type headache mimics. Curr Pain Headache Rep. 2011;15:459–66.
283. Kaniecki RG. Tension-type headache. Continuum Lifelong Learning Neurol. 2012;18(4):823–34.
284. Rains JC, Davis RE, Smitherman TA. Tension-type headache and sleep. Curr Neurol Neurosci Rep. 2015;15(2):1–9.

285. Rains JC, Poceta JS. Sleep and headache. Curr Treat Options Neurol. 2010;12(1):1–15. https://doi.org/10.1007/s11940-009-0056-y.
286. Rains JC, Poceta JS. Sleep-related headaches. Neurol Clin. 2012;30(4):1285–98. https://doi.org/10.1016/j.ncl.2012.08.014.
287. American Academy of Sleep Med. International Classification of Sleep Disorders. 3rd ed. Dairen: American Academy of Sleep Medicine; 2014.
288. Wang J, Huang Q, Li N, et al. Triggers of migraine and tension-type headache in China: a clinic-based survey. Eur J Neurol. 2013;20:689–96. https://doi.org/10.1111/ene.12039.
289. Kikuchi H, Yoshiuchi K, Yamamoto Y, Komaki G, Akabayashi A. Does sleep aggravate tension-type headache? An investigation using computerized ecological momentary assessment and actigraphy. Biopsychosoc Med. 2011;5:10. https://doi.org/10.1186/1751-0759-5-10.
290. Alvaro PK, Roberts RM, Harris JK. A systematic review assessing bidirectionality between sleep disturbances, anxiety, and depression. Sleep. 2013;36(7):1059–68. https://doi.org/10.5665/sleep.2810.
291. Lisotto C, Mainardi F, Maggioni F, Zanchin G. The comorbidity between migraine and hypothyroidism. J Headache Pain. 2013;1:138.
292. Steiner TJ, Stovner LJ, Vos T. GBD 2015: migraine is the third cause of disability in under 50s. J Headache Pain. 2016;17(1):104.
293. Khan HB, Shah PA, Bhat MH, Imran A. Association of hypothyroidism in patients with migraine and tension type headache disorders in Kashmir, North India. Neurology Asia. 2015;20(3):257–26.
294. Yener A, Korucu O. Visual field losses in patients with migraine without aura and tension-type headache. Neuroophthalmology. 2017;41:59–67.
295. Flammer J, Pache M, Resink T. Vasospasm, its role in the pathogenesis of diseases with particular reference to the eye. Prog Retin Eye Res. 2001;20:319–49.
296. Reddy SM, Vergo MT, Paice JA, Kwon N, Helenowski IB, Benson AL, et al. Quantitative sensory testing at baseline and during cycle 1 oxaliplatin infusion detects subclinical peripheral neuropathy and predicts clinically overt chronic neuropathy in gastrointestinal malignancies. Clin Colorectal Cancer. 2016;15(1):37–46.
297. Kitaj MB, Klink M. Pain thresholds in daily transformed migraine versus episodic migraine headache patients. Headache. 2005;45(8):992–8.
298. Komiyama O, De Laat A. Tactile and pain thresholds in the intra- and extra-oral regions of symptom-free subjects. Pain. 2005;115:308–15.
299. Komiyama O, Obara R, Iida T, Wang K, Svensson P, Arendt-Nielsen L, de Laat A, Kawara M. Influence of age and gender on trigeminal sensory function and magnetically evoked masseteric exteroceptive suppression reflex. Arch Oral Biol. 2012;57:995–1002.
300. Rolke R, Magerl W, Campbell KA, Schalber C, Caspari S, Birklein F, Treede RD. Quantitative sensory testing: a comprehensive protocol for clinical trials. Eur J Pain. 2006;10:77–88.
301. Bag B, Hacihasanoglu R, Tufekci F. Examination of anxiety, hostility and psychiatric disorders in patients with migraine and tension-type headache. Int J Clin Pract. 2005;59(5):515–21.
302. Öze A, Nagy A, Benedek G, Bodosi B, Kéri S, Pálinkás É, et al. Acquired equivalence and related memory processes in migraine without aura. Cephalalgia. 2017;37(6):532–40.
303. Gil-Gouveia R, Oliveira AG, Martins IP. Cognitive dysfunction during migraine attacks: a study on migraine without aura. Cephalalgia. 2015;35(8):662–74.
304. Qu P, Yu JX, Xia L, Chen GH. Cognitive performance and the alteration of neuroendocrine hormones in chronic tension-type headache. Pain Pract. 2018;18:8–17.
305. Joëls M, Baram TZ. The neuro-symphony of stress. Nat Rev Neurosci. 2009;10(6):459.
306. Row BW, Dohanich GP. Post-training administration of corticotropin-releasing hormone (CRH) enhances retention of a spatial memory through a noradrenergic mechanism in male rats. Neurobiol Learn Mem. 2008;89(4):370–8.

307. Heinrichs S, Stenzel-Poore M, Gold L, Battenberg E, Bloom F, Koob G, et al. Learning impairment in transgenic mice with central overexpression of corticotropin-releasing factor. Neuroscience. 1996;74(2):303–11.

308. Chen Y, Brunson K, Adelmann G, Bender R, Frotscher M, Baram T. Hippocampal corticotropin releasing hormone: pre-and postsynaptic location and release by stress. Neuroscience. 2004;126(3):533–40.

309. Sandström A, Peterson J, Sandström E, Lundberg M, Nystrom ILR, Nyberg L, et al. Cognitive deficits in relation to personality type and hypothalamic-pituitary-adrenal (HPA) axis dysfunction in women with stress-related exhaustion. Scand J Psychol. 2011;52(1):71–82.

310. Ackermann S, Hartmann F, Papassotiropoulos A, de Quervain DJ-F, Rasch B. Associations between basal cortisol levels and memory retrieval in healthy young individuals. J Cogn Neurosci. 2013;25(11):1896–907.

311. Chen G, Xia L, Wang F, Li XW, Jiao CA. Patients with chronic insomnia have selective impairments in memory that are modulated by cortisol. Psychophysiology. 2016;53(10):1567–76.

312. Beydoun M, Beydoun H, Kitner-Triolo M, Kaufman J, Evans M, Zonderman A. Thyroid hormones are associated with cognitive function: moderation by sex, race, and depressive symptoms. J Clin Endocrinol Metab. 2013;98(8):3470–81.

313. Bagger YZ, Tankó LB, Alexandersen P, Qin G, Christiansen C, Group PS. Early postmenopausal hormone therapy may prevent cognitive impairment later in life. Menopause. 2005;12(1):12–7.

314. MacLennan AH, Henderson VW, Paine BJ, Mathias J, Ramsay EN, Ryan P, et al. Hormone therapy, timing of initiation, and cognition in women aged older than 60 years: the REMEMBER pilot study. Menopause. 2006;13(1):28–36.

315. Ghazvini H, Khaksari M, Esmaeilpour K, Shabani M, Asadi-Shekaari M, Khodamoradi M, et al. Effects of treatment with estrogen and progesterone on the methamphetamine-induced cognitive impairment in ovariectomized rats. Neurosci Lett. 2016;619:60–7.

316. Diagnostic and statistical manual of mental disorders. 5th ed. Arlington: American Psychiatric Association; 2013.

317. Alders EEA, Hentzen A, Tan CT. A community-based prevalence study on headache in Malaysia. Headache. 1996;36:379–84.

318. Wöber C, Wöber-Bingöl C. Triggers of migraine and tension-type headache. Handb Clin Neurol. 2010;97:161–72.

319. Andress-Rothrock D, King W, Rothrock J. An analysis of migraine triggers in a clinic-based population. Headache. 2010;50:1366–70. https://doi.org/10.1111/j.1526-4610.2010.01753.x.

320. Wöber C, Holzhammer J, Zeitlhofer J, Wessely P, Wöber-Bingöl C. Trigger factors of migraine and tension-type headache: experience and knowledge of the patients. J Headache Pain. 2006;7(4):188–95.

321. Carod-Artal FJ, Ezpeleta D, Martín-Barriga ML, Guerrero AL. Triggers, symptoms, and treatment in two populations of migraneurs in Brazil and Spain. a cross-cultural study. J Neurol Sci. 2011;304(1–2):25–8.

322. Finocchi C, Sivori G. Food as trigger and aggravating factor of migraine. Neurol Sci. 2012;33(Suppl 1):S77–80.

323. Holzhammer J, Wöber C. Non-alimentary trigger factors of migraine and tension-type headache. Schmerz. 2006;20(3):226–37.

324. Rasmussen BK. Migraine and tension-type headache in a general population: precipitating factors, female hormones, sleep pattern and relation to lifestyle. Pain. 1993;53(1):65–72.

325. Spierings EL, Ranke AH, Honkoop PC. Precipitating and aggravating factors of migraine versus tension-type headache. Headache. 2001;41(6):554–8.

326. Chabriat H, Danchot J, Michel P, Joire JE, Henry P. Precipitating factors of headache. A prospective study in a national control-matched survey in migraineurs and nonmigraineurs. Headache. 1999;39:335–8.

327. Turner L, Molgaard C, Gardner C, Rothrock J, Stang P. Migraine trigger factors in a non-clinical Mexican-American population in San Diego County: implications for etiology. Cephalalgia. 1995;15:523–30.
328. Zarifoglu M, Siva A, Hayran O. The Turkish Headache Epidemiology Study Group. An epidemiological study of headache in Turkey: a nationwide survey. Neurology. 1998;50(Suppl 4):80–5.
329. Schwaiger J, Kiechl S, Seppi K, Sawires M, Stockner H, Erlacher T, et al. Prevalence of primary headaches and cranial neuralgias in men and women aged 55–94 years (Bruneck Study). Cephalalgia. 2009;29:179–87.
330. Nappi RE, Terreno E, Tassorelli C, Sances G, Allena M, Guaschino E, Antonaci F, Albani F, Polatti F. Sexual function and distress in women treated for primary headaches in a tertiary university center. J Sex Med. 2012;9:761–9.
331. Sicuteri F, Del Bene E, Fonda C. Sex, migraine and serotonin interrelationships. Monogr Neural Sci. 1976;3:94–101.
332. Lifting the Burden in Collaboration with the European Headache Federation. Aids to management of common headache disorders in primary care. J Headache Pain. 2007;8(Suppl 1):S3.
333. Lifting the Burden. The Global Campaign against Headache. www.l-t-b.org.
334. Affaitati G, Martelletti P, Lopopolo M, et al. Use of nonsteroidal anti-inflammatory drugs for symptomatic treatment of episodic headache. Pain Pract. 2017;17:392–401.
335. Dowson A. The burden of headache: global and regional prevalence of headache and its impact. Int J Clin Pract Suppl. 2015;182:3–7.
336. Steiner TJ, Stovner LJ, Katsarava Z, Lainez JM, Lampl C, Lantéri-Minet M, et al. The impact of headache in Europe: principal results of the Eurolight project. J Headache Pain. 2014;15(1):31.
337. Palacios-Ceña M, Wang K, Castaldo M, et al. Variables associated with the use of prophylactic amitriptyline treatment in patients with tension-type headache. Clin J Pain. 2019;35:315–20.
338. Bendtsen L, Bigal ME, Cerbo R, et al. Guidelines for controlled trials of drugs in tension-type headache: second edition. Cephalalgia. 2010;30:1–16.
339. Cathcart S, Bhullar N, Immink M, Della Vedova C, Hayball J. Pain sensitivity mediates the relationship between stress and headache intensity in chronic tension-type headache. Pain Res Manag. 2012;17:377–80. https://doi.org/10.1111/j.1468-2982.2009.01917.x.
340. Sillanpaa M, Piekkala P, Kero P. Prevalence of headache at preschool age in an unselected child population. Cephalalgia. 1991;11(5):239–42.
341. Claar RL, Baber KF, Simons LE, et al. Pain coping profiles in adolescents with chronic pain. Pain. 2008;140:368–75.
342. Weiss AJ, et al. Overview of emergency department visits in the United States, 2011: statistical brief #174. Rockville, MD: Healthcare Cost and Utilization Project (HCUP) Statistical Briefs; 2006.
343. Levin M. Approach to the workup and management of headache in the emergency department and inpatient settings. Semin Neurol. 2015;35(6):667–74.
344. Penzien DB, Irby MB, Smitherman TA, Rains JC, Houle TT. Well-established and empirically supported behavioral treatments for migraine. Curr Pain Headache Rep. 2015;19(7):34.
345. Nicholson RA, Buse DC, Andrasik F, Lipton RB. Nonpharmacologic treatments for migraine and tension-type headache: how to choose and when to use. Curr Treat Options Neurol. 2011;13(1):28–40.
346. Haddock CK, Rowan AB, Andrasik F, Wilson PG, Talcott GW, Stein RJ. Home-based behavioral treatments for chronic benign headache: a meta-analysis of controlled trials. Cephalalgia. 1997;17(2):113–8.
347. Holroyd KA, O'Donnell FJ, Stensland M, Lipchik GL, Cordingley GE, Carlson BW. Management of chronic tension-type headache with tricyclic antidepressant medication, stress management therapy, and their combination: a randomized controlled trial. JAMA. 2001;285(17):2208–15.

348. Smitherman TA, Wells RE, Ford SG. Emerging behavioral treatments for migraine. Curr Pain Headache Rep. 2015;19(4):13.
349. Petter M, McGrath PJ, Chambers CT, Dick BD. The effects of mindful attention and state mindfulness on acute experimental pain among adolescents. J Pediatr Psychol. 2014;39(5):521–31.
350. Garland EL, Baker AK, Larsen P, Riquino MR, Priddy SE, Thomas E, et al. Randomized controlled trial of brief mindfulness training and hypnotic suggestion for acute pain relief in the hospital setting. J Gen Intern Med. 2017;32(10):1106–13. A recent RCT of 2 brief psychological interventions delivered by social workers for acute pain relief in hospitalized patients, showing benefit in both interventions compared to an active control condition.
351. Ernst MM, O'Brien HL, Powers SW. Cognitive-behavioral therapy: how medical providers can increase patient and family openness and access to evidence-based multimodal therapy for pediatric migraine. Headache. 2015;55(10):1382–96.
352. Lenssinck MLB, Damen L, Verhagen AP, Berger MY, Passchier J, Koes BW. The effectiveness of physiotherapy and manipulation in patients with tension-type headache: a systematic review. Pain. 2004;112:381–8.
353. Chaibi A, Russell MB. Manual therapies for primary chronic headaches: a systematic review of randomized controlled trials. J Headache Pain. 2014;15(1):67.
354. Posadzki P, Ernst E. Spinal manipulations for cervicogenic headaches: a systematic review of randomized clinical trials. Headache. 2011;51:1132–9.
355. Chaibi A, Russell MB. Manual therapies for cervicogenic headache: a systematic review. J Headache Pain. 2012;13:351–9.
356. Falsiroli Maistrello L, Geri T, Gianola S, Zaninetti M, Testa M. Effectiveness of trigger point manual treatment on the frequency, intensity, and duration of attacks in primary headaches: a systematic review and meta-analysis of randomized controlled trials. Front Neurol. 2018;9:254.
357. Luedtke K, Allers A, Schulte LH, et al. Efficacy of interventions used by physiotherapists for patients with headache and migraine—systematic review and meta-analysis. Cephalalgia. 2015;0:1–19.
358. Abu Bakar N, Tanprawate S, Lambru G, Torkamani M, Jahanshahi M, Matharu M. Quality of life in primary headache disorders: a review. Cephalalgia. 2016;36(1):67–91.
359. Andrasik F, Lipchik GL, McCrory DC, et al. Outcome measurement in behavioral headache research: headache parameters and psychosocial outcomes. Headache. 2005;45:429–37.
360. Berggreen S, Wiik E, Lund H. Treatment of myofascial trigger points in female patients with chronic tension-type headache—a randomized controlled trial. Adv Physiother. 2012;14:10–7.
361. Castien RF, van der Windt DAWMWM, Grooten A, et al. Effectiveness of manual therapy for chronic tension-type headache: a pragmatic, randomised, clinical trial. Cephalalgia. 2011;31:133–43.
362. Voigt K, Liebnitzky J, Burmeister U, Sihvonen-Riemenschneider H, Beck M, Voigt R, et al. Efficacy of osteopathic manipulative treatment of female patients with migraine: results of a randomized controlled trial. J Altern Complement Med. 2011;17:225–30.
363. Higgins JP, Green S. In: Higgins JP, Green S, The Cochrane Collaboration, editors. Cochrane handbook for systematic reviews of interventions. Version 5.1.0. Wiley; 2011.
364. Ferragut-Garcías A, Plaza-Manzano G, Rodríguez-Blanco C, et al. Effectiveness of a treatment involving soft tissue techniques and/or neural mobilization techniques in the management of the tension-type headache: a randomized controlled trial. Arch Phys Med Rehabil. 2016;98:211–219.e2. A very well conducted RCT that used quality of life as primary outcome.
365. Espí-López GV, Rodríguez-Blanco C, Oliva-Pascual-Vaca A, Benítez-Martínez JC, Lluch E, Falla D. Effect of manual therapy techniques on headache disability in patients with tension-type headache. Randomized controlled trial. Eur J Phys Rehabil Med. 2014;50(6):641–7.

366. Cerritelli F, Ginevri L, Messi G, Caprari E, di Vincenzo M, Renzetti C, et al. Clinical effectiveness of osteopathic treatment in chronic migraine: 3-armed randomized controlled trial. Complement Ther Med. 2015;23:149–56.
367. Espí-López GV, Gómez-Conesa A, Gómez AA, Martínez JB, Pascual-Vaca ÁO, Blanco CR. Treatment of tension-type headache with articulatory and suboccipital soft tissue therapy: a double-blind, randomized, placebo-controlled clinical trial. J Bodyw Mov Ther. 2014;18:576–85.
368. Espí-López GV, Rodriguez-Blanco C, Oliva-Pascual-Vaca A, et al. Effect of manual therapy techniques on headache disability in patients with tension-type headache. Randomized controlled trial. Eur J Phys Rehabil Med. 2014;50:641–7.
369. Smelt AFH, Assendelft WJJ, Terwee CB, Ferrari MD, Blom JW. What is a clinically relevant change on the HIT-6 questionnaire? An estimation in a primary-care population of migraine patients. Cephalalgia. 2014;34:29–36.
370. Castien RF, Blankenstein AH, van der Windt DA, et al. Minimal clinically important change on the Headache Impact Test-6 questionnaire in patients with chronic tension-type headache. Cephalalgia. 2012;32:710–4.
371. Coeytaux RR, Kaufman JS, Chao R, Mann JD, DeVellis RF. Four methods of estimating the minimal important difference score were compared to establish a clinically significant change in Headache Impact Test. J Clin Epidemiol. 2006;59:374–80.
372. Lozano López C, Mesa Jiménez J, de la Hoz Aizpurúa JL, et al. Efficacy of manual therapy in the treatment of tension-type headache. A systematic review from 2000-2013. Neurologia. 2016;31(6):357–69.
373. Uthaikhup S, Assapun J, Watcharasaksilp K, Jull G. Effectiveness of physiotherapy for seniors with recurrent headaches associated with neck pain and dysfunction: a randomized controlled trial. Spine J. 2017;17:46–55.
374. World Health Organization. Global recommendations on physical activity for health. Geneva: WHO; 2010.
375. Anheyer D, Leach MJ, Klose P, Dobos G, Cramer H. Mindfulness-based stress reduction for treating chronic headache: a systematic review and meta-analysis. Cephalalgia. 2019; https://doi.org/10.1177/0333102418781795.
376. Gu Q, Hou JC, Fang XM. Mindfulness meditation for primary headache pain: a meta-analysis. Chin Med J (Engl). 2018;131(7):829–38.
377. Harris P, Loveman E, Clegg A, Easton S, Berry N. Systematic review of cognitive behavioural therapy for the management of headaches and migraines in adults. Br J Pain. 2015;9(4):213–24. https://doi.org/10.1177/2049463715578291.
378. Lee HJ, Lee JH, Cho EY, Kim SM, Yoon S. Efficacy of psychological treatment for headache disorder: a systematic review and meta-analysis. J Headache Pain. 2019;20(1):17. https://doi.org/10.1186/s10194-019-0965-4.
379. Sjaastad O, Fredriksen TA, Pfaffenrath V. Cervicogenic headache: diagnostic criteria. The Cervicogenic Headache International Study Group. Headache. 1998;38(6):442–5. https://doi.org/10.1046/j.1526-4610.1998.3806442.x.
380. Centre NCG. Headaches: diagnosis and management of headaches in young people and adults: Commissioned by the National Institute for Health and Clinical Excellence. London: National Clinical Guideline Centre (UK); 2012.
381. Wackenfors A, Jarvius M, Ingemansson R, Edvinsson L, Malmsjo M. Triptans induce vasoconstriction of human arteries and veins from the thoracic wall. J Cardiovasc Pharmacol. 2005;45:476–84.
382. Botox for migraine. American Migraine Foundation. https://americanmigrainefoundation.org/understanding-migraine/botox-for-migraine/.
383. Diener HC, Dodick DW, Aurora SK, Turkel CC, DeGryse RE, Lipton RB, et al. OnabotulinumtoxinA for treatment of chronic migraine: results from the double-blind, randomized, placebo-controlled phase of the PREEMPT 2 trial. Cephalalgia. 2010;30(7):804–14.

384. Ching LM. Research into osteopathic manipulative medicine: steps on the evidence pyramid. J Am Osteopath Assoc. 2016;116(3):133–4. https://doi.org/10.7556/jaoa.2016.029. Evidence of a lymphatic system in the brain.
385. Lee-Wong M, Karagic M, Doshi A, Gomez S, Resnick D. An osteopathic approach to chronic sinusitis. J Aller Ther. 2011;2(2):109. https://doi.org/10.4172/2155-6121.1000109. Evidence of OMT relieving sinus headache symptoms.
386. Meyer PM, Gustowski SM. Osteopathic manipulative treatment to resolve head and neck pain after tooth extraction. J Am Osteopath Assoc. 2012;112(7):457–60.
387. Franke H, et al. Osteopathic manipulative treatment for chronic nonspecific neck pain: a systematic review and meta-analysis. Int J Osteopath Med. 2015;18(4):255–67. Evidence of OMT relieving headache symptoms related to a tooth extraction.
388. Watson DH, Drummond PD. Head pain referral during examination of the neck in migraine and tension-type headache. Headache. 2012;52:1226–35.
389. Watson DH, Drummond PD. Cervical referral of head pain in migraineurs: effects on the nociceptive blink reflex. Headache. 2014;54:1035–45.
390. Satpute K, Bedekar N, Hall T. Headache symptom modification: the relevance of appropriate manual therapy assessment and management of a patient with features of migraine and cervicogenic headache—a case report. J Man Manip Ther. 2020;28:181–8.
391. Kjaergaard M. Vitamin D, depression and headache—results from the Tromso study and from an intervention study with vitamin D. Dissertation for the Degree of Philosophiae Doctor, Faculty of Health Sciences, Department of Clinical Medicine, 2012.
392. Ahmad M, Qaisy M. Assessing stress among university students. Am Int J Contemp Res. 2012;2:110.
393. Söderberg E. Chronic tension-type headache treatment with acupuncture, physical training and relaxation training. Göteborg: Institute of Neuroscience and Physiology. Sahlgrenska Academy at University of Gothenburg; 2012.
394. Milde A, Blaschek A, Heinen F, Borggrafe I, Koerte I, Straube A, et al. Associations between stress and migraine and tension-type headache: results from a school-based study in adolescents from grammar schools in Germany. Cephalalgia. 2011;31:774–85.
395. Senthil C, Gunasekaran N. Clinical profile of patients with chronic headache in a tertiary care hospital. Int J Adv Med. 2016;3(3):721–6.
396. Steiner TJ, Jensen R, Katsarava Z, et al. Aids to management of headache disorders in primary care (2nd edition). J Headache Pain. 2019;20:57.
397. Vidor LP, Torres IL, Custódio de Souza IC, Fregni F, Caumo W. Analgesic and sedative effects of melatonin in temporomandibular disorders: a double-blind, randomized, parallel-group, placebo-controlled study. J Pain Symptom Manag. 2013;46(3):422–32.
398. Stefani LC, Muller S, Torres IL, et al. A phase II, randomized, double-blind, placebo controlled, dose-response trial of the melatonin effect on pain threshold of healthy subjects. PLoS One. 2013;8(10):e74107.
399. Mistraletti G, Umbrello M, Sabbatini G, et al. Melatonin reduces the need for sedation in ICU patients: a randomized controlled trial. Minerva Anestesiol. 2015;81(12):1298–310.
400. Hussain SA, Al-Khalifa II, Jasim NA, Gorial FI. Adjuvant use of melatonin for treatment of fibromyalgia. J Pineal Res. 2011;50(3):267–71.
401. Wilhelmsen M, Amirian I, Reiter RJ, Rosenberg J, Gögenur I. Analgesic effects of melatonin: a review of current evidence from experimental and clinical studies. J Pineal Res. 2011;51(3):270–7.
402. Long R, Zhu Y, Zhou S. Therapeutic role of melatonin in migraine prophylaxis: a systematic review. Medicine (Baltimore). 2019;98(3):e14099.

# Chapter 2
# Trigeminal Autonomic Cephalalgias

## 2.1 Introduction

Trigeminal autonomic cephalalgias are a group of headache disorders not epidemiologically relevant but extremely demanding for their clinical expression. They include cluster headache, paroxysmal hemicrania, hemicrania continua, SUNCT and SUNA and have been studied a lot over the decades and only recently they have found an application of innovative drugs for prevention. As for the acute treatment, we are still on drugs from a few decades ago. The importance of these forms of headache is given precisely by their relative rarity, as the clinician is often challenged by diagnoses that are not complex, but an adequate background often leads diagnostic delays and errors. This chapter allows immediate access to relevant and referenced literature for clinical aspects and pathophysiology, and above all for an adequate and immediate management of these extremely painful and overwhelming forms of headache. Furthermore, a series of experimental approaches to the trigeminal autonomic cephalalgias are present and must be left at the disposal of researchers.

## 2.2 Machine-Generated Summaries

Machine generated keywords: cluster, cch, cluster headache, hemicrania, cgrp, gene, ech, indomethacin, tac, migraine cluster, score, attack, stimulation, network, hypothalamus

© The Author(s), under exclusive license to Springer Nature Switzerland AG 2023
P. Martelletti (ed.), *Non-Migraine Primary Headaches in Medicine*,
https://doi.org/10.1007/978-3-031-20894-2_2

## Cluster Headache

Machine generated keywords: cluster, cch, cluster headache, gene, ech, cgrp, migraine cluster, score, attack, stimulation, network, control, receptor, hypothalamus, risk

### Public Health

Machine generated keywords: burden, cch, cost, leave, ech, control, work, impact, disease, productivity, questionnaire, period, family, compare control, remission

## Chronic Cluster Headache Update and East–West Comparisons: Focusing on Clinical Features, Pathophysiology, and Management

DOI: https://doi.org/10.1007/s11916-020-00902-7

### Abstract-Summary

This review provides an update on chronic cluster headache (CH) focusing on clinical features, pathophysiology, and management as well as comparisons between Eastern and Western populations.

Chronic CH in Eastern populations was relatively rare, compared to that in Western populations.

Advances have emerged in neuromodulatory therapies for chronic CH, but treatment with calcitonin gene-related peptide (CGRP) monoclonal antibodies has been unsuccessful.

Recent evidence shows divergence of chronic CH between Eastern and Western populations.

Extended:

This review provides an update of CH, focusing on chronic CH, and it compares the similarities and differences of how Eastern and Western populations experience chronic CH in terms of epidemiology, pathophysiology, and management.

### Introduction

Cluster headache (CH) is considered the most severe primary headache disorder, characterized by attacks of excruciating unilateral headache or facial pain lasting 15–180 min and is the most common form of trigeminal autonomic cephalalgias [1].

CH also exhibits circadian and circannual rhythmicity, with attacks often occurring at the same time(s) each day during sustained episodes lasting weeks or months (in-bout period), separated by periods of remission (out-of-bout period) [2].

10–15% of CH patients have the chronic form, in which remission periods are either absent or last <3 months within 1 year [1, 3].

Current neuroimaging studies support that the hypothalamus, as well as pain-modulating circuitry, is involved in CH pathophysiology with dynamic alterations during in- and out-of-bout periods.

## Clinical Similarities and Differences in Chronic CH Between Eastern and Western Countries

In Western countries, the reported prevalence of CH ranges from 0.1 to 0.4%, with chronic CH accounting for 15.2–25.9% of cases [4–7].

In Western studies, nocturnal CH attacks were common (58–73%) and most often occurred in spring and autumn [8–11].

In Asian studies, lacrimation was the most common cranial autonomic symptom accompanying CH, followed by conjunctival injection and rhinorrhea [12–16].

In Asian patients, few data could be found concerning chronic CH, but in Western patients, lacrimation and/or conjunctival injection were the most concurrent symptoms.

Auras more commonly occur in Western patients (14–23%), and visual auras was the most common type reported in those experiencing chronic or episodic CH [6, 9, 10, 17].

In Western studies, the prevalence of depression in episodic CH patients ranged from 6.3 to 24% and occurred with greater prevalence in chronic CH patients [10, 18, 19].

## Pathophysiological Similarities and Differences in Chronic CH Between Eastern and Western Countries

Recent studies conducted both in Western and Eastern (Taiwan) countries showed common changes in GMV nonspecifically involved in pain-processing areas such as the frontal, cingulate and insular cortex, temporal lobe, hippocampus, and cerebellum in CH [20–22].

Other VBM studies on CH in both Western and Eastern countries suggest potential alternations in pain-processing regions.

A Taiwanese study recognized that CH pathophysiology and dynamic changes between bouts involved not only the hypothalamus but also pain-related circuits.

A subsequent UK study enrolled nine chronic CH patients and revealed exclusive gray matter activation during nitroglycerin-induced CH attacks within the ipsilateral inferior hypothalamus as well as increased regional CBF in the contralateral ventroposterior thalamus, anterior cingulate cortex, and bilateral insula [23].

The first fMRI study on CH demonstrated that activation of the hypothalamus and other pain-processing regions occurred during headache attacks on the side ipsilateral to the pain [24].

## Similarities and Differences in Management of Chronic CH Between Eastern and Western Countries

A recent Italian study disclosed absence of electrocardiogram abnormalities or serious adverse effects in 53 chronic CH patients receiving more than twice daily administrations of sumatriptan for 2 years [25].

A double-blind crossover RCT enrolled 30 Italian chronic CH patients and compared the prophylactic effects of verapamil to lithium.

The most recent British open-labeled verapamil trial disclosed headache alleviation in 10 (55%) of 18 chronic CH patients [26].

A retrospective study included eight chronic CH patients and showed a beneficial effect in the first 2 weeks after lithium treatment.

A recent prospective open-label trial in Taiwan reported one chronic CH patient who did not achieve remission until the daily dose was increased to 400 mg and experienced a recurrence of symptoms within a few days of drug discontinuation [27].

## Conclusions

CH patients (and those with chronic CH) from Eastern and Western populations share similarities and differences.

The prevalence of chronic CH is higher in Western populations.

Recent evidence indicates that midbrain dopaminergic systems may be involved in the chronicization process of CH.

Clinical trials of CGRP monoclonal antibodies failed to alleviate symptoms in chronic CH patients despite previous studies suggesting CGRP involvement in CH pathophysiology.

## Acknowledgement

*A machine generated summary based on the work of Tsai, Chia-Lin; Lin, Guan-Yu; Wu, Sheng-Kai; Yang, Fu-Chi; Wang, Shuu-Jiun. 2020 in Current Pain and Headache Reports.*

# *Cluster Headache Is Still Lurking in the Shadows*

DOI: https://doi.org/10.1007/s40122-021-00278-5

## Abstract-Summary

Cluster headache, apart from its legendary reputation as the most violent headache that can exist, suffers from an average 60-month delay in diagnosis.

The simplicity of the clinical manifestations, although dramatic, makes this delay inexplicable.

The education of emergency department physicians and various specialists not specifically dedicated to headaches allows cluster headache to remain in a lurking position with flourishing periods of disease that are often unpredictable in both onset and disappearance.

**Digital Features**

This article is published with digital features, including a summary slide, to facilitate understanding of the article.

To view digital features for this article go to https://doi.org/10.6084/m9.figshare.14687217.

**Cluster Headache, the Cinderella Among the Primary Headaches**

Further multiple basic and clinical research approaches have added important information on the role of neurosteroids, neuroimaging and neurophysiology data, sleep disorders, and psychiatric comorbidities in this still not completely clear pathophysiological picture of CH [28–31].

One of the well-known criticalities in the treatment of CH is the aged drugs used for the control of the brutal attacks and for the suppression of the active and thriving phases of the disease or its prevention [32, 33].

Beyond this criticality, it has recently been highlighted that the transition from randomized control trials (RCTs), which offer a mathematical view of drugs applied to a specific pathology, should be weighed against the flexibility of clinical practice as observed by real-world evidence (RWE) data [34].

The paucity of therapeutic approaches towards CH has over time stimulated researchers to reapply innovative therapies already used in migraine, such as neurostimulation and botulinum toxin with RWE, unfortunately far from the original results of the RCTs [35, 36].

**Old and Novel Treatments for CH**

The problems for CH do not end here because only part of these suffering patients can take advantage of a new therapy that has been extended from migraine also to CH in the USA and immediately abates the crises.

On February 28, 2020, the European Medicines Agency (EMA) rejected the approval of galcanezumab (100 mg × 3/monthly subcutaneously) for the prevention of episodic and chronic cluster headache, a highly effective therapy currently available in USA after the Food Drug and Administration approval [37–40].

Just to give an example, among the currently available preventative therapies, verapamil at high dosage (360 mg and more up to 720 mg/day) offers good efficacy [41].

Recent valuable estimates of the direct and indirect costs of episodic and chronic CH in the specific setting of a tertiary headache center confirmed the high economic impact of CH on both the National Health System and patients [42].

**Acknowledgement**

*A machine generated summary based on the work of Martelletti, Paolo; Curto, Martina. 2021 in Pain and Therapy.*

# *Prevalence of Familial Cluster Headache: A Systematic Review and Meta-analysis*

DOI: https://doi.org/10.1186/s10194-020-01101-w

## Abstract-Summary

The population rate of familial cluster headache (CH) has been reported to be as high as 20% however this varies considerably across studies.

To obtain a true estimate of family history in CH, we conducted a systematic review and meta-analysis of previously published data.

To further ameliorate the accuracy of our analysis we included an additional unpublished cohort of CH patients recruited at a tertiary referral centre for headache, who underwent detailed family history with diagnostic verification in relatives.

Data was extracted and meta-analysis conducted to provide a true estimation of family history.

The estimated true prevalence of CH patients with a positive family history was 6.27% (95% CI: 4.65–8.40%) with an overall $I^2$ of 73%.

Fitted models for gender subgroups showed higher estimates 9.26% (95% CI: 6.29–13.43%) in females.

Our findings estimate a rate of family history in CH to be approximately 6.27% (95% CI: 4.65–8.40%).

## Background

Those with a family history of CH appear to have an increased risk of developing the condition [43–46].

Estimations of the presence of a positive family history amongst sufferers varies across studies.

Inter-familial clinical variability has also been observed, with an earlier age of onset reported in the offspring of parents with CH, inferring the possibility of anticipation [47].

The purpose of this study was to perform a systematic appraisal and meta-analysis of all studies in addition to presenting original data reporting a prevalence of familial CH.

## Methods

All studies reporting the prevalence of familial CH within a defined cohort of CH patients were included in the analysis.

To avoid an over representation of familial history, only studies that confirmed a diagnosis of CH in an affected relative were included in the systematic review.

In cases where relatives were uncontactable or deceased, only those with a diagnosis of CH confirmed by a neurologist were deemed eligible. A total of 645 patients were included in the study.

Due to high inter-study variation and high $I^2$, a random-effects model was fitted for estimation of family history in CH.

We performed a gender-segregated analysis that included all studies from our initial analysis which also reported the prevalence for males and females separately.

We represented each study with a male and female estimate of family history prevalence.

## Results

The remaining full texts consisted of 7 cohort studies with an estimated prevalence of family history of CH ranging from 4.9% to 26.3%.

In order to estimate the true prevalence of family history in patients with CH, we selected studies that had quantified the number of first and/or second degree relatives suffering from CH and had also confirmed these clinical diagnoses.

Despite the overall prevalence of CH being higher in males, a number of the identified studies reported an increased prevalence of family history of CH in females compared to males.

We therefore conducted a separate analysis including only those studies which reported family history in males and females separately.

This may potentially explain the heterogeneity seen in the female-only estimates as overall there were fewer females across studies The year of publication did not significantly influence the estimates (p = 0.2186).

## Discussion

A number of studies have attempted to report the prevalence of family history in CH patients.

Several epidemiology studies have reported higher prevalence of familial CH, possibly reflecting inflated estimations [10, 48, 49].

Clinical verification of a presumed diagnosis of CH in a relative should be a critical requirement in any study reporting family history.

The high degree of variance in the reported estimates was illuminated further by a gender segregated analysis, which revealed that although the prevalence of family history was higher in females than in male probands, this difference was not significantly different.

An explanation for this seemingly increased prevalence of family history in females is that CH is more common in males, therefore published studies tend to have larger numbers of male probands.

## Conclusion

In this systematic review and meta-analysis, we predict the prevalence of family history in CH to be approximately 6.27%.

These results provide a robust estimation of the prevalence of familial CH and support the hypothesis of a potential genetic risk factors predisposing to the condition.

## Acknowledgement

*A machine generated summary based on the work of O'Connor, Emer; Simpson, Benjamin S.; Houlden, Henry; Vandrovcova, Jana; Matharu, Manjit. 2020 in The Journal of Headache and Pain.*

# Cluster Headache: Clinical Characteristics and Opportunities to Enhance Quality of Life

DOI: https://doi.org/10.1007/s11916-021-00979-8

## Abstract-Summary

People with cluster headache often endorse depressive symptoms, are more likely than the general population to report suicidal ideation and behaviors, and experience significantly decreased quality of life.

Psychological treatments such as Acceptance and Commitment Therapy may be particularly valuable for patients with cluster headache given that they are transdiagnostic in nature and can therefore simultaneously address the disease burden and common psychiatric comorbidities that present.

Greater understanding of the debilitating nature of cluster headache and behavioral interventions that seek to reduce the burden of the disease and improve the quality of life of people with cluster headache is paramount.

## Introduction

Cluster headache is characterized by attacks of severe, unilateral, periorbital pain that last between 15 and 180 min, and occur up to eight times per day [1].

Cluster headache attacks also involve ipsilateral autonomic symptoms including nasal congestion, miosis, and eyelid edema and are accompanied by a sense of restlessness or agitation [1].

As attacks occur most often at night, many people with cluster headache endorse anticipatory anxiety related to going to bed due to fear of triggering a cluster attack [50].

Even with the best currently available treatment, people with cluster headache experience significant burden.

Psychological treatments, including behavioral interventions, hold a promise to improve the quality of life of people with cluster headache through increasing knowledge about the disease, maximizing adherence to effective medical treatment options, and decreasing functional impairments related to cluster headache.

## Cluster Headache and Psychological Factors

Depressive symptoms, burden of current pain, and fear of future painful attacks are all potential treatment targets for psychological interventions for cluster headache.

It is concerning that the rates of suicidal ideation and behaviors continue to be high in people with cluster headache; there is a necessity for adequate management of cluster headache symptoms both in the ictal and interictal periods.

The high rates of suicidal ideation and behaviors reveal an urgent need to develop strategies to mitigate the burden of cluster headache on patients' lives.

Given the substantial impact cluster can have on quality of life, depression, and even suicidal behavior, it is surprising so little research has examined psychological and behavioral treatments to improve the lives of people with cluster headache.

Given the observed associations between cluster headache, psychiatric comorbidities, suicidality, and quality of life impairments, there is a substantial need to develop treatments that have long-lasting effects to reduce the burden of this disease.

## Conclusions

Given high comorbidity of affective disease, poor quality of life, and high suicidality in these patients, there are many behavioral and psychological factors to consider, but there are no current recommendations for psychological interventions in treating people with cluster headache.

Third-wave behavioral interventions such as Acceptance and Commitment Therapy may show promise for improving the quality of life of people living with cluster headache.

Greater understanding of the debilitating nature of cluster headache [51] and behavioral treatments that provide opportunities and seek to reduce the burden of the disease and improve the quality of life of people with cluster headache is paramount.

## Acknowledgement

*A machine generated summary based on the work of Grinberg, Amy S.; Best, Rachel D.; Min, Kathryn M.; Schindler, Emmanuelle A. D.; Koo, Brian B.; Sico, Jason J.; Seng, Elizabeth K. 2021 in Current Pain and Headache Reports.*

# *Cluster Headache in Relation to Different Age Groups*

DOI: https://doi.org/10.1007/s10072-019-03767-w

## Abstract-Summary

Recent studies carried out in large case series of patients with CH show that not infrequently it may set in also after age 50; by contrast, onset before adolescence is very rare.

When onset occurs before age 14 or from the sixth decade of life onward, male predominance decreases to the point that in chronic forms CH predominantly affects the female sex.

This particular pattern of the gender ratio in relation to onset in different age groups suggests that hormonal factors may actually play a role in the genesis of CH.

## Introduction

Epidemiologically, cluster headache (CH) is generally considered a disorder characterized by low prevalence in the general population, male predominance, and onset in early and medium adulthood [52–54].

While literature reports historically indicated a prevalence rate of 1‰ in the general population [52, 54], more recent data confirm that CH is a rather rare type of primary headache but demonstrate that it occurs more frequently, at a rate of about 3‰ [4, 55].

This trend is the result of an actual increase in the disorder rate among women, even though we cannot exclude that it might be due to improved knowledge of CH by the medical community.

## Age at Onset: Classical Literature Data

Mean age at onset of CH, as long since reported by several authors, is about 29–30 years [52–54, 56–58].

While it is believed that patients may continue to suffer from CH also in older age, possibly presenting an episodic form that has evolved into chronic or vice versa [59], there is a great lack of data on CH onset in the elderly.

In the literature, there is a lack of data on the possible onset of CH in the different stages of the first and especially of the second decade of life.

This enabled us to identify more accurately different features that characterize age at CH onset.

## Age at Onset: Recent Data

When we applied the diagnostic criteria of the latest international classifications of headache disorders [1, 60], we found that 686 (503 men and 183 women) had an episodic form of CH (ECH), 103 (66 men and 37 women) a chronic form (CCH), and 19 (16 men and three women) a form with an undefined temporal pattern, because its recent onset did not make it possible to attribute it to either form.

Mean age at onset was 30.2 years (30.1 in men and 30.4 in women).

Patients with ECH had a mean age at onset of 29.7 years (29.5 in men and 29.0 in women), while those with CCH had a mean age at onset of 33.9 years (32.0 in men and 37.2 in women).

Women with primary CCH, i.e., chronic ab initio, had a mean age at onset of 42.8 years, while those with secondary CCH, i.e., chronic evolved from episodic, did not differ from those with ECH.

## Late-Onset CH

A recent study carried out at the University of Parma Headache Centre [61] showed 73 patients (43 men and 30 women) with CH onset after age 50, including 56 with an episodic form and 17 with a chronic form.

Over 20% of patients with CH onset after age 50 had a chronic form.

In accordance with Ekbom and others [53], we observed that late onset of CH occurs more frequently in women with chronic forms.

If we consider that our female patients suffering from episodic forms with onset after age 50 had significantly longer cluster periods than those with onset at a younger age, we can conclude that late onset of CH in women is a negative prognostic factor.

## Pediatric-Onset CH

Compared with cases with adult onset (AO), PO cases reported a significantly greater family history of CH in females and of non-CH headache in males.

In PO males, CH by adulthood was characterized by clinical features that were significantly different from those of AO cases: increased frequency and duration of attacks and greater presence of symptoms accompanying pain, such as conjunctival injection and forehead and facial flushing, and of migraine-like features and nausea.

In three of the seven cases in which it was easier to trace back the clinical features of CH at onset because they were first observed before age 18, the duration of attacks was at the lower limit (15–30 min) of the range set by the international classifications [1, 60], and in five of them, cluster periods consisted of mini-bouts (3–7 days).

**Conclusions**
Both in early and late-onset cases, we did not observe the male predominance typically associated with this type of primary headache; by contrast, we even saw an increased frequency of CH among female patients when we considered only CCH cases.

The investigators' attention focused on testosterone levels.

The current findings of increased CH frequency in females with onset before age 14, its increased frequency in males with onset between age 14 and age 50, and, again, its increase frequency in females with onset after age 50, corroborate the idea that hormonal factors may be involved in this type of headache.

It would be interesting to investigate a possible protective role played by estrogen.

**Acknowledgement**
*A machine generated summary based on the work of Manzoni, Gian Camillo; Camarda, Cecilia; Genovese, Antonio; Quintana, Simone; Rausa, Francesco; Taga, Arens; Torelli, Paola. 2019 in Neurological Sciences.*

# *Cluster Headache Impact Questionnaire (CHIQ)—A Short Measure of Cluster Headache Related Disability*

DOI: https://doi.org/10.1186/s10194-022-01406-y

**Abstract-Summary**
There is little research on CH-related disability, and most of it is based on non CH-specific questionnaires.

The aim of this study was to develop a short, CH-specific disability questionnaire.

The questionnaire was tested in 254 CH patients (171 males; $47.5 \pm 11.4$ years; 111 chronic CH, 85 active episodic CH, 52 episodic CH in remission) from our tertiary headache center or from a German support group.

Reliability and validity of the CHIQ was evaluated in active episodic and chronic CH patients (n = 196).

CHIQ scores significantly differentiated between chronic CH ($25.8 \pm 6.5$), active episodic CH ($23.3 \pm 6.9$) and episodic CH patients in remission ($13.6 \pm 11.9$, $p < 0.05$ for all 3 comparisons).

                                                          

The CHIQ is a short, reliable, valid, and easy to administer measure of CH-related disability, which makes it a useful tool for clinical use and research.

## Background

Due to the lack of CH-specific questionnaires, generic or migraine-specific questionnaires like the Headache Impact Test™ (HIT-6™), Migraine Disability Assessment (MIDAS), SF-12v2® Health Survey (SF-12v2®) or Migraine Specific Quality of Life Questionnaire Version 2.1 (MSQ v2.1) have mostly been used [62].

One disadvantage of generic questionnaires is that they don't evaluate CH-specific characteristics like frequent daily or nocturnal attacks or agitation.

Two CH-specific questionnaires concerning quality of life (QoL) and psychosocial factors have been developed and validated, the 28-item Cluster Headache Quality of Life Scale (CHQ) and the 36-item Cluster Headache Scales (CHS), with the latter including an 11-item disability subscale [63, 64].

The objective of this study was to develop a short questionnaire to specifically assess the current impact of CH on daily life and to demonstrate reliability and validity of this instrument.

## Methods

The survey comprised five questionnaires: the CHIQ, a customized questionnaire assessing demographics, medical history and clinical characteristics of CH (including headache characteristics, attack abortive and prophylactic treatment), the HIT-6, the DASS and the SF-12v2.

The follow-up survey comprised the CHIQ, a short customized questionnaire assessing the current status of CH and treatment, HIT-6, DASS and SF12v2.

This short-term follow-up was aimed to address stability of the items and the questionnaire, therefore only participants with active CH at both surveys and a stable attack frequency (a change $\leq 2$ attacks per week from first to follow-up survey) were included in the analysis of test-retest reliability (n = 41).

Convergent validity between the CHIQ, CH characteristics and the results of other questionnaires were assessed using Spearman correlations, and the same correlations were later also calculated with the HIT-6 score.

## Results

Average CHIQ values of the test (24.56 ± 6.5) and retest (23.71 ± 7.61) were not significantly different (Z = −1.56, p = 0.12).

Similar to the CHIQ, Kruskal-Wallis ANOVA detected significant group differences for the HIT-6 scores (cCH: 63.78 ± 6.83, n = 106, active eCH: 62.28 ± 5.72, n = 79, eCH in remission: 52.67 ± 6.44, n = 49, H [65] = 70.8, p < 0.001) and posthoc tests with Bonferroni correction revealed significant differences between eCH in remission and both, cCH and active eCH (both p < 0.001).

Different from CHIQ scores, HIT-6 scores were not significantly different between active eCH and cCH (p = 0.192).

## Discussion

The CHIQ was also positively correlated with the DASS depression, anxiety and stress scores and negatively correlated with the SF12v2 PCS and MCS, showing the expected relations to psychosocial factors and QoL. Previous studies have used non-CH-specific questionnaires like HIT-6, MIDAS, HDI or MSQ 2.1 to measure disability in CH patients [62, 66].

The CHIQ correlates with CH attack and medication intake frequency, and is rated by patients as appropriate to capture disability related to CH.

Compared to the HIT-6, the CHIQ received better suitability ratings from participants, showed larger correlations with clinical CH characteristics (attack and acute medication frequency and CH pain AUC) and detected a difference between cCH and active eCH patients that was not detected by the HIT-6.

### Conclusions

The CHIQ has a couple of advantages making it a convenient measure of CH-related disability in both clinical routine and research.

The one week timeframe reduces recall bias and helps assessing the current impact of CH in patients with often rapidly changing attack frequencies.

The CHIQ includes CH-specific items and is validated for the use in CH patients.

In clinical routine, patients may be asked to fill the questionnaire immediately before their appointment, giving the physician individual information about current burden and therapeutic needs.

### Acknowledgement

*A machine generated summary based on the work of Kamm, Katharina; Straube, Andreas; Ruscheweyh, Ruth. 2022 in The Journal of Headache and Pain.*

## *The Economic and Personal Burden of Cluster Headache: A Controlled Cross-sectional Study*

DOI: https://doi.org/10.1186/s10194-022-01427-7

### Abstract-Summary

We investigated both the personal and societal disease burden and cost in 400 patients with well-classified cluster headache according to the ICHD-criteria and 200 sex- and age matched controls.

Patients with chronic cluster headache constituted 146 out of 400 (37%).

Even in remission, nine times as many episodic patients rated their health as poor/very poor compared to controls (9% vs 1%, p = 0.002).

For chronic patients, the odds of rating health as good/very good were ten times lower compared to controls (OR: 10.10, 95% CI :5.29–18.79.

p < 0.001) and three times lower compared to episodic patients in remission (OR: 3.22, 95% CI: 1.90–5.47, p < 0.001).

Chronic cluster headache patients were 5 times more likely to receive disability pension compared to episodic (OR: 5.0, 95% CI: 2.3–10.9, p < 0.001).

The mean direct annual costs amounted to 9158€ and 2763€ for chronic and episodic patients, respectively (p < 0.001).

We identified a substantial loss of productivity due to absence from work resulting in a higher indirect cost of 11,809 €/year/patient in the chronic population and 3558 €/year/patient in the episodic population.

Presenteeism could not be quantified but productivity was reduced in patients by 65% in periods with attacks compared to controls.

Cluster headache has a major negative impact on personal life, self-perceived health, and societal cost.

## Background

This raises the question whether CH patients in remission can be regarded as "healthy" or as sufferers from a chronic disease with some symptoms manifesting cyclically and others permanently.

Our first hypothesis was that eCH patients in remission were more burdened compared to controls.

Per definition, chronic CH (cCH) patients do not go into meaningful remission periods [1] and intuitively this group should be more burdened by the disease.

We aimed to explore the impact on both personal and societal parameters to compile a comprehensive assessment of the disease burden in a large cohort of eCH and cCH patients compared to controls.

## Methods

Participants were asked if they received fulltime or part-time disability pension and if they received full-time disability pension, whether it was based on their CH diagnosis.

For direct cost of acute treatment, only patients with attacks within the last year were included.

In the indirect cost analysis, we included absenteeism (sick days and disability pension) but not presenteeism.

Participants could indicate if the fulltime disability pension had been approved due to CH, and only patients who indicated this were included in the indirect cost analysis.

We could not determine if the part-time disability pension was approved due to CH or to comorbidities, but it is assumed that CH at least in part contributed to the decision.

We explored the literature on sociodemographic and CH specific factors of receiving disability pension and three variables was selected: sex, educational level and phenotype (cCH or eCH).

## Results

Health was rated as poor/very poor by one-fifth of the eCH patients in bout compared to more than one-third of the cCH patients (26 out of 127 (20%) vs 49 out of 144 (34%), p = 0.0009).

Compared to a cCH patient, the odds to rate health as good/very good were 3 times higher for an eCH patient in remission (OR 3.22, 95% CI 1.90–5.47, p < 0.001) and 10 times higher for a control (OR 10.10, 95% CI 5.29–18.79.

Among currently employed participants, cCH patients had 31.9 ± 68.5 annual sick days (N = 48), eCH patients had 13.6 ± 23.8 (N = 165), and controls had 4.1 ± 9.3 (N = 200), p < 0.001.

If excluding CH related absenteeism, cCH patients had 6.9 additional sick days compared to the control group whereas the eCH patients had 1.5 more sick days than controls (p = 0.011).

**Discussion**

Amongst the 400 CH patients we also identified a mean annual direct cost of 5178 €/patient and substantial loss of productivity resulting in a higher mean annual indirect cost of 6561 €/patient.

Self-rated health was significantly reduced in periods with attacks and cCH patients had ten-fold lower odds of rating their health as good or very good compared to controls.

From Denmark, Italy and the USA, 10–17% of the patients had reported loss of a job due to CH [10, 42, 67] whereas this only occurred in 3% in a recent Korean study [68].

It was found that CH patients had higher employment rates compared to their unaffected family relatives, but this study only included eCH patients [69].

The direct and indirect cost of CH were high especially in cCH patients where the total cost was three times that of the eCH patients.

The direct costs of eCH patients were slightly higher in a German study (1819 €/ half year vs 2763 €/year) from 2011 [70].

**Acknowledgement**
*A machine generated summary based on the work of Petersen, Anja Sofie; Lund, Nunu; Snoer, Agneta; Jensen, Rigmor Højland; Barloese, Mads. 2022 in The Journal of Headache and Pain.*


# *Direct and Indirect Costs of Cluster Headache: A Prospective Analysis in a Tertiary Level Headache Centre*

DOI: https://doi.org/10.1186/s10194-020-01115-4


**Abstract-Summary**
CH can manifest as episodic (ECH) or chronic cluster headache (CCH) causing significant burden of disease and requiring attack therapy and prophylactic treatment.

This prospective study aimed to quantify the total direct and indirect cost of ECH and CCH over a cluster period, both for the patient and for the National Health System (NHS), using data from subjects who consecutively attended an Italian tertiary headache centre between January 1, 2018 and December 31, 2018.

A total 108 patients (89 ECH, 19 CCH) were included.

Mean total cost of a CH bout was €4398 per patient and total cost of CCH was 5.4 times higher than ECH (€13,350 vs. €2487, p < 0.001).

The costs for any item of expense were higher for CCH than for ECH (p < 0.001).

Mean indirect costs for a CH bout were €1226 per patient and were higher for CCH compared to ECH (€3.538 vs. €732), but the difference was not significant.

Our results provide a valuable estimate of the direct and indirect costs of ECH and CCH in the specific setting of a tertiary headache centre and confirm the high economic impact of CH on both the NHS and patients.

Extended:

Governments and decision-makers should strongly support these investigations to reveal the true economic and social impact of this devastating pain disease, particularly when it is chronic.

## Introduction

CH is characterized by excruciating unilateral pain lasting from 15 min to 3 h, with attacks occurring every other day up to eight times a day for weeks or months during active cluster periods, followed by periods of remission.

According to the third edition of the International Classification of Headache Disorders (ICHD3) [1], patients with ECH suffer from headache attacks that occur in periods ranging from 7 days to 1 year, separated by pain-free periods lasting at least 3 months.

CH has often been referred to as "suicide headache" due to the excruciating pain of the attacks and although these are periodic in most cases, the personal burden can be considerable due to lifestyle restrictions during the bouts, increased use of health care and the negative impact on work [10].

This study was conducted in a tertiary headache centre to estimate the total cost (direct and indirect) of treating ECH and CCH over a cluster period and to determine the economic burden for patients and the National Health System (NHS).

## Methods

Patients' electronic medical records (EMRs) were used to collect further information, such as the number of visits to our headache centre, other specialist visits, diagnostic tests, therapeutic procedures performed at our clinic (e.g. steroid suboccipital injections) and admissions to the emergency department (ED).

The data collected included demographic characteristics, medical history of CH, number of specialist visits, number of diagnostic tests (e.g. electrocardiogram and brain magnetic resonance), medication consumption (acute, transitional and preventive drugs) and number of ED admissions.

Indirect costs due to days of absence from work and days with reduced work efficiency were assessed analyzing the data recorded by participants in their diaries.

The demographic and clinical characteristics, the number of specialist visits, the number of diagnostic tests, the consumption of drugs (reimbursed and not reimbursed by the NHS) and the number of ED visits have been assessed in a descriptive way.

## Results

The mean number of ECG per patient was higher for CCH (2.5 ± 1.2) than ECH (0.6 ± 0.7; p < 0.0001).

The mean cost of preventive medications for CH bout was €102 ± €138 (range: €0–537) per patient and was significantly higher for CCH (€357 ± €74) than ECH (€48 ± €70; p < 0.0001).

The mean cost of transitional treatments for CH bout was €20 ± €34 (range: €0–92) per patient and was significantly higher for CCH (€66 ± €35) than ECH (€10 ± €24; p < 0.0001).

The mean cost attributed to days with reduced productive capacity for CH bout was €792 ± €3541 (range: €0–29,501) per patient and was higher for CCH (€2659 ± €7818) then ECH (€393 ± €1352), but the difference was not significant.

## Discussion

Our study provides a detailed quantification of the mean direct and indirect costs associated with ECH and CCH (assessed with the ICHD-3 [1]) in a large population of patients attending an Italian tertiary level headache centre.

The total cost of CCH was 5.4 times higher than that of ECH.

They estimated the total costs of a 6-month period in €10,985 per patient with CCH and €2583 per patient with ECH.

As regard to indirect costs, in our study they represented 27.9% of the total cost of CH bout and, as expected, they were higher for CCH than ECH (€3.538 vs. €732), although not significantly.

CCH patients made significantly more absences from work than ECH patients (15.2 ± 11.8 vs. 5.6 ± 7.9) and, although the cost of days off work was higher for CCH then ECH (€879 vs. €339), the difference was not significant.

## Methodological Considerations

Our study was conducted on a sample of patients attending a tertiary headache centre and our results may therefore not be representative of CH patients in the general population as specialist clinics usually see most disabled patients with a history of treatment failures and treatment attempts by general practitioners.

Most previous studies of CH have been conducted on patients from headache clinics.

The higher proportion of CCH patients in a tertiary headache centre compared than in the general population may result in more people refractory to conventional treatment.

Recall bias is usually a major problem in retrospective clinical studies, even for highly debilitating diseases such as CH, for which one might expect most patients to be able to remember their attacks accurately.

## Conclusions

Our results provide a valuable estimate of the direct and indirect costs of patients with ECH and CCH in the specific setting of a tertiary level headache centre and confirm the high economic impact of CH on both the NHS and patients.

CCH Patients had more visits, diagnostic tests and drug use than patients with ECH, which led to a total cost of 5.4 times that of ECH.

Cost of illness studies become obsolete due to changing healthcare systems and new treatments become available.

**Acknowledgement**

*A machine generated summary based on the work of Negro, Andrea; Sciattella, Paolo; Spuntarelli, Valerio; Martelletti, Paolo; Mennini, Francesco Saverio. 2020 in The Journal of Headache and Pain.*

# Burden of Migraine in Finland: Multimorbidity and Phenotypic Disease Networks in Occupational Healthcare

DOI: https://doi.org/10.1186/s10194-020-1077-x

**Abstract-Summary**

Electronic medical records (EMR) of patients with migraine (n = 17,623) and age- and gender matched controls (n = 17,623) were included in this retrospective analysis.

EMRs were assessed for the prevalence of ICD-10 codes, those with at least two significant phi correlations, and a prevalence >2.5% in migraine patients were included to phenotypic disease networks (PDN) for further analysis.

The diagnosis-wise connectivity based on the PDNs was compared between migraine patients and controls to assess differences in morbidity patterns.

The mean number of diagnoses per patient was increased 1.7-fold in migraine compared to controls.

1337 different ICD-10 codes were detected in EMRs of migraine patients.

Monodiagnosis was present in 1% and 13%, and the median number of diagnoses was 12 and 6 in migraine patients and controls.

The number of significant phi-correlations was 2.3-fold increased, and cluster analysis showed more clusters in those with migraine vs. controls (9 vs. 6).

Migraine patients were more likely affected by multiple conditions compared to controls, even if no notable differences in morbidity patterns were identified through connectivity measures.

Frequencies of ICD-10 codes on a three character and block level were increased across the whole diagnostic spectrum in migraine.

A systematic increase in the morbidity across the whole spectrum of ICD-10 coded diagnoses, and when interpreting PDNs, were detected in migraine patients.

Extended:

1337 different ICD-10 codes were detected in EMRs, but all were not included in the further analyses due to low abundancy.

The number of distinct diagnoses per person was assessed from ICD-10 codes for controls and patients with migraine.

The number of significant phi-correlations (p < 0.05) was greater in patients with migraine than among controls (4752 vs. 2804).

These findings strongly point at a significant multimorbidity among migraine patients that may reflect the polygenic nature of migraine but also complex representation of migraine symptoms in ICD-10 coded clinical praxis.

## Introduction

Multimorbidity, defined as the co-occurrence of two or more diseases or conditions in an individual, has been described in migraine [71–74].

Although multimorbidity generally increases with age, comorbidities are present already in pediatric migraine [75].

Global burden of disease repeatedly identifies migraine as one of the top conditions resulting in years lived with disability, likely attributable to the multimorbid strain on individuals [76, 77].

PDNs have been used to study the multimorbidity patterns underlying depression as well as heart failure, migraine, diabetes and dementia in elderly patients [73, 78].

The aim of the current study was to further investigate comprehensive patterns of morbidity based on ICD-10 coded phenotypic diseasomes in migraine patients compared to age- and gender-matched controls.

Migraine was associated with significant increase in overall morbidity seen both as increased multimorbidity across the ICD-10 coded diagnostic spectrum and in the larger PDN, in which diagnoses clustered differentially between migraine patients and controls.

## Material and Methods

Phi-correlations were calculated between 205 and 105 diagnostic codes in migraine patients and controls, respectively.

Phi correlation is calculated like the regular Pearson correlation, but between two binary variables, here if a patient was or was not recorded with a given diagnosis code.

Phi correlation − 1 between two diagnosis codes mean that exactly the patients that were recorded with the diagnosis code 1 were not recorded with the diagnosis code 2, and conversely for the diagnosis code 2.

Phi correlation 1 means that exactly the same patients were recorded with both diagnosis code 1 and 2.

Phi correlation 0 means that there was no correlation between the diagnosis codes.

One random walk consists of first selecting a diagnosis code at random and then again randomly selecting another diagnosis code that has a phi correlation with the current diagnosis code.

## Results

The study provides new insight on increased multimorbidity across all diagnosis codes in migraine and shows that diagnoses cluster differentially between migraine patients and controls in phenotypic disease networks.

The mean number of diagnoses per patient was increased 1.7-fold in migraine compared to controls.

The median number of distinct diagnoses per person was 12 for migraine patients and 6 for controls.

The number of significant phi-correlations ($p < 0.05$) was greater in patients with migraine than among controls (4752 vs. 2804).

There were 197 potential co-existing morbidities in migraine patients and 148 morbidities in controls with at least two significant phi-correlations.

The median number of significant phi-correlations per diagnosis code was 12 and 9 for migraine patients and controls, respectively.

Migraine patients had an increase in overall diagnoses that were distributed across multiple ICD-10 code blocks.

## Discussion

The most important results of the current study include 1) demonstrating that large datasets collected as a part of routine clinical praxis can be useful in naturally clustering diseasomes in an untargeted fashion; 2) diagnostic codes clustered differently into 9 and 6 clusters for migraine patients and controls, respectively; 3) the migraine PDN was larger and denser and exhibited one large cluster with functional-disorder-like symptoms including fatigue, respiratory, sympathetic nervous system, gastrointestinal, infection, mental and mood disorder diagnoses; 4) elucidating holistic and substantial multimorbidity for migraine seen as a holistic increase in prevalences of diagnoses across the whole ICD-10 coded diagnostic spectrum.

The study provided new insight to the migraine related diseasome, and we detected a global holistic increase in frequencies in more abundant diagnostic codes or blocks in migraine patients when compared to controls.

## Acknowledgement

*A machine generated summary based on the work of Korolainen, Minna A.; Tuominen, Samuli; Kurki, Samu; Lassenius, Mariann I.; Toppila, Iiro; Purmonen, Timo; Santaholma, Jaana; Nissilä, Markku. 2020 in The Journal of Headache and Pain.*

# Impact of Cluster Headache on Employment Status and Job Burden: A Prospective Cross-sectional Multicenter Study

DOI: https://doi.org/10.1186/s10194-018-0911-x

## Abstract-Summary

Cluster headaches (CH) are recurrent severe headaches, which impose a major burden on the life of patients.

Patients with CH were enrolled from September 2016 to February 2018 from 15 headache clinics in Korea.

We also enrolled a headache control group with age-sex matched patients with migraine or tension-type headache.

All participants responded to a questionnaire that included questions on employment status, type of occupation, working time, sick leave, reductions in productivity, and satisfaction with current occupation.

We recruited 143 patients with CH, 38 patients with other types of headache (migraine or tension-type headache), and 52 headache-free controls.

The proportion of employees was lower in the CH group compared with the headache and headache-free control groups (CH: 67.6% vs. headache controls: 84.2% vs. headache-free controls: 96.2%; p = 0.001).

The CH group more frequently experienced difficulties at work and required sick leave than the other groups (CH: 84.8% vs. headache controls: 63.9% vs. headache-free controls: 36.5%; p < 0.001; CH: 39.4% vs. headache controls: 13.9% vs. headache-free controls: 3.4%; p < 0.001).

Among the patients with CH, sick leave was associated with younger age at CH onset (25.8 years vs. 30.6 years, p = 0.014), severity of pain rated on a visual analogue scale (9.3 vs. 8.8, p = 0.008), and diurnal periodicity during the daytime (p = 0.003).

Most patients with CH experienced substantial burdens at work.

Extended:

The proportion of individuals who had retired was higher in the CH group than in the other groups (CH: 7.7%, Migraine/TTH: 5.3%, Control: 0%; p = 0.029).

The proportion of employees was lower in the CH group than in the other groups (CH: 67.6%, Migraine/TTH: 84.2%, Control: 96.2%; p = 0.001).

Among the patients with CH, 25 were employers or self-employed, 96 were employees, and 22 were freelancers.

## Background

Previous studies have shown that patients with CH report restrictions in daily living, difficulties in social-activity participation, family life, and housework; and overall life changes [67, 79].

A previous study showed that 30% of patients experienced absenteeism due to CH [67].

Migraine headaches can cause serious problems; however, CH is also severe and can be expected to cause many work-related difficulties.

We analyzed the effect of CH on employment status, type of occupation, working time, difficulties including sick leave and decreases in productivity, and satisfaction with current employment.

We compared patients with CH to patients with migraine or tension-type headaches (TTH) and a headache-free control group.

## Methods

The Korean Cluster Headache Registry Study is a prospective, cross-sectional, multicenter registry study that enrolled consecutive patients with CH from 15 hospitals (13 university hospitals: eight tertiary and five secondary referral hospitals and two secondary referral general hospitals) in Korea.

Patients with migraine or TTH were enrolled as headache controls.

Investigators assessed and recorded clinical information regarding the current incidence and previous history of CH in the patients.

We compared difficulties at work due to headaches between patients with CH and migraine or TTH, and difficulties at work were generally assessed in the headache-free controls.

Each patient completed a self-administered questionnaire assessing depression with the Patient Health Questionnaire-9 (PHQ-9), anxiety with the Generalized Anxiety Disorder-7 (GAD-7), and stress with the Short Form Perceived Stress Scale-4 (PSS 4) [80–83].

Logistic regression was performed adjusting for age, sex, and PHQ-9, GAD-7, and PSS-4 scores as predictors for any difficulty at work or sick leave.

## Results

We initially enrolled 159 patients with CH, 40 patients with migraine or TTH, and 53 headache-free controls.

Following this, the questionnaires of 143 patients with CH (CH, n = 19, episodic CH, n = 100; chronic CH, n = 5; probable CH, n = 19), 38 patients with migraine or TTH (chronic migraine, n = 5; episodic migraine, n = 25; chronic TTH, n = 4; episodic TTH, n = 4), and 52 controls were analyzed.

The proportion of individuals who had retired was higher in the CH group than in the other groups (CH: 7.7%, Migraine/TTH: 5.3%, Control: 0%; p = 0.029).

The proportion of employees was lower in the CH group than in the other groups (CH: 67.6%, Migraine/TTH: 84.2%, Control: 96.2%; p = 0.001).

## Discussion

The main findings of this study were follows: 1) more patients were self-employed and less were employees in the CH group than in the other groups; 2) patients with CH had a 8.26× increased risk of having difficulties at work and a 15.12× increased risk of requiring sick leave compared with headache-free controls after adjusting for age, sex, and depression, anxiety, and stress levels; 3) and, in the CH group, the patients requiring sick leave were younger at CH onset and had more severe pain than those who did not require sick leave.

Although the significance of younger age at CH onset was decreased with multivariable logistic analysis, the association between younger age at onset and increased risk for sick leave suggested that the headaches in this subgroup started before they had the opportunity to secure meaningful employment and thus these patients were more disabled by their condition when they started working and/or less able to adapt to the working environment.

## Conclusions

We revealed that CH were an important predictor of work disability and need for sick leave after adjusting for psychiatric comorbidities.

We revealed that severity of pain, younger age at CH onset, and diurnal periodicity during the daytime were associated with sick leave of CH patients.

**Acknowledgement**

*A machine generated summary based on the work of Choi, Yun-Ju; Kim, Byung-Kun; Chung, Pil-Wook; Lee, Mi Ji; Park, Jung-Wook; Chu, Min Kyung; Ahn, Jin-Young; Kim, Byung-Su; Song, Tae-Jin; Sohn, Jong-Hee; Oh, Kyungmi; Lee, Kwang-Soo; Kim, Soo-Kyoung; Park, Kwang-Yeol; Chung, Jae Myun; Moon, Heui-Soo; Chung, Chin-Sang; Cho, Soo-Jin. 2018 in The Journal of Headache and Pain.*

## *Cluster Headache and the Comprehension Paradox*

DOI: https://doi.org/10.1007/s42399-021-01083-z

### Abstract-Summary

Participants self-reported their number of sick days, the number of days on which leisure activities were missed and whether they felt understood by colleagues and family.

We then investigated the correlation between the number of sick days and the proportion of patients feeling understood by colleagues and friends.

We found that feeling understood by colleagues and friends decreases with a growing number of sick days.

When sick days accrue further, this proportion increases again.

The number of sick days correlates similarly with both colleagues' and friends' understanding.

The number of cluster headache patients feeling understood by others decreases with an increasing number of sick days.

With a growing number of sick days, however, the portion of patients feeling understood rises again despite patients meeting others' expectations even less.

We suspect that growing numbers of sick days foster understanding as the disability of the disease becomes increasingly apparent.

Extended:

The number of CH patients feeling understood by others decreases with an increasing number of sick days.

With a growing number of sick days, however, the portion of patients feeling understood rises again.

### Introduction

Patients with primary headache disorders such as migraine or cluster headache (CH) cycle between being entirely healthy and almost completely incapacitated [67, 84].

The challenge of headache patients is to find ways of meeting personal or professional obligations despite the pain.

Patients' sick leave or reduced performance due to headache attacks demands flexibility by their social counterparts [85].

Presumably, headache patients cause frustration that grows with the times colleagues have to take over their work.

## Methods

We will focus on the number of days employed patients had been unable to go to work ('sick days'), as well as on the number of days patients had missed social activities ('missed leisure days').

We assessed the former with the following question, 'On how many days in the last 3 months could you not go to work or school because of your headaches?'; the latter was assessed asking, 'On how many days in the last 3 months did you miss family, social or leisure activities because of your headaches?'.

We will include the answers to the following two questions into the analysis. (i) 'Do you feel that your family and friends understand and accept your headaches?' (ii) 'Do you feel that your employer and work colleagues understand and accept your headaches?'

We calculated the proportion of patients who had reported feeling understood by colleagues and employers as well as family and friends, respectively, for each subset.

## Results

In that period, patients with episodic CH had 11 ± 17 (median: 4 days) sick days and patients with chronic CH had 23 ± 30 days (median: 8 days); all participants taken together were absent from work on 14 ± 22 days (median: 5 days).

Patients with episodic CH had reached an average score of 8 ± 4 points (median 8 points); 151 (151/286, 52.8%, 13 n.r.) had scored eight or more points.

Patients with episodic CH had reached an average score of 6 ± 4 points (median 6 points); 107 (107/282, 37.9%, 17 n.r.) had scored eight or more points.

Patients with episodic CH had missed 17 ± 21 days (median: 9 days), and patients with chronic CH had missed 30 ± 27 days (median: 21 days); all participants taken together had missed 21 ± 24 days (median: 10 days).

## Discussion

We analysed the correlation between feeling understood and both sick days and missed leisure days in patients suffering from CH.

With a certain number of missed days—between one-third and half of the highest possible numbers, a paradoxical increase in perceived understanding occurs despite patients meeting others' expectations even less (hence the 'comprehension paradox').

Similar to migraineurs [86], patients generally experienced family members and friends as more understanding than colleagues and employers.

A holistic therapeutic approach taking into account not just the patients but also their families might help patients feel understood even when the number of sick days or missed leisure days does not make their suffering evident to others, yet.

We would like to encourage further research on the perspectives of headache patients' social circles; in future studies, colleagues, employers, friends and family members should be inquired directly.

## Conclusion

The number of CH patients feeling understood by others decreases with an increasing number of sick days.

With a growing number of sick days, however, the portion of patients feeling understood rises again.

We suspect that growing numbers of sick days foster understanding as the disability of the disease becomes increasingly apparent.

**Acknowledgement**
*A machine generated summary based on the work of Pohl, Heiko; Gantenbein, Andreas R.; Sandor, Peter S.; Schoenen, Jean; Andrée, Colette. 2022 in SN Comprehensive Clinical Medicine.*

**Mechanisms**

Machine generated keywords: gene, cluster headache, cluster, receptor, network, hypothalamus, migraine cluster, structural, susceptibility, association, genetic, functional, connectivity, casecontrol, cortex

## *Cluster Headache*

DOI: https://doi.org/10.1038/nrdp.2018.6

**Abstract-Summary**
Cluster headache is an excruciating, strictly one-sided pain syndrome with attacks that last between 15 minutes and 180 minutes and that are accompanied by marked ipsilateral cranial autonomic symptoms, such as lacrimation and conjunctival injection.

The past decade has seen remarkable progress in the understanding of the pathophysiological background of cluster headache and has implicated the brain, particularly the hypothalamus, as the generator of both the pain and the autonomic symptoms.

Anatomical connections between the hypothalamus and the trigeminovascular system, as well as the parasympathetic nervous system, have also been implicated in cluster headache pathophysiology.

Extended:

Cluster headache is probably the most severe pain known and is characterized by ipsilateral headache, with pain localized to the orbit, supraorbital and/or temporal regions and associated autonomic features.

**Introduction**
Based on the ICHD-3 criteria, diagnosis of episodic cluster headache requires at least two cluster periods (also known as cluster bouts), each lasting from 7 days to 1 year [1].

Diagnosis of chronic cluster headache requires cluster attacks that occur for >1 year without remission periods or with remission periods of <3 months in duration.

The trigeminal-autonomic cephalalgias (TACs) are a group of headache disorders characterized by unilateral headaches with autonomic symptoms ipsilateral to the pain, such as miosis (constriction of the pupil), ptosis (drooping of the upper eyelid), lacrimation (tearing) and conjunctival injection (redness of the sclera).

In the most current International Classification of Headache Disorders (ICHD-3), the following syndromes are classified as TACs: Episodic and chronic cluster headaches Episodic and chronic paroxysmal hemicrania Hemicrania continua Short-lasting unilateral neuralgiform headache attacks with cranial autonomic symptoms (SUNA-syndrome) Short-lasting unilateral neuralgiform headache attacks with conjunctival injection and tearing (SUNCT-syndrome)

## Epidemiology

These patients (up to 46% in a large Italian study) also show a relatively younger age of onset and attacks that are longer in duration than cluster headache attacks without migraineous features [87].

In the United States, cluster headache onset has been shown to occur before 20 years of age in 35% of patients and between 21 years and 30 years of age in 36% of patients [10].

Other studies conducted in the United States and Italy have shown an onset of cluster headache before 50 years of age in 83.3% of women and 91.3% of men [52, 88].

A recent genome-wide association study in a cohort of 99 Italian patients with cluster headache and 360 age-matched, cigarette-smoking, healthy controls demonstrated that ADCYAP1R1 (encoding pituitary adenylyl cyclase-activating polypeptide type I receptor, also known as PACAP) and MME (encoding membrane metalloendopeptidase, also known as neprilysin) variants were associated with cluster headache susceptibility, suggesting roles for genes implicated in pain processing [89].

## Mechanisms/Pathophysiology

Studies using $^{18}$F-fluorodeoxyglucose PET showed increased glucose metabolism in frontal brain areas (such as the perigenual anterior cingulate and prefrontal cortices) in addition to the thalamus, posterior cingulate, insular cortex and temporal cortex during cluster-bout periods compared with out-of-bout periods in patients with episodic cluster headache, suggesting that dynamic functional differences in central descending pain modulation between cluster-bout (interictally between headaches) and out-of-bout periods may facilitate attacks [90].

White matter microstructural differences have been reported in frontal pain modulation areas during the cluster-bout period in patients with cluster headache compared with healthy controls, and these changes mostly persisted during out-of-bout periods [91].

A decrease in functional co-activation of the hypothalamus and salience network areas in patients with cluster headache has been observed, suggesting the association with the defective central pain control pathway and autonomic nervous system dysregulation [92].

**Diagnosis, Screening and Prevention**

In a questionnaire-based study of 275 individuals with cluster headache, 80% reported sleep as a trigger for their attacks [93].

Data from a population-based, cross-sectional study of 462 patients showed the lifetime prevalence of depression was 2.8-fold higher in those with cluster headache compared with healthy individuals [94].

The 2.5-year incidence of depression was 5.6-fold higher in patients with cluster headache than healthy individuals in a population-based follow-up study using the Taiwan National Health Insurance database, and more cluster-bout periods per year was a risk factor for depression [95].

As cluster headache attacks are frequently initiated during sleep, several studies have evaluated patients with cluster headache for sleep disorders [93, 96–98].

In one study, the rate of obstructive sleep apnoea was not higher in patients with cluster headache compared with healthy controls; however, sleep-disordered breathing was present in 80% of patients (using an apnoea-hypopnea index cut-off of $\geq 5$) [97, 98] and in 44% of patients (using an apnoea-hypopnea index cut-off of $\geq 10$) [97].

**Management**

In one study, sumatriptan administered orally was not effective in preventing attacks in a placebo-controlled trial [99], although in open-label trials, eletriptan [100] or naratriptan [101] reduced the number of attacks in patients with episodic cluster headache.

Oral melatonin was effective in reducing attack frequency in a single double-blind, placebo-controlled study in patients with episodic cluster headache [102] but did not provide any additional efficacy when used as an adjunctive therapy to standard treatment in patients with refractory disease [103].

Warfarin was reported to effectively reduce attack frequency in a small controlled trial and in case reports of patients with episodic cluster headache [104, 105] but should not be used as a treatment given its adverse effect profile (including bleeding).

The Pathway CH-1 study was followed by an open-label trial involving 33 patients with chronic cluster headache who had 5956 cluster attacks over 24 months [106].

In the ACT-1 randomized controlled trial, 133 patients (of whom two-thirds had episodic cluster headache), were asked to use noninvasive VNS to treat five attacks each [107].

**Quality of Life**

Given the intense pain of cluster headaches, surprisingly few studies have investigated the effect of the disorder on quality of life.

Some studies suggest that patients have a poorer quality of life during active cluster bouts than the general population and that the impairment is greater in patients with an older age of onset [108].

No difference was reported in the quality of life of patients during cluster-bout periods in those with episodic compared with chronic cluster headache [108].

During the out-of-bout period in patients with episodic cluster headache, quality-of-life scores tended to improve and were similar to scores in those who are headache-free [109, 110], although other studies have reported high levels of disability in patients with episodic chronic headache during out-of-bout periods [67, 111].

One study in Denmark reported that 16% of patients had lost their job, and 8% needed early retirement; this occurred in episodic and chronic cluster headache [67].

Using the Headache Impact Test-6 (HIT-6) scale, 74% of patients with cluster headache were classified as severely affected (HIT-6 grade IV disability) [112], with 78% of patients reporting restrictions in daily living and 96% needing to make a lifestyle change [67].

**Outlook**

Hypothalamic DBS has been used for the treatment of drug-refractory chronic cluster headache and can decrease attack frequency in 60% of patients.

Several selective CGRP receptor antagonists are under development and seem to be effective in inhibiting nociceptive trigeminal processing in both animal models and patients [113, 114].

The more recent and promising development of monoclonal antibodies targeting free CGRP and CGRP receptors has enabled clinicians to circumvent these adverse effects.

These antibodies have promising efficacy in patients with migraine [115, 116] and are likely to be effective in cluster headache, although these trials are still ongoing.

Future development of monoclonal antibodies and pharmacological agents targeting CGRP and possibly PACAP might improve the clinical management of cluster headache.

**Acknowledgement**

*A machine generated summary based on the work of May, Arne; Schwedt, Todd J.; Magis, Delphine; Pozo-Rosich, Patricia; Evers, Stefan; Wang, Shuu-Jiun. 2018 in Nature Reviews Disease Primers.*


# *Cluster Headache: Pathophysiology, Diagnosis and Treatment*

DOI: https://doi.org/10.1007/s00415-018-9007-4

**Abstract-Summary**

Cluster headache (CH) is characterized by attacks of severe, strictly unilateral pain that is orbital, supraorbital, temporal, or any combination of these, lasts 15–180 min, and occurs from once every other day to eight times a day.

The diagnosis of CH is based on a careful history that elicits the clinical features of attacks, ipsilateral autonomic phenomena, and the cyclical nature of the bouts in which the attacks occur.

Alternative interventions in patients with CH who have not experienced any meaningful benefit from preventive drugs are well defined.

Although there have been advances in the diagnosis and therapy of CH, a significant number of CH patients experience misdiagnoses and diagnostic delay, which stalls the possibility of the timely application of adequate abortive and preventive therapy.

Extended:

Although there have been advances in the diagnosis and therapy of CH, a significant number of patients still have a delayed diagnosis of CH, which postpones the possibility of a timely application of adequate abortive and preventive therapy.

## Definition

Trigeminal autonomic cephalalgia (TAC) is a type of primary headache disorder characterized by pain in the distribution of the first division of the trigeminal nerve in parallel with cranial autonomic features on the same side of the head.

CH is characterized by attacks of severe, strictly unilateral pain that is orbital, supraorbital, temporal, or any combination of these, lasts 15–180 min, and occurs from once every other day to eight times a day.

## Epidemiology

Although patients can be affected at any age, CH attacks typically start between the 20 and 40 s [117].

One study showed that patients with CH onset after 40 years of age reported a lower number of autonomic features and less frequently had conjunctival injection and nasal congestion/rhinorrhea phenomena during their attacks; the diagnostic delay was the longest in the patients with CH onset before 20 years of age [117].

Increasing evidence suggests an association between CH and smoking, with around 65% of patients being active smokers or reporting a history of smoking [118].

Recent published data suggest higher smoking rate of 88% among CH patients [119].

The clinical phenotype of CH is a more severe based on attack frequency, cycle duration, headache related disability and chronification in smoking exposed patients, while nonexposed smoking CH patients have an earlier age of onset, higher rate of familial migraine, and less circadian periodicity and daytime entrainment [119].

## Pathophysiology

The endogenous circadian control by the hypothalamus, actually by its structures such as the suprachiasmatic nuclei stimulated by light conditions via a retino-hypothalamic pathway, etc., represents the strongest trigger for the pathogenesis of CH.

Reduced hypocretin-1 level concentrations in CH patients were considered as an insufficient antinociceptive activity of the hypothalamus in CH pathogenesis [120].

A positron emission tomography study performed to visualize regional cerebral blood flow in CH patients both in and out of cluster showed significant activation of the ipsilateral, posterior, and hypothalamic gray matter, but only in CH patients in a cluster period [121].

A voxel-based, morphometric, magnetic resonance study found a significantly increased density and volume of the gray matter region in the inferior posterior hypothalamus in CH patients compared to healthy controls [122].

A functional magnetic resonance imaging study of CH patients also showed significant hypothalamic activation ipsilaterally, attributable to cluster attacks [123].

## Diagnosis

The diagnosis of CH is based on a careful history that elicits the clinical features of attacks: severe, strictly unilateral pain that is orbital, supraorbital, temporal, or any combination of these, duration, ipsilateral autonomic phenomena, and the cyclical nature of the bouts in which the attacks occur.

The local painful and painless pre-attack symptoms occur in CH.

The pain of CH is unilateral in almost all patients with episodic CH.

Pain can shift sides between bouts of CH attacks (less commonly during a bout; never during the attack itself).

CH attacks often occur during the night, waking patients from sleep [96].

CH attacks may present with migraine-like features such as nausea, vomiting, phono/photophobia, and aura phenomena similar to those experienced during migraine, as well as symptoms often limited to the same side as the pain; slightly fewer patients report an aversion to loud noise or strong smells during an attack [124, 125].

## Differential Diagnosis

Brain MRI with detailed study of the pituitary area and cavernous sinus, is recommended for all TACs including CH, because even clinically typical CH can be caused by structural lesions [126, 127].

Pituitary function testing should be considered in all refractory CH patients.

Comorbidity with trigeminal neuralgia (TN) (CH-tic syndrome) should be ruled out in cases of refractory CH.

As in other TAC [128], some CH patients have been described having both CH and TN (sometimes referred to as cluster-tic syndrome).

Misdiagnoses at the first consultation were recorded in more than two-third of CH patients (trigeminal neuralgia, migraine without aura, sinusitis, etc); in the majority, instrumental and laboratory investigations were conducted, and the diagnostic delay was more than 5 years [129].

Migraine patients prefer not to move during the episode, in contrast to the agitation and restlessness experienced during CH.

## Comorbidities

The rate of bipolar disorder in CH patients is largely unknown [130].

There is study which results suggest the rate for suicide ideations is 55% among CH patients, and the rate for CH patients who have actually tried to commit suicide is 2% [10].

Some results suggest a higher incidence of obstructive sleep apnea in CH patients [131].

Reports indicate that CH and obstructive sleep apnea are associated with an improvement in CH upon following treatment for sleep apnea [132].

**Therapy**
There is consensus that high-dose and high-flow-rate oxygen is effective for the abortive treatment of episodic or chronic CH acute attacks [133].

There is consensus that subcutaneous octreotide is effective for abortive treatment of CH.

The effectiveness of intranasal lidocaine and hyperbaric oxygen for abortive treatment of CH is unknown [133].

Preventive treatment aims to suppress the attacks for the duration of the bout, or over longer periods in those with chronic CH, with the fewest possible side effects [134].

There is evidence that greater occipital nerve injections (betamethasone plus xylocaine) are effective for preventive treatment of CH.

There are results for the effective treatment with onabotulinum toxin A in refractory CH patients [36].

Percutaneous radiofrequency ablation of the sphenopalatine ganglion has been shown to be an effective modality of treatment for patients with intractable chronic CH [135].

**Conclusion**
CH presents a relatively rare primary headache disorder, but it should be considered in all clinical settings when pain occurs in the disturbance of the first branch of the trigeminal nerve associated with ipsilateral autonomic phenomena with a circadian and circannual rhythm.

The secondary causes of CH must be excluded particularly in cases with atypical presentation, late onset, debut of chronic CH and abnormal neurological examination.

**Acknowledgement**
*A machine generated summary based on the work of Ljubisavljevic, Srdjan; Zidverc Trajkovic, Jasna. 2018 in Journal of Neurology.*


# *Olfactory Dysfunction in Patients with Cluster Headache*

DOI: https://doi.org/10.1007/s00405-021-06738-0


**Abstract-Summary**
Our study aimed to determine whether CH patients had olfactory dysfunction and to correlate it with clinical characteristics.

The CH patients had significantly lower threshold scores than healthy controls $(6.9 \pm 1.70$ vs. $7.8 \pm 1.08$, $p = 0.007$).

The mean threshold scores of CH patients during in-bout (n = 9) were significantly lower than CH patients during out-of-bout (n = 11) in subgroup analysis (5.9 ± 1.16 vs. 7.6 ± 1.76, p = 0.038).

CH patients with left-sided headache had significantly lower discrimination scores compared to CH patients with right-sided headache (12.8 ± 1.24 vs. 14.4 ± 1.51, p = 0.03).

There is marked impairment in olfactory function in CH patients compared to healthy controls.

Extended:

Lower threshold scores during in bout and lower discrimination scores with left-sided headaches in CH patients were also among the significant findings of this study.

## Introduction

Cluster headache (CH) is a primary headache characterized by strictly unilateral, short-lasting severe headache attacks accompanied by at least one ipsilateral autonomic symptom, such as conjunctival injection, lacrimation, forehead/facial sweating, miosis, ptosis and/or eyelid edema, and/or restlessness or agitation besides autonomic symptoms related to nose including nasal congestion and rhinorrhea [1].

Several studies have demonstrated physical and chemical changes, including gray matter volume change [122, 136], cortical thickness [137], microstructural brain tissue changes [138], and brain metabolism [121, 139] in CH patients compared to controls.

Considering the aforementioned nasal autonomic symptoms and these structural alterations, olfaction in CH patients is expected to be affected.

Our study aimed to determine whether CH patients had olfactory dysfunction compared to healthy controls by using the Sniffin' Sticks test and to correlate it with clinical characteristics.

## Material and Methods

The Sniffin' Sticks test is a psychophysical tool allowing detailed, semi-objective evaluation of a patient's olfactory performance, and it has been validated in various countries, including Turkey [140].

For the patient group, olfactory testing was performed either during the "bout" period (but without acute pain during the testing, the last attack >6 h prior to testing) or during when the patients were out of bout' (last attack >6 weeks before testing).

All testing was performed by two trained neurology residents who were blinded to other clinical data and were strictly performing previously described test instructions.

All CH patients and healthy controls were examined in the otorhinolaryngology outpatient clinic to exclude other clinical problems causing olfactory dysfunction like sinonasal disease, trauma, and upper respiratory tract infection.

Spearman's correlation test and linear regression analysis were conducted between olfactory scores and demographic/clinical parameters.

## Results

There were no significant differences between the two groups regarding age (35.4 ± 14.75 vs. 37.6 ± 11.55, p = 0.349) and smoking (p = 0.194).

Five CH patients (25%) had hyposmia, and none of the patients tested was diagnosed as having complete anosmia based on population norms [140].

CH patients with left-sided headache had significantly lower discrimination scores compared to CH patients with right-sided headache (12.8 ± 1.24 vs. 14.4 ± 1.51, p = 0.03).

**Discussion**

This is the first study investigating whether CH patients have olfactory dysfunction compared with healthy controls.

The Sniffin' Sticks test was performed in 20 CH patients and 57 healthy controls, and we demonstrated significantly lower threshold scores in CH patients than controls.

These data are consistent with our findings that patients during out-of-bout also had lower olfactory testing scores than healthy controls.

Despite these structural changes reported in the literature, discrimination and identification scores were only mildly and insignificantly impaired in CH patients compared with healthy controls in our study.

Threshold scores, which are believed to be more specific to peripheral elements of the olfactory system, were significantly lower in CH patients compared to healthy controls in our study.

The major strength of our study was that it is the first study investigating whether CH patients have olfactory dysfunction than healthy controls.

**Conclusion**

The current study investigating the olfactory status of CH patients demonstrated significantly lower threshold scores in CH patients compared to healthy controls, indicating marked impairment in olfactory function.

Lower threshold scores during in bout and lower discrimination scores with left-sided headaches in CH patients were also among the significant findings of this study.

**Acknowledgement**

*A machine generated summary based on the work of Samancı, Bedia; Şahin, Erdi; Şen, Cömert; Samancı, Yavuz; Sezgin, Mine; Emekli, Serkan; Kocasoy Orhan, Elif; Orhan, Kadir Serkan; Baykan, Betül. 2021 in European Archives of Oto-Rhino-Laryngology.*

## The Role of Neurotransmitters and Neuromodulators in the Pathogenesis of Cluster Headache: A Review

DOI: https://doi.org/10.1007/s10072-019-03768-9

**Abstract-Summary**

The pathogenesis underlying cluster headache remains an unresolved issue.

Although both the autonomic system and the hypothalamus play a central role, the modality of their involvement remains largely unknown.

Extended:

The pathogenesis underlying the chronicity in episodic CH is unknown as is the pathogenesis of CCH itself.

## Introduction

The first demonstration that anomalies in catecholamines occur in CH patients derives from the measurement of the circulating platelet levels of DA and NE in both remission and active periods.

Utilizing a new HPLC method, we measured the levels of Tyr, Oct, and Syn in plasma and platelets of the two groups of episodic CH patients in the remission and in the active periods.

Whether the anomalies in the synthesis of catecholamines and elusive amines, found in episodic CH patients, play a role in the pathogenesis of CCH is also unknown.

The plasma levels of DA were found, as in episodic CH, several folds higher in CCH patients with respect to controls.

In order to verify this, we assessed the plasma levels of Try, Tyr, NE, and E, together with the products of arginine metabolism such as arginine, homoarginine, citrulline, $N^G$, $N^G$-asymmetric dimethyl-l-arginine (ADMA), and $N^G$-monomethyl-l-arginine (NMMA), all products related to the synthesis and release of NO in the circulation [141], in a group of CCH patients and controls.

## Discussion

This is supported by several evidences: (i) the hypothalamus and locus coeruleus contain the highest levels of elusive amines, and these areas are connected with the autonomic system [142]; (ii) voxel-based morphometry MRI analysis has shown an enlarged volume of posterior part of hypothalamus in CH patients [143]; (iii) a treatment based on stereotactic stimulation of the same enlarged area significantly reduces the number of pain attacks in intractable chronic CH patients [144]; (iv) the high levels of DA found in CH and CCH patients suggest an activation of the dopaminergic system.

The high plasma levels of elusive amines and DA that are $TAAR_1$ agonists and the low plasma levels of NE that are $\alpha_1$-receptor agonists, widely distributed in the same areas, may interfere with the synaptic function of the hypothalamus and perhaps other subcortical circuitries potentially implicated in CH [145].

It is possible to conceive that the very high levels of NE and the low circulating levels of Oct and Syn, that constitute the major biochemical differences between episodic and chronic CH, may play a role in CCH.

The very high levels of NE in CCH patients may derive from the loss of the inhibitory presynaptic function of $TAAR_1$ receptors.

## Acknowledgement

*A machine generated summary based on the work of D'Andrea, G.; Gucciardi, A.; Perini, F.; Leon, A. 2019 in Neurological Sciences.*

# *Migraine and Cluster Headache Show Impaired Neurosteroids Patterns*

DOI: https://doi.org/10.1186/s10194-019-1005-0

## Abstract-Summary
We measured plasma levels of four neurosteroids, i.e., allopregnanolone, epiallo-pregnanolone, dehydroepiandrosterone and deydroepiandrosterone sulfate, in patients affected by episodic migraine, chronic migraine, or cluster headache.

Nineteen female patients affected by episodic migraine, 51 female patients affected by chronic migraine, and 18 male patients affected by cluster headache were recruited to the study.

We found disease-specific changes in neurosteroid levels in our study groups.

Allopregnanolone levels were significantly increased in episodic migraine and chronic migraine patients than in control subjects, whereas they were reduced in patients affected by cluster headache.

Dehydroepiandrosterone and dehydroepiandrosterone sulfate levels were reduced in patients affected by chronic migraine, but did not change in patients affected by cluster headache.

We have shown for the first time that large and disease-specific changes in circu-lating neurosteroid levels are associated with chronic headache disorders, raising the interesting possibility that fluctuations of neurosteroids at their site of action might shape the natural course of migraine and cluster headache.

This might also be matter for further investigation because stress is a known trig-gering factor for headache attacks in both migraineurs and cluster headache patients.

## Introduction
Neurosteroids are endogenous steroids synthesized in the central nervous system (CNS) that modulate neuronal excitability by interacting with either $\gamma$-aminobutyric acid A or N-methyl-d-aspartate receptors [146–148].

The association between serum $\gamma$-aminobutyric acid levels and the clinical char-acteristics of migraine suggests a causal link between changes in $\gamma$-aminobutyric acid mediated neurotransmission and the pathophysiology of migraine [149].

The aim of our study was to measure for the first time circulating levels of neurosteroids in patients with ICHD3-beta confirmed diagnosis [60] of episodic or chronic migraine (EM, CM), medication overuse headache (MOH) and cluster headache (CH), and to explore possible associations with their clinical characteristics.

Migraine and cluster headache are complex and multifaceted clinical diseases, whose conceptual framework has been recently organized by the International Classification of Headache Disorders 3rd Edition beta classification [60].

## Materials and Methods
Patients of both sexes, aging 18–80 years and referring to the Headache Unit at Azienda Ospedaliera-Universitaria S. Andrea, Rome, were recruited for the study.

After signing the informed consent, patients were enrolled and the following information collected and registered: age, sex, education, comorbidities, actual drug therapy, the presence of a concurrent migraine/headache attack, number of attacks/month, day of the menstrual cycle (women only).

Patients were asked to fill the Beck Depression Inventory (BDI), the Migraine Disability Assessment Test (MIDAS; only migraine patients), the Headache Impact test (HIT-6), and the Self-rating Anxiety Scale (SAS).

A mobile phase of formic acid (0.1%) in water and methanol through a gradient of composition and a flow rate of 0.3/mL/min was used since we demonstrated that results in good separations of the analytes [150].

## Results

No changes in DHEAS levels and in the ratio between AP and EAP were found in patients affected by EM with respect to healthy controls ($1.9 \pm 0.9$ vs $1.8 \pm 1.2$; $p = $ n.s.).

Knowing that the ovarian cycle has a strong impact on neurosteroid synthesis [151], we also examined AP, EAP, DHEA, and DHEAS levels in pre- and post-menopausal patients and healthy controls.

No significant associations were found between blood neurosteroids and BDI, SAS, HIT-6 and MIDAS scores, and educational level in EM patients and controls.

The AP/EAP ratio was higher In the overall population of CM patients with respect to healthy control ($3.0 \pm 1.7$ vs $1.8 \pm 1.2$, respectively; $p < 0.01$), whether or not blood samples were collected during the headache attack or in the interictal period.

## Discussion

Activation of γ-aminobutyric acid A receptors restrains synaptic excitation, and, therefore, the increase in AP found in EM and CM patients might be considered as a defensive mechanism aimed at limiting the enhanced neuronal excitability associated with migraine.

The reduction in DHEA (in EM and CM patients) and DHEAS (only in CM patients) levels might contribute to restrain neuronal excitation and neurogenic edema because both steroids behave as weak negative allosteric modulators or γ-aminobutyric acid A receptors [152].

And counterintuitively, the drop in DHEA and DHEAS levels was more substantial in CM patients, suggesting that adaptive mechanisms that reinforce γ-aminobutyric acid mediated transmission are more prominent in CM with respect to EM.

Only EM patients showed increases in the levels of EAP, a neurosteroid that is devoid of intrinsic efficacy and behaves as competitive antagonist at the AP site of γ-aminobutyric acid A receptors [153].

## Conclusion

We have shown for the first time that large and disease-specific changes in circulating neurosteroid levels are associated with chronic headache disorders, raising the interesting possibility that fluctuations of neurosteroids at their site of action might shape the natural course of migraine and CH.

This might also be matter for further investigation because stress is a known triggering factor for headache attacks in both migraineurs and CH patients.

Our findings may lay the groundwork for novel neurosteroid-based therapeutic strategies in the treatment chronic headache disorders.

Our data encourage the experimental use of ganoxolone particularly in CH patients, where AP levels were found to be largely reduced.

**Acknowledgement**

*A machine generated summary based on the work of Koverech, Angela; Cicione, Claudia; Lionetto, Luana; Maestri, Marta; Passariello, Francesco; Sabbatini, Elisabetta; Capi, Matilde; De Marco, Cristiano Maria; Guglielmetti, Martina; Negro, Andrea; Di Menna, Luisa; Simmaco, Maurizio; Nicoletti, Ferdinando; Martelletti, Paolo. 2019 in The Journal of Headache and Pain.*

## *Cluster Headache: Insights from Resting-State Functional Magnetic Resonance Imaging*

DOI: https://doi.org/10.1007/s10072-019-03874-8

**Abstract-Summary**

Clinical, neuroendocrinological, and neuroimaging studies strongly suggested the involvement of the hypothalamus as the generator of cluster headache attacks.

The latency of the improvement and the inefficacy of the hypothalamic deep brain stimulation (DBS) in the acute phase suggested that the hypothalamus might play a modulating role, pointing to the presence of some dysfunctional brain networks, normalized or modulated by the DBS.

Despite the great importance of possible dysfunctional hypothalamic networks in cluster headache pathophysiology, only quite recently the scientific community has begun to explore the functional connectivity of these circuits using resting-state functional magnetic resonance imaging.

We present a review of the few resting-state functional magnetic resonance imaging studies investigating the hypothalamic network contributing to a deeper comprehension of this neurological disorder.

These studies seem to demonstrate that both the hypothalamus and the diencephalic-mesencephalic junction regions might play an important role in the pathophysiology of CH.

Future studies are needed to confirm the results and to clarify if the observed dysfunctional networks are a specific neural fingerprint of the CH pathophysiology or an effect of the severe acute pain.

**[Section 1]**

In the first RS-fMRI study investigating episodic CH patients in out-of-bout condition, Rocca and others [154] showed an increased functional connectivity, in comparison to control subjects, between the hypothalamus (seed in the diencephalic-mesencephalic junction) and the anterior cingulate cortex, the secondary somatosensory cortex and the occipital regions, indicating therefore possible stable alterations of this functional circuit.

Two observations are important in this regard: (1) the central processing of the parasympathetic activity occurs in the regions of the default mode network; therefore, the typical autonomic symptoms of the CH during the attack well explain the dysfunctional connectivity in regions belonging to the default mode network; (2) the observed abnormal functional connectivity of the hypothalamus with some default mode network regions occurs in areas involved in the recalling of the past experience, namely the posterior cingulate cortex/precuneus, the parietal cortex, and the hippocampus.

**Acknowledgement**

*A machine generated summary based on the work of Ferraro, Stefania; Nigri, Anna; Bruzzone, Maria Grazia; Demichelis, Greta; Pinardi, Chiara; Brivio, Luca; Giani, Luca; Proietti, Alberto; Leone, Massimo; Chiapparini, Luisa. 2019 in Neurological Sciences.*

# *Population-Based Analysis of Cluster Headache-Associated Genetic Polymorphisms*

DOI: https://doi.org/10.1007/s12031-018-1103-5

**Abstract-Summary**

Associations between cluster headache and polymorphism rs2653349 of the HCRTR2 gene have been demonstrated.

The polymorphism rs5443 of the GNB3 gene positively influences triptan treatment response.

The frequency of the wild-type G allele was 88.7%.

The frequencies for rs5443 were C:C = 44.0%, C:T = 42.6%, and T:T = 13.4%.

The frequency of the wild-type C allele was 65.3%.

The frequency distribution of rs2653349 in the Southeastern European Caucasian population differs significantly when compared with other European and East Asian populations, and the frequency distribution of rs5443 showed a statistically significant difference between Southeastern European Caucasian and African, South Asian, and East Asian populations.

For rs2653349, a marginal statistically significant difference between genders was found (p = 0.080) for A:A versus G:G and G:A genotypes (OR = 2.78), indicating a higher representation of male homozygotes for the protective mutant A:A allele than female.

No statistically significant difference was observed between genders for rs5443.

**Background**

Two G-protein-coupled orexin receptors have been identified, HCRTR1 and HCRTR2.

A G1246A SNP on the HCRTR2 gene, rs2653349, which is responsible for an amino acidic substitution (Val308Iso) within the receptor sequence, has been reported to be related to CH [155].

According to a meta-analysis of three studies which were conducted in Caucasian populations, a relationship between the G1246A polymorphism (rs2653349) in the HCRTR2 gene and CH was found (fixed effect OR: 1.58 (CI 95% 1.27–1.95), random effect OR: 1.55 (CI 95% 1.14–2.12)) [156].

Triptans are G-protein-linked serotonergic (5-HT) receptor selective agonists, commonly used for acute CH therapy as injectable or intranasal preparation [157].

A population-based frequency distribution analysis of the HCRTR2 gene (rs2653349) and GNB3 (rs5443) gene polymorphism was performed in an attempt to evaluate potential biomarkers for CH susceptibility and triptans' efficacy in CH, respectively.

**Materials and Methods**

SEC origin and aged >18 years was considered for inclusion in the study.

Volunteers without SEC origin, obese, and aged <18 years were excluded.

The genotypes were classified as homozygote for wild type (G:G or C:C) allele, heterozygote (G:A or C:T), and homozygote mutated (A:A or T:T) for rs2653349 or rs5443 polymorphisms, respectively.

Chi square (Pearson and Fischer exact) tests were used to compare the frequencies of genotypes and alleles in SEC and other populations.

All statistical tests were performed at a significance level of $\alpha = 0.05$.

**Results**

For polymorphism rs2653349 of the HCRTR2 gene, 79.1% volunteers were homozygous for the wild-type genotype (G:G); 19.2% were heterozygous (G:A), and 1.7% were homozygous for the rare allele (A:A).

HWE applied for the HCRTR2 gene polymorphism rs2653349 in SEC population of this study.

The Chi square statistics of 1.27 gives sufficient statistical significance that the population is in HWE for the polymorphism rs2653349 of the HCRTR2 gene (p = 0.260).

**Discussion**

The rs2653349 (G1246A) polymorphism of the HCRTR2 gene reduces the chance of developing CH, meaning that genetic predisposition for developing CH is lower for those individuals carrying the protective rare allele A. The rare A allele occurs in 12.1% of the global population, in 10.7% of the AFR, in 13.4% of the SAS, in 18.4% of the EUR, in 6.2% of the EAS, and in 12.4% of the American population.

Chi square test was conducted between the AFR, SAS, EUR, EAS, AMR, and SEC populations in order to determine significant differences between the allele frequency distribution regarding the rs2653349 polymorphism.

The heterozygous genotypes appear in the 41.3% of the global population, in 28.9% of the AFR, in 44.4% of the SAS, in 41.9% of the EUR, in 51.4% of the EAS, in 44.7% of the AMR, and in 42.6% of the SEC population.

**Limitations of the Study**

Further, larger scale investigations may be needed, in order to precisely determine CH-associated polymorphism incidence rates.

Novel CH-associated gene polymorphisms may be necessary in order to form an algorithm capable to reveal CH susceptibility as well as to predict individual drug response.

Further studies should be initialized to investigate the frequency distribution of these polymorphisms in patients experiencing CH.

**Acknowledgement**

*A machine generated summary based on the work of Katsarou, Martha-Spyridoula; Papasavva, Maria; Latsi, Rozana; Toliza, Ioanna; Gkaros, Alfrent-Pantelis; Papakonstantinou, Stylianos; Gatzonis, Stylianos; Mitsikostas, Dimos-Dimitrios; Kovatsi, Leda; Isotov, Boris N.; Tsatsakis, Aristides M.; Drakoulis, Nikolaos. 2018 in Journal of Molecular Neuroscience.*


# *Analysis of HCRTR2, GNB3, and ADH4 Gene Polymorphisms in a Southeastern European Caucasian Cluster Headache Population*

DOI: https://doi.org/10.1007/s12031-019-01439-0

**Abstract-Summary**

The frequency of the mutated A allele was 11.0% for patients and 11.3% for controls.

The frequencies for rs5443 were CC = 44.7%, CT = 44.7%, and TT = 10.5% for patients and CC = 43.9%, CT = 42.6%, and TT = 13.5% for controls.

The frequency of the mutated T allele was 32.9% for patients and 34.8% for controls.

For rs1800759, the frequencies were CC = 36.0%, CA = 43.0%, and AA = 21.0% for patients and CC = 34.0%, CA = 50.2%, and AA = 15.8% for controls.

The frequency of the mutated A allele was 42.5% and 40.9% for patients and controls, respectively.

The mutated T allele of GNB3 rs5443 polymorphism was more prevalent in patients with better triptan treatment response, indicating a possible trend of association between this polymorphism and triptan treatment response in SEC population.

According to our observation, no association of HCRTR2 rs2653349 and ADH4 rs1800759 polymorphisms and cluster headache in SEC population could be documented.

Extended:

The frequency of the wild-type G allele was 203 for CH subjects (89.0%) and 1011 for controls (88.7%), and the frequency of the rare A allele was 25 (11.0%) and 129 (11.3%) for CH subjects and controls, respectively.

The frequency of the wild-type C allele was 153 (67.1%) for CH subjects and 743 (65.2%) for controls and that of the mutated T allele was 75 (32.9%) for CH subjects and 397 (34.8%) for controls.

The frequency of the wild-type C allele was 131 (57.5%) for CH subjects and 674 (59.1%) for controls and that of the mutated A allele was 97 (42.5%) for CH subjects and 466 (40.9%) for controls.

**Background**

The episodic (ECH) versus chronic cluster headache (CCH) ratio, with a higher male preponderance in CCH (15:1) versus ECH (3.8:1), was found to be 6:1 [55, 158]. Pathophysiology of CH has been only partially understood, although its clinical features are well defined [159–161]. Any theory that explains the pathophysiology of CH should incorporate the concomitant presentation: distribution of pain in the trigeminal area, cranial autonomic symptoms ipsilateral to the pain, and circadian pattern of attacks [159, 160]. The pain in CH is likely due to the activation of the ophthalmic branch of the trigeminal nerve whereas the cranial autonomic symptoms are due to the activation of cranial parasympathetic outflow from the facial nerve [162]. The inheritance of CH was confirmed by findings in monozygotic twins and by the increased risk of developing the disease in first- and second-degree relatives of CH patients.

The rs2653349 polymorphism (G1246A) in exon 5 of HCRTR2 gene has been associated with CH susceptibility [163]. This polymorphism is responsible for the substitution at position 308 of valine with isoleucine within the receptor sequence (Transmembrane helix 6-TM6) [155, 156, 164]. Studies found that homozygosity for the wild-type G allele of rs2653349 is associated with an increased risk of developing CH, although others did not find an association [163, 165–169]. The GNB3 gene, that encodes $\beta$3 subunit of the G protein, is located on 12p13 and consists of 11 exons and 10 introns [170]. The rs5443 polymorphism is responsible for the substitution at position 825 of thymidine with cytosine in exon 10 of GNB3 gene without modifying the amino acid sequence [171]. C825T has been associated with alternative splicing in exon 9 of the GNB3 gene, causing deletion of 123 base pairs that encode a WD40 region in the G$\beta$3 subunit.

This ADH subunit contributes significantly to the oxidation of ethanol when at higher concentrations [172, 173]. The ADH4 is located on chromosome 4 (4q22) and consists of 9 exons [174]. The rs1800759 polymorphism, in the promoter region of ADH4, increases the promoter activity thereby affecting the expression of $\pi$ subunit [175, 176]. Zarrilli and others showed with statistical significance a more frequent occurrence of the rs1800759 mutated A allele in patients with CH compared with controls (P = 0.03) [177]. Other studies did not support these findings [174, 178, 179]. A recent study in a general SEC population (n = 636) undertook a frequency distributions analysis of rs2653349 and rs5443 polymorphisms (HCRTR2 and GNB3 genes, respectively) [180]. The aim of this study was to determine if rs2653349, rs5443, and rs1800759 polymorphisms of HCRTR2, GNB3, and ADH4 genes, respectively, are associated with the susceptibility to develop CH in a SEC case-control population.

## Materials and Methods

Seventy-eight case subjects met the diagnostic criteria for ECH and 36 for CCH.

Responder rates to subcutaneous sumatriptan were assessed for 48 case subjects. Informed consent was obtained from all subjects.

The Hardy-Weinberg equilibrium (HWE) was verified for the genotypic distribution of each polymorphism in control subjects (P > 0.05) [181]. Chi square (Pearson and Fischer exact) tests were used to compare the frequencies of genotypes and alleles in CH subjects and controls.

## Results

HCRTR2 gene polymorphism (rs2653349) revealed 79.8% CH subjects and 79.1% controls homozygous (GG) for the wild-type G allele, 18.4% CH subjects and 19.1% controls heterozygous (GA), and 1.8% CH subjects and 1.8% controls homozygous (AA) for the rare A allele.

For polymorphism rs5443, 44.7% CH subjects and 43.9% controls were homozygous (CC) for the wild-type C allele, 44.7% CH subjects and 42.6% controls were heterozygous (CT), and 10.5% CH subjects and 13.5% controls were homozygous (TT) for the rare T allele.

For the rs1800759 polymorphism, 36.0% CH subjects and 34.0% controls were homozygous wild type (CC), 43.0% CH subjects and 50.2% controls were heterozygous (CA), and 21.0% CH subjects and 15.8% controls were homozygous for the mutated A allele (AA).

## Discussion

Two single nucleotide polymorphisms (SNPs) in HCRTR2 (rs2653349) and ADH4 (rs1800759) genes, associated with CH and rs5443 polymorphism in GNB3 gene, correlated with triptan treatment response, were examined.

The GNB3 rs5443 polymorphism is associated with triptan treatment response.

The data of the current study did not provide supportive evidence for statistically significant association between CH in SEC population and HCRTR2 gene polymorphism rs2653349, GNB3 gene polymorphism rs5443, and ADH4 gene polymorphism rs1800759.

The mutated T allele of rs5443 polymorphism was more prevalent in CH patients with better triptan treatment response, indicating a possible trend associating this polymorphism with triptan treatment response.

This is the first study investigating the association between HCRTR2, GNB3, and ADH4 gene polymorphisms and CH susceptibility in a Southeastern European Caucasian population.

**Limitations of the Study**

The small sample size of CH subjects' response to triptan treatment is a limitation.

Most of the case subjects included in this study have a positive triptan treatment response.

The effect of the mutated T allele on triptan treatment response is difficult to be evaluated conclusively due to the small sample size of the mutated T allele carriers.

**Acknowledgement**

*A machine generated summary based on the work of Papasavva, Maria; Katsarou, Martha-Spyridoula; Vikelis, Michail; Mitropoulou, Euthymia; Dermitzakis, Emmanouil V.; Papakonstantinou, Stylianos; Arvaniti, Chryssa; Mitsikostas, Dimos-Dimitrios; Gozes, Illana; Tsatsakis, Aristides M.; Drakoulis, Nikolaos. 2019 in Journal of Molecular Neuroscience.*


# *Genetic Association of HCRTR2, ADH4 and CLOCK Genes with Cluster Headache: A Chinese Population-Based Case-Control Study*

DOI: https://doi.org/10.1186/s10194-017-0831-1

**Abstract-Summary**

A large numbers of genetic association studies have confirmed that the HCRTR2 (Hypocretin Receptor 2) SNP rs2653349, and the ADH4 (Alcohol Dehydrogenase 4) SNP rs1126671 and rs1800759 polymorphisms are linked to CH.

The purpose of this study was to evaluate the association between CH and the HCRTR2, ADH4 and CLOCK genes in a Chinese CH case–control sample.

We genotyped polymorphisms of nine single nucleotide polymorphisms (SNPs) in the HCRTR2, ADH4 and CLOCK genes to perform an association study on a Chinese Han CH case-control sample (112 patients and 192 controls),using Sequenom MALDI-TOF mass spectrometry iPLEX platform.

The GA genotypes was associated with a higher CH risk (OR = 1.483, 95% CI: 0.564–3.387, p = 0.038), however, after Bonferroni correction, the association lost statistical significance.

Haplotype analysis of the HCRTR2 SNPs showed that among eight haplotypes, only H1-GTGGGG was linked to a reduced CH risk (44.7% vs. 53.1%, OR = 0.689, 95% CI = 0.491~0.966, p = 0.030).

No significant association of ADH4, CLOCK SNPs with CH was statistically detected in the present study.

Association between HCRTR2, ADH4,CLOCK gene polymorphisms and CH was not significant in the present study, however, haplotype analysis indicated H1-GTGGGG was linked to a reduced CH risk.

Extended:

The purpose of this study was to evaluate the association between CH and the HCRTR2 (rs10498801, rs2653342,rs2653349, rs3122156, rs3800539, rs9357855), ADH4(rs1126671, rs1800759) and CLOCK (rs1801260) genes, estimating the frequency of different gene haplotypes in a Chinese case–control cohort population.

The GA genotypes was associated with a higher CH risk (OR = 1.483, 95% CI: 0.564–3.387, p = 0.038), However, there was no significant association after the correction for multiple tests ($p^{corr}$ = 0.114).

Haplotype analysis of the HCRTR2 SNPs revealed that only H1-GTGGGG had significant lower frequency in cases than in controls (44.7% vs. 53.1%, OR = 0.689, 95% CI = 0.491~0.966, p = 0.030).

No significant association of CLOCK rs1801260 with CH was statistically detected in the present study, consistent with the previous results.

Although a significant association with CH in Chinese case–control group was not found, CLOCK as a candidate gene for screening CH could not be excluded in the future study.

## Background

Four studies revealed significant association of HCTR gene polymorphism with CH.

A significant association between a 1246G-A polymorphism (rs2653349) in the HCRTR2 gene and CH has been independently reported by two research groups [165–168].

Four studies have been conducted to investigate the association of the polymorphism of the human CLOCK gene (rs1801260) with CH, however, no consistent evidence for association of CLOCK with CH was observed yet [177, 182–184].

There is a limited number of the research on genetic association of polymorphisms in the HCRTR2, ADH4 and CLOCK genes with CH with contradictory results.

The purpose of this study was to evaluate the association between CH and the HCRTR2 (rs10498801, rs2653342, rs2653349, rs3122156, rs3800539, rs9357855), ADH4(rs1126671, rs1800759) and CLOCK (rs1801260) genes, estimating the frequency of different gene haplotypes in a Chinese case–control cohort population.

## Methods

The candidates in the control group were matched with the candidates in the case group by age and gender, and recruited from physical examination center of the same geographic areas, consisting of 192 unrelated non-headache healthy volunteers (170 men and 22 women).

Both CH patients and controls were from the Chinese Han population according to the selection criteria as follows: 1) registered as the ethic Han, 2) their parents were registered as the ethnic Han, and 3) the families have settled in China for more than 5 generations without marrying other ethics and intermarrying with other nationalities.

Single nucleotide polymorphism (SNP) genotyping was performed by using MassARRAY Analyzer 4 System (http://agenabio.com/products/massarray-system/).

SHEsis was used to construct the single body of 6 SNPs in the HCRTR2 gene and compare the distribution differences between the control and the case groups.

## Results

All the genes showed the polymorphisms of SNPs except for rs1126671 that was excluded from the statistical analysis.

The allele frequency at each locus and the genotype distributions of all SNPs were in the Hardy–Weinberg equilibrium in both patients and controls (P > 0.05).

The frequency of the rs3800539 GA genotypes was significantly higher in cases than in controls (48.2% vs.37.0%).

The GA genotypes was associated with a higher CH risk (OR = 1.483, 95% CI: 0.564–3.387, p = 0.038), However, there was no significant association after the correction for multiple tests ($p^{corr}$ = 0.114).

## Discussion

As far as we are aware, the present study is the first to explore molecular evidence for association of different genotypes of SNPs in HCRTR2, ADH4 and CLOCK genes with CH in Chinese Han population.

No statistically significant association of the polymorphism of HCRTR2 rs2653349 with CH was found in several case-control studies in Denmark, Sweden and the UK populations.

Rainero and others (2010) found that the rs1126671 located in exon 7 of the ADH4 gene was associated with an increased risk for CH in Italian case-control study, and the carriers with homozygous rs1126671 AA genotype had more than 2-fold CH risk than those with GG/GA genotypes (OR = 2.33, 95% CI = 1.25–4.37, P = 0.006) [174].

The present study did not provide supportive evidence for significant association of CLOCK gene rs1801260 with CH in Chinese Han population.

## Conclusion

This study is the first report to evaluate the association between CH and the HCRTR2, ADH4 and CLOCK genes in Chinese Han population.

The results suggest that the HCRTR2 (rs10498801, rs2653342, rs2653349, rs3122156, rs3800539, rs9357855), ADH4 (rs1126671, rs1800759) and CLOCK (rs1801260) are not genetic risk factors for CH in the Chinese Han population.

## Acknowledgement

*A machine generated summary based on the work of Fan, Zhiliang; Hou, Lei; Wan, Dongjun; Ao, Ran; Zhao, Dengfa; Yu, Shengyuan. 2018 in The Journal of Headache and Pain.*

## *VDR Gene Polymorphisms and Cluster Headache Susceptibility: Case–Control Study in a Southeastern European Caucasian Population*

DOI: https://doi.org/10.1007/s12031-021-01892-w

**Abstract-Summary**

Cluster headache (CH) is a severe primary headache disorder with a genetic component, as indicated by family and twin studies.

The aim of the present case–control study was to investigate the association of cluster headache susceptibility and clinical phenotypes with the VDR gene polymorphisms FokI, BsmI and TaqI in a Southeastern European Caucasian population.

Linkage disequilibrium (LD) analysis confirmed that BsmI and TaqI, both located in the 3′UTR of the VDR gene, are in strong LD.

Genotype and allele frequency distribution analysis of the VDR FokI, BsmI, and TaqI polymorphisms showed no statistically significant difference between cases and controls, whereas haplotype analysis indicated that the TAC haplotype might be associated with decreased cluster headache susceptibility.

Intra-patient analysis according to diverse clinical phenotypes showed an association of the BsmI GG and TaqI TT genotypes with more frequent occurrence of CH attacks in this cohort.

A possible association was observed between VDR gene polymorphisms BsmI and TaqI or a linked locus and susceptibility for cluster headache development and altered clinical phenotypes in the Southeastern European Caucasian study population.

Extended:

Cluster headache (CH) is a relatively rare neurovascular disorder, with a complex pathophysiology that is not completely understood [185].

Cluster headache (CH) is a primary headache disorder and represents the most common type of the trigeminal autonomic cephalalgias (TACs) [1, 49].

Linkage disequilibrium (LD) and haplotype analysis was performed using SHEsis online software (http://analysis.bio-x.cn).

**Introduction**

The occurrence of VDR and other enzymes and proteins related to the vitamin D metabolic pathway in brain areas implicated in the pathophysiology of primary headaches, and particularly the hypothalamus [186, 187], suggests that vitamin D may be involved in the pathogenesis of these disorders [188].

Considering the crucial role of nuclear VDR in mediating the majority of $1,25(OH)_2D_3$ genomic effects and its occurrence in brain areas, particularly the hypothalamus, VDR might represent a candidate gene for susceptibility to primary headaches, including CH.

The implication of VDR gene polymorphisms in CH pathogenesis has not been previously investigated, although one study in an Iranian population investigated the association between VDR polymorphisms and migraine susceptibility [189].

The aim of the current case–control study was to investigate the possible association of three common SNPs of the gene encoding for the vitamin D receptor (VDR), i.e., rs2228570 (FokI), rs1544410 (BsmI) and rs731236 (TaqI), with susceptibility to developing CH and its clinical characteristics, in a Southeastern European Caucasian (SEC) population.

## Subjects and Methods

The population of this prospective, case–control study consisted of 131 unrelated cluster headache patients of SEC origin, aged 22 to 68 years (mean ± standard deviation age: 41.56 ± 10.24 years; 74.0% male), and 281 unrelated non-headache control subjects, aged 21 to 85 years (mean ± standard deviation age: 57.30 ± 13.20 years; 49.5% male), matched with the case subjects for geographical origin.

During patients' regular clinic visit, buccal swab samples and detailed information on demographics and clinical characteristics of CH, including age at diagnosis, frequency of attacks, family history of CH, alcohol consumption, and smoking habits were collected.

The genotype and allele frequency distribution of VDR polymorphisms in CH patients and control subjects were compared using chi-square ($\chi^2$) (Pearson and Fischer's exact) tests under co-dominant, dominant, over-dominant, recessive genotypic and allelic inheritance models.

Accordance of each polymorphism genotype frequency distribution with the Hardy–Weinberg equilibrium (HWE) in control subjects was assessed using the web-based Online Encyclopedia for Genetic Epidemiology studies software [181].

## Results

In the episodic CH group of patients (N = 90), 43 subjects (47.8%) were homozygous (CC) for the C allele, 35 (38.9%) were heterozygous and 12 (13.3%) were homozygous (TT) for the T allele, whereas 23 (56.1%) subjects were CC homozygous, 17 (41.5%) were heterozygous and 1 (2.4%) subject was TT homozygous in the chronic CH group (N = 41).

The FokI TT genotype was more prevalent in episodic compared to chronic CH patients (TT vs. TC + CC: OR 6.326 95% CI 0.792–50.523, P = 0.082; CC vs. TT: OR 0.151, 95% CI 0.018–1.242, P = 0.079).

A more frequent occurrence of CH attacks (≥ 4 attacks/day) was observed in patients carrying the BsmI GG genotype (GG vs. GA + AA: OR 0.343, 95% CI 0.144–0.816, P = 0.016).

## Discussion

The current case–control study examined the association of the three most widely studied SNPs in the gene encoding for VDR, FokI (rs2228570), BsmI (rs1544410), and TaqI (rs731236), with susceptibility to developing CH and diverse clinical phenotypes of this primary headache disorder in a SEC population.

The results of the stratified analysis according to clinical characteristics indicated that BsmI GG and TaqI TT genotypes were associated with more frequent occurrence of CH attacks, thus these VDR polymorphisms may serve as genetic susceptibility factors for altered CH phenotypes.

Several recent studies indicate an association between low serum vitamin D levels and headache disorders, particularly migraine, but only one recent study has examined the correlation between serum vitamin D levels and CH, despite its characteristic seasonal periodicity.

Vitamin D/VDR may be implicated in CH pathological mechanisms due to its ability to regulate the transcription activity of various genes by controlling the epigenetic landscape of gene promoters and affect phenotypic stability [190].

## Conclusion

The data of the current study provide supportive evidence that VDR may serve as a disease modifier gene in CH patients with SEC origin, although did not support the hypothesis for an association between the examined VDR gene polymorphisms and CH susceptibility, at a statistically significant threshold.

This is the first study examining the relationship between common VDR gene polymorphisms and CH susceptibility and clinical phenotypes in a Southeastern European Caucasian population.

Studies investigating additional VDR gene polymorphisms, considering gene–gene and gene–environment interactions as well as vitamin D levels, are needed to further understand the role of vitamin D/VDR signaling in CH pathogenesis and progression, in SEC and other populations.

## Acknowledgement

*A machine generated summary based on the work of Papasavva, Maria; Vikelis, Michail; Siokas, Vasileios; Katsarou, Martha-Spyridoula; Dermitzakis, Emmanouil; Raptis, Athanasios; Dardiotis, Efthimios; Drakoulis, Nikolaos. 2021 in Journal of Molecular Neuroscience.*

# *Implications for the Migraine SNP rs1835740 in a Swedish Cluster Headache Population*

DOI: https://doi.org/10.1186/s10194-018-0937-0

## Abstract-Summary

Genetic factors have been implicated in both migraine and cluster headache.

In order to determine whether or not migraine and cluster headache share genetic risk factors, we screened two genetic variants known to increase the risk of migraine in Sweden in a Swedish cluster headache case-control study population.

We found a trend for association between rs1835740, which is reported to affect MTDH mRNA levels, and cluster headache in our Swedish case-control material ($p = 0.043$, $X^2 = 4.102$).

This association was stronger in a subgroup of patients suffering from both cluster headache and migraine ($p = 0.031$, $X^2 = 6.964$).

In this Swedish cluster headache cohort we did not find an association with the rs2651899 variant.

We conclude that rs1835740 is a potential risk factor for cluster headache in Sweden.

Our data indicates that rs1835740 and MTDH might be involved in neurovascular headaches in general whilst rs2651899 is specifically related to migraine.

Extended:

We conclude that rs1835740 in MTDH is associated not only with migraine but also with CH, whilst rs2651899 in PRDM16 seems to be specifically related to migraine in Sweden.

## Background

Migraine and cluster headache (CH) are two primary headache disorders that share pathological features and a majority of CH patients are successfully treated with drugs used for migraine, such as triptans [1, 29, 96, 191].

There are also phenotypic similarities between CH and migraine, such as recurring attacks of headache, lateralized pain and associated autonomic symptoms [1, 29].

There are marked differences in the clinical manifestations and associated symptoms between migraine and CH.

Genetic factors are likely to influence the risk of developing both migraine and CH [192].

The aim of this study was to investigate whether migraine and CH might share genetic determinants since similar pathophysiological events occur in both disorders.

Analysis of the distribution of the genetic migraine markers rs2651899 and rs1853740 has not previously been performed in CH.

We therefore screened a large Swedish CH case-control population and performed an association analysis of these two markers that have been shown to increase the risk for migraine in Sweden.

## Material and Methods

The material consisted of 541 CH cases and 581 controls where 571 of the controls were anonymous healthy blood donors, these samples were obtained from local blood donation centres in 2003–2005.

Medical journals of all 541 CH patients were reviewed by a neurologist (one of the co-authors A.S., E.W. or C.S.) in order to confirm the diagnosis according to the International Classification of Headache Disorders (ICHD-II) [193].

23 of the CH cases were obtained from the TwinGene study, conducted between 2004 and 2008, the procedure of identifying individuals with cluster headache, blood sampling, genotyping and quality control of the array data has been described in previous publications [5, 194].

Primary fibroblast cell lines derived from 12 CH patients and 12 control subjects were obtained from skin biopsies performed on the inside of research subjects' upper arm.

## Results

Both the TT and the CT genotypes were more common in patients than controls, but there was no significant genotypic association.

Since these two SNPs are known to influence the risk of migraine, and many CH patients in our material also suffer from migraine, we performed a stratified analysis with respect to migraine.

When comparing the allele and genotype frequencies, the mutated allele became increasingly more common in the group of patients suffering from both CH and migraine; 21.1% in CH patients and 26.2% in CH patients with migraine, as compared to the control group where the MAF was 18.5%.

The genetic association discovered here between CH and rs1835740, in combination with the discovery study reporting that rs1835740 potentially affects the expression levels of the MTDH gene lead us to also investigate the MTDH mRNA expression levels in a subset of patients and controls [195].

## Discussion and Conclusion

A more detailed analysis of rs1835740 revealed that the association was even stronger in a subgroup of patients that have both CH and migraine.

In a former GWAS suggesting MTDH as a candidate gene for migraine, the effect of the rs1835740 association was stronger in a subgroup of patients suffering from migraine with aura (MA) than in patients with migraine without aura (MO), which is also an indication of this SNP being associated with more complex headache phenotypes [195].

In a study on rs1835740 and migraine by Azimova and others (2015) small groups of CH patients (n = 9) and chronic tension type headache patients (n = 20) were used as control groups.

We studied the MTDH mRNA levels in individuals with different rs1835740 genotype, and also analyzed expression with respect to CH diagnosis.

## Acknowledgement

*A machine generated summary based on the work of Ran, Caroline; Fourier, Carmen; Zinnegger, Margret; Steinberg, Anna; Sjöstrand, Christina; Waldenlind, Elisabet; Belin, Andrea Carmine. 2018 in The Journal of Headache and Pain.*

# Clinical Symptoms of Androgen Deficiency in Men with Migraine or Cluster Headache: A Cross-sectional Cohort Study

DOI: https://doi.org/10.1186/s10194-021-01334-3

## Abstract-Summary

To compare symptoms of clinical androgen deficiency between men with migraine, men with cluster headache and non-headache male controls.

We performed a cross-sectional study using two validated questionnaires to assess symptoms of androgen deficiency in males with migraine, cluster headache, and non-headache controls.

As secondary outcome we assessed the percentage of patients reporting to score below average on four sexual symptoms (beard growth, morning erections, libido and sexual potency) as these items were previously shown to more specifically differentiate androgen deficiency symptoms from (comorbid) anxiety and depression.

Patients reported more severe symptoms of clinical androgen deficiency compared with controls, with higher AMS scores (Aging Males Symptoms; mean difference ± SE: migraine $5.44 ± 0.90$, $p < 0.001$; cluster headache $5.62 ± 0.99$, $p < 0.001$) and lower qADAM scores (quantitative Androgen Deficiency in the Aging Male; migraine: $−3.16 ± 0.50$, $p < 0.001$; cluster headache: $−5.25 ± 0.56$, $p < 0.001$).

Both patient groups more often reported to suffer from any of the specific sexual symptoms compared to controls (18.4% migraine, 20.6% cluster headache, 7.2% controls, $p = 0.001$).

Men with migraine and cluster headache more often suffer from symptoms consistent with clinical androgen deficiency than males without a primary headache disorder.

Extended:
We performed a cross-sectional questionnaire study among men with migraine, men with cluster headache and male controls without headache.

Men with migraine (episodic or chronic) or cluster headache (episodic or chronic) that fulfilled the International Classification of Headache Disorders (ICHD-3) criteria, and men without a primary or secondary headache disorder (apart from an occasional episodic tension-type headache), who gave written informed consent to be contacted in case of future research, were identified.

## Introduction

With migraine being a predominantly female disease, a limited number of studies has investigated sex hormones in men, but one small scale study showed a decreased testosterone/estradiol ratio in males with migraine [196].

Recent studies show that cluster headache occurs in women more often than previously assumed with a male to female ratio of 2:1 [197].

Calcitonin gene-related peptide (CGRP) is known to be involved in the pathophysiology of migraine and cluster headache.

As relative androgen deficiency has been suggested in men with migraine, but may play a role in cluster headache as well, we aimed to compare symptoms of clinical androgen deficiency between male migraine and cluster headache patients and controls.

## Methods

Migraine and cluster headache patients were first asked to fill out a validated web-based screening questionnaire with a sensitivity of 0.93 and specificity of 0.36 for migraine, and a sensitivity of 1.00 and specificity of 0.58 for cluster headache [198, 199].

Patients who fulfilled the screening criteria for migraine or cluster headache, were sent a validated web-based extended migraine or cluster headache questionnaire, based on the International Classification of Headache Disorders criteria (previously ICHD-2, now ICHD-3 version) criteria [1].

As both the AMS and qADAM questionnaire contain multiple items associated with anxiety and depression, which are more prevalent in chronic headache disorders, we performed a secondary analysis determining the number of patients reporting to score below average ($\geq 4$) on four selected items of the AMS scale regarding sexual symptoms (beard growth, morning erections, libido and sexual potency).

## Results

The mean AMS scores were higher in patients with migraine compared to controls (mean difference $\pm$ SE: $5.44 \pm 0.90$, $p < 0.001$), and cluster headache compared to controls ($5.62 \pm 0.99$, $p < 0.001$).

Mean qADAM scores were lower in patients with migraine compared to controls ($-3.16 \pm 0.50$, $p < 0.001$), and cluster headache compared to controls ($-5.25 \pm 0.56$, $p < 0.001$).

Men with episodic cluster headache out of bout still scored higher on the AMS ($4.72 \pm 1.04$, $p < 0.001$) and lower on qADAM ($-4.62 \pm 0.58$, $p < 0.001$) than non-headache controls.

## Discussion

This cross-sectional study shows that men with migraine and cluster headache more often suffer from symptoms consistent with (relative) clinical androgen deficiency than males without a primary headache disorder.

Our study shows that patients with migraine and cluster headache suffer more frequently and more severely from these symptoms than men without headache.

A recent study in male migraine patients showed symptoms of a relative androgen deficiency with a higher estradiol/testosterone ratio compared to controls, which was attributed to higher estradiol levels [196].

These presumed differences in estradiol/testosterone ratios may be responsible for the symptomatology described in the present study, which would strengthen the hypothesis of hormonal imbalances in men with migraine and cluster headache.

Our study shows that men with migraine and cluster headache more frequently report symptomatology consistent with androgen deficiency than males without a primary headache disorder.

## Acknowledgement

*A machine generated summary based on the work of Verhagen, Iris E.; Brandt, Roemer B.; Kruitbosch, Carlijn M. A.; MaassenVanDenBrink, Antoinette; Fronczek, Rolf; Terwindt, Gisela M. 2021 in The Journal of Headache and Pain.*

# *Alterations of Thalamic Nuclei Volumes in Patients with Cluster Headache*

DOI: https://doi.org/10.1007/s00234-022-02951-8

## Abstract-Summary

This study aimed to compare the alterations of thalamic nuclei volumes and the intrinsic thalamic network in patients with cluster headache and healthy controls.

We calculated the thalamic nuclei volumes in the patients with cluster headache and healthy controls based on three-dimensional T1-weighted imaging with automated segmentation using the FreeSurfer program.

We compared the thalamic nuclei volumes and intrinsic thalamic networks in patients with cluster headaches and healthy controls.

The right and left whole thalamic volumes did not differ in the patients with cluster headaches and healthy controls (0.4199 vs. 0.4069%, p = 0.2008; 0.4386 vs. 0.4273%, p = 0.3437; respectively).

There were significant alterations of right and left medial geniculate nuclei volumes in the patients with cluster headaches and the healthy controls.

The right and left medial geniculate nuclei volumes of the patients with cluster headaches were greater than those of the healthy controls (0.0088 vs. 0.0075%, p < 0.0001; 0.0086 vs. 0.0072%, p < 0.0001; respectively).

This study demonstrates significant alterations in the bilateral medial geniculate nuclei volumes in patients with cluster headache compared to healthy controls.

Extended:

The right and left medial geniculate nuclei volumes of the patients with cluster headache were greater than those of the healthy controls (0.0088 vs. 0.0075%, p < 0.0001; 0.0086 vs. 0.0072%, p < 0.0001; respectively).

There were significant differences between the right and left medial geniculate nuclei volumes of the groups.

The right and left whole thalamic volumes of the patients with cluster headache and healthy controls were not different (0.4199 vs. 0.4069%, p = 0.2008; 0.4386 vs. 0.4273%, p = 0.3437; respectively).

## Introduction

Although the exact pathophysiology of cluster headache is unknown, several studies have demonstrated that the trigeminovascular system, parasympathetic system, hypothalamus, and pain network all play a role in cluster headache pathogenesis [121, 200–204].

Although the results of each study are slightly different, numerous findings have been reported in patients with cluster headache, including the following: (1) structural and functional changes in the pain network, which are dynamic during the in-bout and out-of-bout phases [20, 138, 139]; (2) hypothalamic activation during acute headache attacks, which tends to reverse outside of acute attacks [205]; and (3) extensive brain network changes outside of the hypothalamus, including the forebrain, cerebellum, and occipital cortex [206].

Structural and functional changes in the pain network, which includes the thalamus, sensorimotor cortex, and parietal lobe, may contribute significantly to the pathophysiology of cluster headache [20, 207].

The purpose of this study was to compare the volume of thalamic nuclei and the intrinsic thalamic network in cluster headache patients and healthy controls.

We hypothesized that patients with cluster headache would have significant changes in the volume of thalamic nuclei or the intrinsic thalamic network compared to healthy controls.

## Methods

We previously described the detailed method for calculating the whole and individual thalamic nuclei volumes using the FreeSurfer program, version 7.0 [208].

We defined the nodes as individual thalamic nuclei volumes and edges as their partial correlation after controlling for the effects of age and sex on them.

We performed correlation analysis between the thalamic nuclei volumes showing abnormalities in volumes and clinical characteristics in patients with cluster headache using Pearson's method.

We set a p-value of 0.001 (0.05/50 = 0.001, 50 numbers of thalamic nuclei, Bonferroni corrections) for the analysis of the thalamic nuclei volume differences between the two groups.

For intrinsic thalamic network analysis, a p-value of 0.004 (0.05/12 = 0.006, 12 numbers of network measures, Bonferroni corrections) was considered to denote statistical significance.

## Results

The age and sex of the patients with cluster headache and healthy controls were not different (40 vs. 40 years, p = 0.865; 19/24 vs. 20/24, p = 1.000; respectively).

The right and left whole thalamic volumes of the patients with cluster headache and healthy controls were not different (0.4199 vs. 0.4069%, p = 0.2008; 0.4386 vs. 0.4273%, p = 0.3437; respectively).

The right and left medial geniculate nuclei volumes of the patients with cluster headache were greater than those of the healthy controls (0.0088 vs. 0.0075%, p < 0.0001; 0.0086 vs. 0.0072%, p < 0.0001; respectively).

There were no differences between the measures of the intrinsic thalamic network of the patients with cluster headache and healthy controls.

## Discussion

This study successfully demonstrated that patients with cluster headache have significant changes in the bilateral medial geniculate nuclei volumes in the thalamus.

The volumes of the right and left medial geniculate nuclei were greater in cluster headache patients than in healthy controls.

This is the first study to examine changes in the volumes of individual thalamic nuclei and intrinsic thalamic networks in patients with cluster headache compared to healthy controls.

We concentrated on the thalamus as one of the subcortical regions associated with pain modulation in this study and discovered significant volume changes in bilateral medial geniculate nuclei in patients with cluster headache.

The volume differences between the bilateral medial geniculate nuclei in the thalamus of patients with cluster headache were successfully demonstrated; however, this study has several limitations.

**Conclusion**
This study demonstrates significant alterations in the bilateral medial geniculate nuclei volumes in patients with cluster headache compared to healthy controls.

These alterations may be related to the pathophysiology of cluster headache.

**Acknowledgement**
*A machine generated summary based on the work of Lee, Dong Ah; Lee, Ho-Joon; Park, Kang Min. 2022 in Neuroradiology.*

# *Alterations of the Structural Covariance Network in the Hypothalamus of Patients with Cluster Headache*

DOI: https://doi.org/10.1007/s00415-021-10629-z

**Abstract-Summary**
This study aimed to analyze the volume of hypothalamic subunits and structural covariance networks in the hypothalamus of patients with cluster headache.

We compared the volumes of hypothalamic subunits and structural covariance networks in the hypothalamus of patients with cluster headache versus those of healthy controls.

There were no significant differences in the structural volumes of the whole hypothalamus and hypothalamic subunits between patients with cluster headache and healthy controls.

Patients with cluster headache had significant alterations of the structural covariance network in the hypothalamus compared to that of healthy controls.

The network measure of small-worldness index in patients with cluster headache was lower than that in healthy controls (0.844 vs. 0.955, p = 0.004).

We demonstrated a significant difference in the structural covariance network in the hypothalamus of patients with cluster headache versus those of healthy controls.

Extended:

This study aimed to analyze the volumes of hypothalamic subunits and evaluate the structural covariance network in the hypothalamus based on its structural volumes in patients with cluster headache compared with those of healthy controls.

These findings could be related to the pathogenesis of cluster headache.

## Introduction

One of the assumptions concerning the pathophysiology of cluster headache is the activation of the trigemino-vascular system, the parasympathetic nervous system, and the hypothalamus.

Previous studies using brain magnetic resonance imaging (MRI) have discovered evidence of a central origin in the pathophysiology of cluster headaches.

We have also identified the alteration of local connectivity in numerous brain structures in patients with cluster headache in a previous study [209].

A lot of studies have suggested that the hypothalamus is one of the key structures involved in the pathophysiology of cluster headaches [121].

A positron emission tomography-based study identified hypothalamic activation during spontaneous and triggered cluster headache attacks [121], while a voxel-based morphometry study found volume alterations of the anterior hypothalamus in patients with cluster headaches [210].

This study aimed to analyze the volumes of hypothalamic subunits and evaluate the structural covariance network in the hypothalamus based on its structural volumes in patients with cluster headache compared with those of healthy controls.

## Methods

We enrolled patients with episodic cluster headache based on the following inclusion criteria: (1) clinical diagnosis of cluster headache according to the ICHD-3 [1], (2) availability of three-dimensional T1-weighted imaging suitable for volumetric analysis; (3) no structural lesions in the brain MRI; and (4) no history of any other neurological or medical diseases except for cluster headache.

It was built for each group as a collection of nodes representing brain regions (individual volumes of the hypothalamic subunits), connected by edges corresponding to the connections between them (calculated as partial correlation coefficients between every pair of brain regions while controlling for the effects of age and sex).

In the comparative analysis of structural volume and structural covariance network in the hypothalamus between the two groups, we applied Bonferroni multiple corrections (right and left hypothalamus, $p = 0.05/2$; right and left five hypothalamic subunits, $p = 0.05/10$; ten structural covariance network measures, $p = 0.05/10$).

## Results

Age and sex did not significantly differ between patients with cluster headache and healthy controls.

No significant differences in the structural volumes of the whole hypothalamus and hypothalamic subunits, including anterior-inferior, anterior-superior, posterior, inferior-tubular, and superior-tubular, were found between the patients with cluster headache and healthy controls.

Patients with cluster headache had significant alterations of the structural covariance network in the hypothalamus compared to that of healthy controls.

The network measure of small-worldness index in patients with cluster headache was lower than that in healthy controls (0.844 vs. 0.955, $p = 0.004$).

**Discussion**

The main finding of this study was that there were statistically significant alterations in the structural covariance network in the hypothalamus of patients with cluster headache, compared to that of healthy controls.

This study is the first to analyze the volumes of the hypothalamic subunits and structural covariance network in the hypothalamus of patients with cluster headache.

Especially using graph theory, we found significant alterations of the structural covariance network in the hypothalamus of patients with cluster headache compared to that of healthy controls.

No significant differences in the structural covariance network of the whole brain were found between patients with cluster headache and healthy controls.

Although we successfully demonstrated the differences in the structural covariance network in the hypothalamus of patients with cluster headache, this study has several limitations.

**Conclusion**

We investigated the differences in volumes of the hypothalamic subunits and the structural covariance network of the hypothalamus between patients with cluster headache and healthy controls.

We successfully demonstrated a significant alteration of the structural covariance network in the hypothalamus of patients with cluster headache compared to that of healthy controls.

**Acknowledgement**

*A machine generated summary based on the work of Lee, Dong Ah; Lee, Ho-Joon; Kim, Hyung Chan; Park, Kang Min. 2021 in Journal of Neurology.*


## *Changes in Grey Matter Volume and Functional Connectivity in Cluster Headache Versus Migraine*

DOI: https://doi.org/10.1007/s11682-019-00046-2

**Abstract-Summary**

Multimodal MRI was acquired in attack-free patients with CH (n = 12), Mig (n = 13) and in normal controls (NC, n = 13).

CH showed lower grey matter (GM) volume, compared to Mig and NC, in frontal cortex regions (inferior frontal gyrus and frontal pole [FP], respectively) and, only compared to Mig, in lateral occipital cortex (LOC).

Functional connectivity (FC) of CH was higher than Mig and NC within working memory and executive control networks and, only compared to Mig, between cerebellar and auditory language comprehension networks.

In the attack-free state, the CH brain seems to be characterized by: (i) GM volume decrease, compared to both Mig and NC, in pain modulation regions (FP) and, only with respect to Mig, in a region of visual processing modulation during pain and working memory (LOC); (ii) increased FC at short range compared to both Mig and NC and at long range only with respect to Mig, in key cognitive networks, likely due to maladaptation towards more severe pain experience.

Extended:

Our results, which are highly significant in statistical terms, are in favor of the occurrence of real differences in GM volumes and connectivity among the three study groups and, therefore, strongly indicate that additional research should be carried out in the future.

## Introduction

Cluster headache (CH) and migraine (Mig) are distinct and potentially disabling primary headaches, accompanied by sensory, cognitive and emotional dysfunction ((IHS) [60]), supporting a diffuse involvement of the brain.

A more severe clinical picture than Mig characterizes CH, with excruciatingly painful, mostly unilateral headache attacks typically accompanied by trigeminal autonomic symptoms.

Except a study assessing hypothalamic GM volume (Arkink and others [210]), no direct comparison has been performed between CH and Mig patients to assess differences in both structural and functional brain changes.

Multimodal and advanced MRI techniques investigating both structural and functional features across the brain could help elucidate whether a different pathophysiology between these two headache types really exists, with the potential to help identify new therapeutic targets.

Using this background, we sought to investigate, at both structural and functional levels, the brain changes explaining the more severe clinical picture in CH compared to Mig.

## Methods

A high-resolution T1-weighted image (TR = 10 ms, TE = 4 ms, voxel size = 1 mm$^3$) was also acquired for image registration, anatomical mapping, and analysis of GM volume.

Voxelwise analysis of GM volumes was performed on 3D T1-weighted images with FSL-voxel based morphometry (VBM), which uses an optimized VBM protocol.

Various preprocessing steps were performed for each resting FMRI image: removal of the first 5 volumes to allow signal stability; initial motion correction by volume-realignment to the middle volume using linear registration MCFLIRT (Jenkinson and Smith [211]); non-brain removal using BET; global 4D mean intensity normalization; spatial smoothing (6 mm FWHM); registration to the T1-weighted image using the affine "boundary-based registration" cost of FLIRT(Jenkinson and Smith [211]), and subsequent transformation to MNI152 standard space using FNIRT nonlinear registration (warp resolution: 10 mm); use of ICA-AROMA (independent component analysis-based automatic removal of motion artifacts) in order to minimize motion-related artifacts (Pruim and others [212]); regression of WM and cerebrospinal fluid (CSF) (both thresholded at a very conservative threshold of 95% tissue probability) in order to remove residual structured noise; application of a high-pass temporal filtering (cut-off frequency = 100 s); final normalization to MNI152 standard space using FNIRT.

## Results

In terms of short-range functional connectivity, this was higher in CH than in NC in various brain networks, including the working memory network (inferior frontal gyrus, $17.2 \pm 13.5$ vs $-2.3 \pm 2.4$, p = 0.001), executive control network (superior frontal gyrus, $8.05 \pm 7.37$ vs $-2.6 \pm 5.07$, p < 0.001) and default mode network (superior parietal lobule, $9.67 \pm 6.2$ vs $-2.6 \pm 5.2$, p < 0.001).

Mig showed, with respect to NC, altered functional connectivity in the default mode network, with lateral increase (angular gyrus, $11.2 \pm 7.8$ vs $-2.49 \pm 5.1$, p < 0.001) and medial decrease (precuneous cortex, $-8.7 \pm 6.76$ vs $6.4 \pm 9.5$, p < 0.001), and lower functional connectivity in the working memory network (middle frontal gyrus, $-0.5 \pm 3.4$ vs $7.6 \pm 7.6$, p = 0.001).

## Discussion

CH, compared to NC and Mig, showed decreased regional GM volume in the frontal cortex, a traditional pain processing area, higher short-range functional connectivity in networks subserving working memory and executive functions and, only compared to Mig, higher long-range functional connectivity in language comprehension networks.

We showed that higher short-range functional connectivity in CH than in both NC and Mig mapped on regions of the prefrontal cortex, which were part of the working memory network (inferior and middle frontal gyrus, respectively) and executive control network (superior frontal gyrus and frontal pole, respectively).

The higher long-range functional connectivity between the cerebellar network and auditory language comprehension network mirror the findings of higher short-range functional connectivity in the working memory network and executive control network of CH compared to Mig and, overall, they may reflect a "maladaptive" (i.e., worsening) process.

## Acknowledgement

*A machine generated summary based on the work of Giorgio, Antonio; Lupi, Chiara; Zhang, Jian; De Cesaris, Francesco; Alessandri, Mario; Mortilla, Marzia; Federico, Antonio; Geppetti, Pierangelo; De Stefano, Nicola; Benemei, Silvia. 2019 in Brain Imaging and Behavior.*

## Diagnosis

Machine generated keywords: depression, cluster, anxiety, registry, ech, cch, state, hit, search, impact, psychological, hospital, aspect, sleep, migraine patient

# Cluster Headache and TACs: State of the Art

DOI: https://doi.org/10.1007/s10072-020-04639-4

## Abstract-Summary

Cluster headache (CH), paroxysmal hemicrania (PH), short-lasting unilateral neuralgiform headache attacks (including SUNCT and SUNA), and hemicrania continua (HC) compose the group of trigeminal autonomic cephalalgias (TACs).

We review the recent advances in the field and summarize the current knowledge about the origin of these headaches.

Similar to the other primary headaches, the pathogenesis is still much obscure.

## Introduction

Trigeminal autonomic cephalalgias (TACs) share the presentation of unilateral head pain associated with ipsilateral autonomic cranial phenomena [1].

Different syndromes are recognized, mainly differentiated by the duration and frequency of the headaches: cluster headache (CH), paroxysmal hemicrania (PH), short-lasting unilateral neuralgiform headache attacks (including the subtypes with both conjunctival injection and tearing (SUNCT), or not (SUNA)), and hemicrania continua (HC) [1].

Components from both the central and the peripheral nervous systems are involved in the generation of headache attacks in TACs.

## Trigeminal Autonomic Cephalalgias

The other TACs, namely PH, SUNCT/SUNA, and HC, are rarer than CH, and proper epidemiological investigations are lacking.

CH attacks have the longest duration, up to 3 h, and a lower frequency compared with SUNCT/SUNA and PH.

PH has an intermediate duration of attacks (from 2 to 30 min) and frequency, and a positive response to indomethacin is a major diagnostic criterion [213].

The duration of attacks can overlap between different TAC forms: as per definition, SUNCT attacks can last up to 10 min, thus far exceeding the lower limit for PH attacks (2 min), which in turn can be longer (up to 30 min) than the briefest CH attacks (15–180 min) [1].

An overlap can be found also in this regard: indomethacin can be of some benefit in CH; verapamil and topiramate might be effective in PH and SUNCT; some patients with HC improve with melatonin [214].

## Genetics

Family and twin studies suggest a heritable component for CH [215].

Most genetic studies in CH used a candidate gene approach, based on clinical observations, and supposed mechanisms of the disease.

As nitric oxide (NO) can induce attacks, and has been implicated in the generation of neurovascular headaches, variants of the genes encoding for NO synthases were tested, but an association with CH was not found [216].

Variants of the P-/Q-type calcium channel alpha 1 subunit (CACNA1A), which can cause various neurological disorders, comprising familial hemiplegic migraine, were not associated with CH [217].

A variant of the hypocretin receptor type 2 (HCRTR2) was associated with increased risk of CH [218], but this result could not be replicated in other studies [166, 179].

Despite epidemiological observations strongly suggesting the presence of shared genetic susceptibility factors, various genetic variants associated with CH have faced lack of reproducibility and conflicting results.

**The Central Nervous System**

Derangements in the secretion of a number of hypothalamus-controlled hormones, including cortisol and thyrotropin, have been reported in CH patients suggesting a hypothalamic dysfunction [202].

The observation of increased metabolic activity in the posterior hypothalamus during CH attacks confirmed its role in CH pathophysiology [121] and gave support for the development of hypothalamic deep brain stimulation (DBS) for the treatment of intractable chronic CH [219] resulting effective in 60–70% of the patients [220].

A peak of activity in local field potentials at around 20 Hz was registered in the posterior hypothalamus at the onset of CH attacks in patients implanted for DBS [221].

Bartsch and others observed the onset of a CH attack during a trial stimulation of the posterior hypothalamus at 130 Hz [222]; on the contrary, the acute stimulation could not terminate ongoing attacks [223].

Imaging studies demonstrated activation of the posterior hypothalamus also during attacks of PH [224], SUNCT [225], and HC [226].

In animals, the posterior hypothalamus modulates nociceptive activity in the trigeminal nucleus caudalis and trigeminocervical complex (TCC) [227] using orexins and GABA as neuromodulators (among the others) [227].

Sumatriptan is able to terminate CH attacks in patients with sectioned trigeminal nerve [228].

**The Peripheral Nervous System**

A painful stimulation in trigeminal territories and nerve induces a reflex activity in the ipsilateral facial parasympathetic system: the trigeminal-autonomic reflex.

Biomarkers of trigeminal and parasympathetic activation are respectively CGRP and VIP, both increased in the ipsilateral to the pain jugular vein during CH attacks [162]; triptans and oxygen reduce the levels of these neurotransmitters while inducing pain relief [162].

Oxygen could relieve CH by inhibiting the parasympathetic efference resulting in decreased autonomic phenomena and reflex trigeminal activation.

The activation of the parasympathetic facial system by either SPG electrical stimulation or by stimulating the nasal mucosa does not provoke CH attacks [229, 230].

The SPG activation is hypothesized to increase the trigeminal activity and pain in CH, but after SPG radiofrequency ablation, some CH patients report improvement of autonomic phenomena without changes of their headaches [231].

PACAP may be of particular interest in TACs, as it co-localizes with VIP in parasympathetic second-order neurons in the SPG and otic ganglia and with CGRP in sensory neurons in the trigeminal ganglia [232].

## Some Considerations About Pain in Cluster Headache

What, where, how, and why originates the pain in CH?

Even if the pain is the fundamental symptom of headache in CH and other TACs, it still remains a mystery and a matter of controversy [233].

Animal studies have shown that the posterior hypothalamus, activated during CH and other TACS, modulates nociception and sensitization at TCC level [227].

Modulation of thresholds in these three systems, trigeminal system, parasympathetic system, and posterior hypothalamus, probably is the key process in CH and other TACs.

It has to be emphasized that the activation of the parasympathetic craniofacial system is not painful per se and does not induce CH attacks [229, 230].

The persistence of CH attacks in patients whose trigeminal and SPG activity have been surgically interrupted suggests that the pain in CH may arise from within the brain itself [228, 234, 235].

## Acknowledgement

*A machine generated summary based on the work of Giani, Luca; Proietti Cecchini, Alberto; Leone, Massimo. 2020 in Neurological Sciences.*

# *Migraine and Cluster Headache—The Common Link*

DOI: https://doi.org/10.1186/s10194-018-0909-4

## Abstract-Summary

Although clinically distinguishable, migraine and cluster headache share prominent features such as unilateral pain, common pharmacological triggers such glyceryl trinitrate, histamine, calcitonin gene-related peptide (CGRP) and response to triptans and neuromodulation.

We review past and current literature shedding light on similarities and differences in phenotype, heritability, pathophysiology, imaging findings and treatment options of migraine and cluster headache.

A continued focus on their shared pathophysiological pathways may be important in paving future treatment avenues that could benefit both migraine and cluster headache patients.

Extended:

Future studies will show whether migraine and CH shares the involvement of PACAP signalling in pathophysiology.

**Background**

In the field of cephalalgias, migraine has a prominent role (35,311 publications retrieved for search terms "migraine" in PubMed, accessed on August 15, 2018), with the recent breakthrough in therapeutics, represented by the successful clinical development of calcitonin gene-related peptide (CGRP) antibodies [236].

In the last 40 years, the number of papers published yearly for cluster headache (CH) has been constantly increasing (3845 publications retrieved for search terms "cluster headache" in PubMed, accessed on August 15, 2018), and new evidence is accumulating about epidemiology, including gender issues, pathophysiology and imaging.

The clinical continuum that unexpectedly but not infrequently characterizes migraine and CH patients increases the value of such a comparison between the two diseases.

**Epidemiology and Genetics in Migraine and Cluster Headache**

The risk of first-degree relatives of patients with CH to develop CH is between five and fifteen times greater than that of the general population [118].

In migraine, first-degree relatives of patients have a 3-fold increase in migraine, compared to the general population [237].

Rare monogenic migraine subtypes can be caused by precise genetic mutations, as in the case of familial hemiplegic migraine; a rare genetic disorder with dominant autosomal transmission due to mutations of three main genes (CACNA1A, ATP1A2 and the sodium channel 1 A SCN1A) [238].

Several studies have failed to identify any association between genetic variants and common forms of migraine indicating that autosomal-dominant inheritance is unlikely, unless the penetrance of the gene is very low.

The mode of inheritance is likely to be different between migraine and CH, and whether some genetic traits are shared between the two disorders is unknown.

**Pathophysiology**

Positron emission tomography (PET) imaging studies showed increased dorsal pons activation in migraine patients during the ictal phase [239].

Functional magnetic resonance imaging (fMRI) studies reported increased functional connectivity between the cortical and subcortical regions involved in nociceptive processing and the PAG [240, 241], having connections coming from the thalamus, hypothalamus, and autonomic nervous system [242].

In cluster headache patients, during active phase, and on the headache side, a pronounced lack of habituation of the brainstem and a general sensitization of pain processing is seen [243].

fMRI studies report a role of the hypothalamus in pain modulation during the pre-ictal phase of attacks in migraine patients.

To the above-mentioned studies involving brainstem and hypothalamus, patients with primary headaches experience dynamic structural [244] and functional [245] changes in cortical-subcortical areas involved in nociception.

In migraine, fMRI and resting-state fMRI studies show marked abnormalities both ictally and interictally in areas involved in nociceptive processing and networks involved in mediating cognitive, attentional, somatosensory and emotional components of pain [240, 246–250], respectively.

## Clinical Picture

Identification and avoidance of attack triggers plays an important role in management of patients with migraine and CH.

The earliest pharmacological provocation studies in migraine and CH patients explored histamine [251–253] and found that histamine infusion, which causes endogenous nitric oxide (NO) formation, induces attacks in both migraine and CH.

In the placebo pretreated group 7 of 10 MwoA patients reported migraine-like attack following histamine infusion compared to 0 of 10 in the mepyramine group.

32 CH patients (9 episodic active phase, 9 episodic remission phase, and 14 chronic) received intravenous infusion of CGRP (1.5 µg/min for 20 min) or placebo in a randomized, double-blind, placebo controlled cross-over study [254].

In episodic remission phase CH patients neither CGRP nor placebo induced any attacks.

## Treatment

A recent randomized placebo-controlled clinical trial on 22 patients reported that high-flow oxygen was significantly more effective than air in the acute treatment of migraine attacks [255], and it has been suggested that this treatment could have greater responses in migraine patients with cranial autonomic symptoms [256] or migraine-cluster and cluster-migraine variants (these rare phenotypes are not included in the ICHD-3).

Different drug categories are effective in the prophylactic treatment of patients affected by episodic or CCH, even though, unlike in migraine, few randomized clinical trials have been conducted [257].

The recent multicenter, double-blind, randomized, sham-controlled PRESTO trial confirmed VNS effective as abortive treatment for migraine attacks, with consistent therapeutic benefit compared to sham stimulation [258].

In a sham controlled randomized trial, single pulse rTMS has been shown to increase in freedom from pain after 2 h when applied early in the treatment of migraine with aura, with substantial benefit for up to 48 h after treatment [259] Although cortical excitability has been implicated in CH [260], to date few data exist on rTMS in CH.

## Conclusions

A key signalling molecule, CGRP, is involved in migraine and CH [261, 262].

The importance of the pituitary adenylate-cyclase activating peptide (PACAP) is well established in migraine [263] and an ongoing phase 2 study is testing the efficacy of a PAC1 receptor antibody for migraine prevention [264].

Future studies will show whether migraine and CH shares the involvement of PACAP signalling in pathophysiology.

## Acknowledgement

*A machine generated summary based on the work of Vollesen, Anne Luise; Benemei, Silvia; Cortese, Francesca; Labastida-Ramírez, Alejandro; Marchese, Francesca; Pellesi, Lanfranco; Romoli, Michele; Ashina, Messoud; Lampl, Christian; on behalf of the School of Advanced Studies of the European Headache Federation (EHF-SAS). 2018 in The Journal of Headache and Pain.*

# Systematic Literature Review on the Delays in the Diagnosis and Misdiagnosis of Cluster Headache

DOI: https://doi.org/10.1007/s10072-018-3598-5

## Abstract-Summary

Patients with cluster headache (CH), the most common trigeminal autonomic cephalalgia, often face delayed diagnosis, misdiagnosis and mismanagement.

To identify, appraise and synthesise clinical studies on the delays in diagnosis and misdiagnosis of CH in order to determine its causes and help the management of this condition.

Nine studies assessed the delays in diagnosis and misdiagnosis of CH, five studies the delays in diagnosis and one study the misdiagnosis of CH.

Delays in diagnosis, misdiagnosis and mismanagement have been reported in many European countries, Japan and in the USA with well-developed health services.

The patients with CH often visited many different clinicians, surgeons and dentists and received multiple diagnosis prior to being correctly diagnosed.

This systematic review shows that the delays in the diagnosis of CH are a widespread problem, the time to diagnosis still vary from country to country and both patients and physicians are responsible for the delays in diagnosis.

Extended:

Delays in diagnosis, misdiagnosis and mismanagement of CH are a widespread problem and have been reported in many countries with well-developed health services, including several European countries, Japan and in the USA.

Future work regarding biomarkers could help in the misdiagnosis and delays in the diagnosis of CH.

## Background

Cluster headache (CH) is the most common of the trigeminal autonomic cephalalgias (TACs) and often described as the most severe pain possible [96].

CH is characterised by attacks of unilateral pain associated with ipsilateral conjunctival injection, lacrimation, nasal congestion, rhinorrhoea, forehead and facial sweating, miosis, ptosis and/or eyelid oedema, and/or with restlessness or agitation [1, 265].

The diagnosis of CH is based entirely on clinical history due to the lack of a diagnostic biomarker.

The aim of this systematic literature review is to identify, appraise and synthesise all relevant clinical studies on the misdiagnosis and delays in the diagnosis of CH.

## Methods

A comprehensive search of different electronic databases was carried out in May 2017 to identify potential studies.

Two authors (AB and JB) independently assessed all titles and abstracts for inclusion.

Two authors (AB and JB) independently assessed all full-text articles and disagreement was resolved by discussion to reach consensus and if needed with the intervention of a third reviewer (FA).

The data was independently extracted by two authors (AB and JB).

The studies were independently assessed by two reviewers (AB and JB) and the discrepancies were resolved through discussion with a third author (FA).

## Results

The studies included a total of 4661 patients, aged 3–81 years, men and women with ECH and CCH.

The articles were excluded as they did not meet the inclusion criteria (the studies were not on delays in diagnosis or misdiagnosis of CH).

In one study performed in the USA, 42% of patients waited more than 5 years to receive a correct diagnosis of cluster headache [10].

Two studies showed a reduction in delay in the diagnosis of CH over time, from 22.3 years (before 1959) to 2.6 years (between 1990 and 1999) in the UK [266] and from 20 years (prior to 1989) to 1 year (between 2010 and 2015) in Greece [49].

Two studies looked at patient's and clinician's delays in the diagnosis of CH [129, 267].

Conducted by Van Vliet and others, the patients with ECH had longer delays in diagnosis compared to CCH patients [268], probably due to longer remission periods.

Patients with CH were often seen by different clinicians before the correct diagnosis was made.

## Discussion

It is evident from the studies that diagnostic delay in CH is not confined to a geographical area.

Only one nationwide survey study performed in the USA that included a sample of 1134 patients was retrieved by our searches and could be considered representative for a large cohort of patients with CH [10].

The studies included in this review showed that patient's delay in diagnosis is as important as clinician's delay [129, 267].

It is possible that clinicians are more aware of trigeminal neuralgia, even though CH is more common (incidence 53/100.000 [158] vs 4.5/100.00 [269]) but there are no studies that validated this.

As CH is a life-long severe and debilitating condition that requires prompt diagnosis and management, it is essential to establish what factors are involved in the diagnostic delay and misdiagnosis.

Future work regarding biomarkers could help in the misdiagnosis and delays in the diagnosis of CH.

## Conclusions

Patients with CH often waited before seeking medical advice and when they did, they visited many clinicians and received multiple misdiagnosis prior to being correctly diagnosed.

The failure to diagnose patients with CH leads to poor management, disability and misuse of healthcare resources.

If a clinician has a suspicion of CH, this should trigger referral to specialised headaches centres for a correct diagnosis and initiation of appropriate treatment and to minimise the wastage of healthcare resources and unnecessary procedures.

## Acknowledgement

*A machine generated summary based on the work of Buture, Alina; Ahmed, Fayyaz; Dikomitis, Lisa; Boland, Jason W. 2018 in Neurological Sciences.*


# *Exploring the Connection Between Sleep and Cluster Headache: A Narrative Review*

DOI: https://doi.org/10.1007/s40122-020-00172-6

## Abstract-Summary

Cluster headache is a rare form of headache associated with sleep and even speculated to be a manifestation of a sleep disorder rather than a primary headache.

While attacks often occur during sleep, the implication that cluster headaches might be involved with rapid eye movement (REM) sleep phases has neither been fully established nor refuted.

While sleep apnea is associated with morning headaches in general, the link between sleep-disordered respiration and cluster headache remains elusive.

Hypoarousal during sleep and periods of hypoxia are associated with cluster headache, the latter likely involving inflammatory processes rather than apnea.

Extended:

Cluster headache is characterized by a paroxysmal onset of severe unilateral typically periorbital pain that often peaks in intensity in a matter of moments; pain can be so severe that the disorder has been nicknamed the "suicide headache" [10, 270].

## Introduction

The International Classification of Sleep Disorders recognizes specific types of sleep-related headache: cluster headache, hypnic headache, chronic paroxysmal hemicrania, and migraine [271].

The relationship between sleep and cluster headache (as well as other headaches) has been known for decades but the underlying neurological mechanisms have yet to be elucidated.

It is particularly challenging to study sleep in cluster headache patients, since prevalence is about 0.1% [272] and attacks are often characterized by wakefulness, agitation, and a desire to pace, making conventional somnographic evaluations very challenging.

The paroxysmal onset of a cluster headache often occurs during sleep [273], and, unlike other forms of sleep-related headaches, cluster headaches exhibit a very pronounced diurnal relationship in addition to a circannual rhythmicitiy [274].

It has been speculated that cluster headache patients may have worse sleep quality than controls or even that cluster headache is the manifestation of a sleep disorder [275].

Unlike migraine headaches, sleep does not relieve cluster headache [276].

## Methods

A few small studies have shown that episodic but not chronic cluster headache patients did indeed suffer attacks during REM sleep, other studies were equivocal or found no evidence of such a relationship [277–279].

In a study of 40 cluster headache patients and 25 matched controls, cluster headache patients had significantly lower REM density (17.3 vs. 23.0%, $p = 0.0037$) and significantly longer sleep latency (2.0 vs. 1.2 h, $p = 0.0012$) although there were no differences in the groups for sleep apnea [98].

Since hypoxia has been observed in cluster headache patients, the role of sleep apnea has been studied with respect to the etiology of cluster headache.

All cluster patients (active and quiet) had a six-fold increased risk for suspected obstructive sleep apnea compared to control patients and changes in autonomic function measured by HRV were detected only in cluster headache patients during active periods; during quiet periods, the cluster headache patients in this study had normal autonomic function [273].

## Discussion

Aura, photophobia, phonophobia, and nausea do not occur with cluster headache, just as lacrimination, rhinorrhea, and seasonal attack patterns do not occur with migraines.

Variations in the circadian rhythm have been associated with migraine as well, although the associations are less pronounced than with cluster headache [280].

Most people with cluster headaches do not get adequate treatment [17].

Misdiagnosis is more likely to occur in women than men because cluster headaches more typically afflict men and migraines women [281].

When women have cluster headaches, onset may be earlier [282, 283], and studies suggest that women with cluster headaches are more prone to develop chronic cluster headaches than men [284].

**Conclusions**
New research into hypothalamic activity suggests that cluster headaches may be more of a disorder of the brain than a sleep disorder, as was once speculated.

More research is required to better understand the etiology and pathogenesis of this severe form of headache.

**Acknowledgement**
*A machine generated summary based on the work of Pergolizzi, Joseph V.; Magnusson, Peter; LeQuang, Jo Ann; Wollmuth, Charles; Taylor, Robert; Breve, Frank. 2020 in Pain and Therapy.*

## *Cluster Headache and Risk of Chronic Transformation*

DOI: https://doi.org/10.1007/s10072-020-04674-1

**[Section 1]**
The disease course was defined as follows: (i) ECH, episodic form throughout all the disease; (ii) pCCH (primary CCH), chronic since the onset of disease; (iii) sCCH (secondary CCH), CCH developing after an episodic onset; (iv) unknown, disease length too short (less than 1 year) to define the clinical course, or clinical course not stated in the available documentation.

We calculated the survival time at the different timepoints: if the state was sCCH (the patient has become chronic within the time period), then the survival corresponded to the chronification latency; if the state was ECH (the patient is still episodic at the end of the time period or hasn't reached the timepoint), then the survival corresponded to the disease length (maximum = time period).

Age at onset affected the evolution of CH: patients with a later onset of CH had a higher risk of becoming chronic within 5 years (p, 0.015 for overall comparison and p, 0.05 for linear trend at log-rank test).

**Acknowledgement**
*A machine generated summary based on the work of Giani, Luca; Proietti Cecchini, Alberto; Leone, Massimo. 2020 in Neurological Sciences.*

## Clinical Features of Cluster Headache in Relation to Age of Onset: Results from a Retrospective Study of a Large Case Series

DOI: https://doi.org/10.1007/s10072-019-03801-x

### [Section 1]

We considered various aspects of clinical features like familiar history of CH or other headache types, frequency and duration of active periods, frequency and duration of attacks, lasting of remissions, site and intensity of pain, cranial autonomic symptoms (CAS) and migraine like features (MLF), lifestyles and personal habits by comparing age of onset, and choosing 50 years old to distinguish the late onset (LO) from the classic onset (CO).

As regards the history of head trauma, the analysis between CO and LO groups showed that the former had a significantly higher proportion of them (38.9% vs 22.8%, p = 0.02), only for the male subgroup; instead, smoking habits resulted in a higher proportion in the male subgroup with LO (p = 0.04).

### Acknowledgement

*A machine generated summary based on the work of Genovese, Antonio; Taga, Arens; Rausa, Francesco; Quintana, Simone; Manzoni, Gian Camillo; Torelli, Paola. 2019 in Neurological Sciences.*

## Clinical Features of Cluster Headache Without Cranial Autonomic Symptoms: Results from a Prospective Multicentre Study

DOI: https://doi.org/10.1038/s41598-021-86408-7

### Abstract-Summary

This study aimed to investigate the frequency and clinical features of CH and PCH without CAS in comparison to those with CAS.

Of the 216 participants with CH and 26 with PCH, 19 (8.8%) and 7 (26.9%), respectively, did not have CAS.

Among participants with PCH, headache intensity was less severe in participants without CAS than in those with CAS (numeric rating scale, 8.0 [7.0–8.0] vs 9.5 [8.0–10.0], p = 0.015).

A significant proportion of participants with CH and PCH did not have CAS.
Some clinical features of CH and PCH differed based on the presence of CAS.
Extended:
This study aimed to assess (1) the frequencies of CH and PCH without CAS among participants with CH and PCH and (2) the differences in the clinical features of participants with CH and PCH with and without CAS.

Of the 216 participants with CH, 19 (8.8%) did not have CAS.

Some clinical features of PCH differ from those of CH.

The findings of the present study may help enhance the understanding of the pathophysiology of CH.

**Introduction**

Some clinical features of PCH differ from those of CH.

The frequency and clinical features of CH without CAS have been reported in only one instance.

A Portuguese study from a single university hospital reported in 2005 that headache intensity was less severe in individuals with CH without CAS than in those with CAS [285].

Since this study did not distinguish between CH and PCH in its analysis, the frequency and clinical features of CH and PCH without CAS compared to those with CAS remain unclear.

This study aimed to assess (1) the frequencies of CH and PCH without CAS among participants with CH and PCH and (2) the differences in the clinical features of participants with CH and PCH with and without CAS.

**Methods**

The KCHR collected data on the following parameters for all participants: sex, age at onset of CH, height, weight, headache intensity on numeric rating scale (from 0 to 10), CH attack frequency per day, mean CH duration since the first cluster period, cluster period duration during the ictal period, total number of cluster periods, smoking status, impact of headache (Headache Impact Test-6 score), circadian and circannual rhythmicity of headache attacks, quality of life (the 3-level version of EuroQol five-dimension scale [EQ-5D-3L]), anxiety (Generalized Anxiety Disorder [GAD-7] score), and depression (Patient's Health Questionnaire-9 [PHQ-9] score) [286, 287].

Participants whose CH or PCH attacks occurred in cluster periods, in whom two or more cluster periods lasted from 7 days to 1 year when untreated, and in whom cluster periods were separated by pain-free remission periods of ≥3 months were classified as having episodic CH (ECH) or episodic PCH.

**Results**

Of the 216 participants with CH, 19 (8.8%) did not have CAS.

Anxiety and depression were less severe in participants with CH without CAS than in those with CAS.

Among the 172 participants with ECH, 15 (8.7%) did not have CAS.

Of the 12 participants with CCH, two (16.7%) did not have CAS.

Of the 26 participants with PCH, 7 (26.9%) did not have CAS.

Headache intensity was less severe in participants with PCH without CAS than in those with CAS.

The frequency of not having CAS was higher in participants with PCH than in those with CH (26.9% [7/26] vs 8.7% [19/216], p = 0.005).

## Discussion

The main findings of the present study were as follows: (1) Approximately one-eleventh of participants with CH and a quarter of those with PCH did not have CAS; (2) Anxiety and depression were less severe in participants with CH without CAS than in those with CAS; and (3) Headache intensity was milder in participants with PCH without CAS than in those with CAS.

CH and PCH without CAS are currently included in the ICHD-3, and our study enrolled participants based on these definitions.

To the best of our knowledge, this study is the first to report that anxiety and depression were less severe in participants with CH without CAS than in those with CAS.

The present study found that approximately 9% of individuals with CH did not have CAS; these individuals had less anxiety and depression, which are closely related with the hypothalamus, compared to those with CAS.

## Acknowledgement

*A machine generated summary based on the work of Chu, Min Kyung; Kim, Byung-Su; Chung, Pil-Wook; Kim, Byung-Kun; Lee, Mi Ji; Park, Jeong Wook; Ahn, Jin-Young; Bae, Dae Woong; Song, Tae-Jin; Sohn, Jong-Hee; Oh, Kyungmi; Kim, Daeyoung; Kim, Jae-Moon; Kim, Soo-Kyoung; Choi, Yun-Ju; Chung, Jae Myun; Moon, Heui-Soo; Chung, Chin-Sang; Park, Kwang-Yeol; Cho, Soo-Jin. 2021 in Scientific Reports.*

# Cluster Headache, Beyond the Pain: A Comparative Cross-sectional Study

DOI: https://doi.org/10.1007/s10072-020-04996-0

## Abstract-Summary

To compare the presence of allodynia, pain catastrophizing, and the impact of headaches on patients with cluster headache (CH) and healthy individuals.

We designed this cross-sectional study to compare various factors among 47 patients diagnosed with CH and 40 healthy controls, and then focus on catastrophism, anxiety, depression, and impact in the CH group.

There were statistically significant differences between CH and the asymptomatic group in Allodynia Symptom Checklist (ASC) (p < 0.001), Pain Catastrophizing Scale (p < 0.001), and HIT-6 (p < 0.001) scores.

We found a correlation among ASC, PCS, anxiety-depression, EuroQoL, and HIT-6 for the CH group.

Our findings reveal significant differences regarding allodynia, pain catastrophism, and impact in CH group compared with controls.

We found a significant relationship between psychological comorbidity, pain catastrophism, and quality of life in CH patients.

Extended:

We found a moderately strong correlation between the presence of depression and quality of life, which confirms our findings from previous studies [288].

These findings suggest the presence of CS signs in CH and reinforce the need for adopting the biopsychosocial model of pain using a complete management involving pharmacological and nonpharmacological therapies to improve the life of patients with CH.

## Introduction

The presence of central sensitization (CS) in CH, as it occurs in other primary headaches, is a subject of controversy [289].

There is a striking lack of studies on catastrophism in patients with CH, although catastrophism is a robust predictor of impaired functioning and reduced quality of life for patients with other primary headaches [290].

The primary objective of this study was to analyze the presence of CA, pain catastrophizing, and the impact of headaches on patients with CH compared with healthy individuals.

Our secondary objective was to analyze the relationship between catastrophism, psychological comorbidities, and the impact of headaches on patients diagnosed with CH.

## Materials and Methods

We designed this study to compare various factors among patients with CH and healthy controls and then focus on certain variables such us catastrophism, anxiety, depression, and headache impact in the CH group.

The pain catastrophizing scale (PCS) is a self-administered Spanish-validated questionnaire for assessing pain-related catastrophic thoughts [291].

The EuroQol-5 Dimensions (EQ-5D) is a standardized, patient-reported, health-related quality-of-life, Spanish-validated questionnaire developed by the EuroQol Group to provide a generic measure of health for clinical and economic assessment [292].

We considered an $\alpha$-error probability of 0.05 and a power ($1$-$\beta$ error probability) of 80% to detect changes in a bilateral comparison of the null hypothesis of the mean and an effect size of 0.36, which we obtained from our previous pilot study with 10 patients per group, considering allodynia, pain catastrophizing, and headache impact as the main variables.

## Results

The results of Student's t test revealed statistically significant differences between the CH group and the asymptomatic group in the ASC ($t = 6.27$; $p < 0.01$), PCS ($t = 8.95$; $p < 0.01$), and HIT-6 ($t = 8.69$; $p < 0.01$).

The regression model for the CH group showed that the combination of anxiety and HIT-6 was a significant covariate of the PCS (adjusted $R^2 = 0.52$; $p = 0.02$).

Same group, the significant covariate of PCS was also a single model with anxiety (adjusted $R^2 = 0.46$; $p < 0.01$).

## Discussion

The results of this study demonstrate that there are significant differences regarding CA, catastrophism, and the impact of headaches in CH patients compared with healthy controls.

A recent South Korean study showed that up to 40% of patients with CH experienced CA during headache attacks but not between headache attacks, which was associated with depression and anxiety [293].

Our study is the first to investigate whether a clinically significant level of pain catastrophizing is associated with psychological comorbidities, quality of life, and headache impact in a CH population.

Our results underline the important role that catastrophism plays in patients with CH, with notable differences compared with healthy controls.

In our model, headache impact and anxiety predicted catastrophizing among patients with CH, findings in line with those of other studies on chronic pain [294].

The present study highlights the relevance of catastrophizing as an important variable associated in patients with CH.

## Conclusions

Pain catastrophism is an important factor that is present in patients with CH and is closely related to headache impact and mood disorders.

There was an important relationship between the presence of psychological comorbidity, pain catastrophism, and quality of life in the patients with CH.

These findings suggest the presence of CS signs in CH and reinforce the need for adopting the biopsychosocial model of pain using a complete management involving pharmacological and nonpharmacological therapies to improve the life of patients with CH.

## Acknowledgement

*A machine generated summary based on the work of Díaz-de-Terán, Javier; Sastre-Real, María; Lobato-Pérez, Luis; Navarro-Fernández, Gonzalo; Elizagaray-García, Ignacio; Gil-Martínez, Alfonso. 2021 in Neurological Sciences.*

# *Pre-attack and Pre-episode Symptoms in Cluster Headache: A Multicenter Cross-sectional Study of 327 Chinese Patients*

DOI: https://doi.org/10.1186/s10194-022-01459-z

## Abstract-Summary

There have been a few studies regarding the pre-attack symptoms (PAS) and pre-episode symptoms (PES) of cluster headache (CH), but none have been conducted in the Chinese population.

The purpose of this study was to identify the prevalence and features of PAS and PES in Chinese patients, as well as to investigate their relationships with pertinent factors.

Among the 327 patients who met the CH criteria (International Classification of Headache Disorders, 3rd edition), 269 (82.3%) patients experienced at least one PAS.

The most common PAS were head and facial discomfort (74.4%).

Multivariable logistic regression analysis depicted that the number of triggers (OR = 1.798, p = 0.001), and smoking history (OR = 2.067, p = 0.026) were correlated with increased odds of PAS.

PAS are quite common in CH patients, demonstrating that CH attacks are not comprised of a pain phase alone; investigations of PAS and PES could help researchers better understand the pathophysiology of CH.

Extended:

The most common PAS was head and facial discomfort (74.4%), followed by neck stiffness (32.3%), anxiety and upset (30.1%), and was unwillingness to talk (29.4%).

The most common PAS was head and facial discomfort (74.4%), followed by neck stiffness (32.3%), anxiety and upset (30.1%), and unwillingness to talk (29.4%).

The most common PAS subtype consisted of local and painless sensory symptoms.

**Introduction**

According to recent studies, some CH patients report pre-episode symptoms (PES) that begin days to weeks before the commencement of cluster episodes, as well as pre-attack symptoms (PAS) that begin minutes before the pain in individual attacks [295, 296].

Because PAS/PES occur before CH, indicating an early and a warning effect for headache attacks and cluster episodes, their identification and recognition may allow for earlier abortive and preventive treatment.

The Chinese population has not yet been examined for PAS and PES of CH.

The purpose of this study was to look into the prevalence and features of PAS and PES in Chinese patients with CH.

**Methods**

General data in the questionnaire included: demographic information (e.g., sex, age, height, weight, education level, occupation, long-term residence, smoking habits, and drinking habits); disease-related information (e.g., diagnosis, course of disease, incidence age, years of misdiagnosis, the family history of CH, and coexisting other types of headache); headache characteristics, including severity (visual analog scale rating from 0 to 10) and nature of headache, locations (frontal, parietal, occipital, temporal, orbital, retro-orbital, facial, nose, ear, teeth, and neck), frequency, attack duration (min), peak time of headache, circadian rhythm, and accompanying cranial autonomic symptoms (CAS); additional features (e.g., nausea, vomiting, photophobia, phonophobia, behaviors during attacks, and aggravation after activity); triggers and alleviating factors; and seasonality, frequency, and duration of the cluster episode.

## Results

327 patients were included in the study, of whom 318 were diagnosed with episodic CH and 9 were diagnosed with chronic CH.

Comparison of the demographic characteristics of patients with and without PAS revealed that more people with PAS smoked (p = 0.037).

In comparing headache characteristics between patients with PAS and those without PAS, a higher number of headache locations (2.0 vs. 3.0; p = 0.009), higher visual analog scale rating (8.5 vs. 9.0; p = 0.025) were observed in patients with PAS.

68 patients (68/327, 20.8%) had PES.

## Discussion

Among CH patients in our study, the strong association between triggers and PAS also supports this speculation that triggers may prompt brain dysfunction in the pre-attack phase.

In patients with PES, the higher number of general symptoms such as local discomfort, anxiety and upset were similar to the PAS.

The poor sleep quality during cluster episode reported by CH patients is most likely associated with frequent nocturnal attacks.

Recall bias is inevitable with a cross-sectional study design; Considering the severity of CH and the high frequency of attacks, most patients presumably had better memories of symptoms.

We did not ask patients about the prevalence of these symptoms without concurrent cluster headache or the frequency of their occurrence outside of the cluster episodes for patients who reported the presence of PAS/PES.

## Conclusions

A greater number of triggers, and a history of smoking were associated with the increased odds of PAS.

Approximately one-fifth of the patients had PES, and the number of triggers was associated with increased odds of PES.

Analyses of PAS and PES can help to better understand the characteristics of the initial stage of CH, thus providing insights regarding the pathophysiological mechanisms of CH.

## Acknowledgement

*A machine generated summary based on the work of Li, Ke; Sun, Shuping; Xue, Zhanyou; Chen, Sufen; Ju, Chunyang; Hu, Dongmei; Gao, Xiaoyu; Wang, Yanhong; Wang, Dan; Chen, Jianjun; Li, Li; Liu, Jing; Zhang, Mingjie; Jia, Zhihua; Han, Xun; Liu, Huanxian; He, Mianwang; Zhao, Wei; Gong, Zihua; Zhang, Shuhua; Lin, Xiaoxue; Liu, Yingyuan; Wang, Shengshu; Yu, Shengyuan; Dong, Zhao. 2022 in The Journal of Headache and Pain.*

# Clinical Factors Influencing the Impact of Cluster Headache from a Prospective Multicenter Study

DOI: https://doi.org/10.1038/s41598-020-59366-9

**Abstract-Summary**

We assessed headache impact using the six-item Headache Impact Test (HIT-6) and evaluated the factors associated with the impact of CH.

Participants with a HIT-6 score $\geq$ 60 were classified into a severe impact group.

These patients were characterized by younger age, earlier onset of CH, longer duration of each headache attack, higher pain intensity, more cranial autonomic symptoms, a higher proportion of depression or anxiety, higher score of stress, and lower score of quality of life.

The anxiety (OR = 1.19, 95% CI: 1.08–1.31, p = 0.006), greater pain intensity (OR = 1.06, 95% CI: 1.02–1.10, p = 0.002), and age (OR = 0.99, 95% CI: 0.99–1.00, p = 0.008) were significant predictors for a severe impact of CH patients.

As pain intensity, anxiety and age modulated CH's impact on their lives.

Extended:

Future research should examine whether treating anxiety may help reduce the impact of headache.

**Introduction**

Cluster headache (CH) is one of the most painful and disabling primary headache disorders, but the severity and rate of disability have not been fully assessed using a headache-specific tool.

The HIT-6 is based on items taken from the Headache Disability Inventory, Headache Impact Questionnaire, MIDAS, and Migraine-specific Quality of Life Questionnaire and measures the overall impact of headache on the patient's life [297, 298].

Unlike the MIDAS, which focuses on migraine patients and assesses disability related to daily life, the HIT-6 can be applied to a variety of headache disorders to measure their impact over a wide range of domains.

The clinical factors associated with disability in CH patients have rarely been reported.

We hypothesized that the majority of patients with CH are severely affected by the disorder and thus examined the clinical factors associated with a severe impact of CH.

**Methods**

This study was based on the multicenter, cross-sectional Korean Cluster Headache Registry (KCHR) and used prospectively collected data from consecutive patients with CH treated at neurology outpatient departments in Korea between September 2016 and December 2018.

The ICHD-3 was published after the initial recruitment phase of the KCHR, so the participants were re-diagnosed using the ICHD-3 based on each patient's clinical history; those who did not meet the criteria for CH were excluded from this analysis [299].

Investigators collected the following clinical data regarding current and previous CH periods: severity of pain on a numeric rating scale, duration and frequency of headache attacks, average duration of a CH bout, and total CH periods.

The information value (IV) statistic was calculated for the variables that differed significantly between the two groups (CH + S and CH − S).

## Results

The HIT-6 scores of the CH patients ranged from 41 to 78, with a mean score of $68.5 \pm 7.9$ (males, $68.2 \pm 8.1$; females, $69.6 \pm 6.9$; p = 0.345).

The HIT-6 score of the patients differed according to the CH subtype (first episode of CH, $66.6 \pm 6.8$; episodic CH, $69.3 \pm 7.6$; chronic CH, $70.9 \pm 4.6$; and probable CH, $64.1 \pm 10.5$; p = 0.006).

In the post-hoc analysis using Tukey's test, the HIT-6 score was lower for the patients with probable CH than those with chronic CH (p = 0.009), but there were no differences among the other groups.

The proportions of patients with anxiety (GAD-7 score $\geq 6$, 68.6% vs. 29.4%, p < 0.001) and depression (PHQ-9 score $\geq 8$, 41.8% vs. 17.6%, p = 0.013) were also higher in the CH + S group.

## Discussion

This group was characterized by a younger age, earlier onset of CH illness, longer duration of individual headache attacks, greater pain intensity, higher stress score, lower score in the quality of life, and more cranial autonomic symptoms compared with the CH − S group.

Although not directly comparable, one study reported that the impact of headache was greatest in chronic CH patients (n = 27), followed by those currently experiencing a bout of episodic CH (n = 26), those currently in remission from episodic CH (n = 22), and those with migraine [111].

One study found no significant difference in the HIT-6 score between 11 patients with episodic CH ($64.60 \pm 4.81$) and 11 patients with chronic CH ($64.60 \pm 11.86$) [108], similar to our findings.

Another study reported higher HIT-6 scores in 72 patients with chronic CH ($61.78 \pm 8.05$) compared with 107 patients with episodic CH ($53.25 \pm 7.57$) [70].

## Conclusions

According to the HIT-6 scores, most of our CH patients were severely affected by their condition, and the impact of episodic CH was as severe as that of chronic CH.

This study identified anxiety, younger age, and greater pain intensity as significant predictors of a severe impact of CH.

These results emphasize the importance of early diagnosis of CH patients suffering from severe effects starting at a younger age.

**Acknowledgement**

*A machine generated summary based on the work of Sohn, Jong-Hee; Park, Jeong-Wook; Lee, Mi Ji; Chung, Pil-Wook; Chu, Min Kyung; Chung, Jae Myun; Ahn, Jin-Young; Kim, Byung-Su; Kim, Soo-Kyoung; Choi, Yun-Ju; Kim, Daeyoung; Song, Tae-Jin; Oh, Kyungmi; Moon, Heui-Soo; Park, Kwang-Yeol; Kim, Byung-Kun; Bae, Dae-Woong; Chung, Chin-Sang; Cho, Soo-Jin. 2020 in Scientific Reports.*

# The Impact of Remission and Coexisting Migraine on Anxiety and Depression in Cluster Headache

DOI: https://doi.org/10.1186/s10194-020-01120-7

**Abstract-Summary**

Our aim was to investigate the relationship between coexisting cluster headache (CH) and migraine with anxiety and depression during active cluster bouts, and how symptoms change during remission.

We assessed for changes in anxiety and depression during CH remission periods.

Among the CH patients, the prevalence of moderate-to-severe anxiety and depression was seen in 38.2% and 34.6%, respectively.

Compared with controls, CH patients were associated with moderate-to-severe anxiety and depression (multivariable-adjusted odds ratio [aOR] = 7.32, 95% confidence intervals [CI] = 3.35–15.99 and aOR = 4.95, 95% CI = 2.32–10.57, respectively).

CH patients with migraine were significantly more likely to have moderate-to-severe anxiety and depression (aOR = 32.53, 95% CI = 6.63–159.64 and aOR = 16.88, 95% CI = 4.16–68.38, respectively), compared to controls without migraine.

Our results indicate that CH patients are at increased risk of anxiety and depression, especially in the presence of coexisting migraine.

Extended:

Further clinical and neuroimaging studies are required to elucidate on the possible mechanisms underlying our findings.

**Introduction**

Given the well-recognized link between migraine and psychiatric comorbidities, coexisting migraine may independently influence the risk for anxiety and depression in CH patients, although this is a relatively unexplored area to date.

Considering the debilitating nature of repetitive CH attacks during an active cluster bout, we hypothesized that CH patients were at an increased risk for anxiety and depression in active bout period, but that their anxiety and depression would reduce during remission.

Given the relationship between migraine and psychiatric comorbidities, we further hypothesized that the risk for anxiety and depression could be influenced by coexisting migraine in CH patients.

To test these hypotheses, we conducted a prospective study based on data from a multicenter CH registry to investigate the associations between CH, coexisting migraine, anxiety, and depression during an active episode of cluster bout (acting as the baseline period) and changes in anxiety and depression during remission periods.

## Methods

During follow-up, CH patients were asked to repeat the tests of GAD-7 and PHQ-9 when their cluster bout status subsided into remission.

GAD-7 and PHQ-9 evaluate the status of anxiety and depression within the last 2 weeks, CH patients performed the follow-up tests of GAD-7 and PHQ-9 after 2 weeks following the end of their cluster bout.

To assess for a change in anxiety and depression scores between active cluster bout and remission periods (remission period analysis), we used the paired t-test for the continuous data and the McNemar test for the dichotomous groups we created, as mentioned above.

Since we expected a reduction in the GAD-7 and PHQ-9 scores during remission, in those with GAD-7 and/or PHQ-9 scores $\geq 5$ during an acute cluster bout we compared the proportion of participants experiencing a more than 50% reduction in the GAD-7 and PHQ-9 scores, according to prespecified subgroups (age $< 40$ years vs. age $\geq 40$ years, male sex vs. female sex, and presence of migraine vs. lack of migraine).

## Results

The prevalence of moderate-to-severe anxiety and depression was highest in the CH with migraine group (51.6% and 45.2%, respectively) relative to the CH without migraine group and the two control groups (with and without migraine).

Those with coexisting CH and migraine had the highest OR for moderate-to-severe anxiety (OR = 32.53, 95% CI = 6.73–157.12).

The CH with migraine group was associated with an extremely high likelihood of moderate-to-severe anxiety (aOR = 32.53, 95% CI = 6.63–159.64).

The CH with migraine group had the highest OR for the presence of moderate-to-severe depression (OR = 16.47, 95% CI = 4.23–64.06).

Using the control without migraine group as a reference, the risk of moderate-to-severe depression was the highest in the group of patients with coexisting CH and migraine (aOR = 16.88, 95% CI = 4.16–68.38).

## Discussion

We assessed for an association between CH and coexisting migraine with anxiety and depression, and for any changes between cluster bouts and remission periods.

Compared to the control group, the CH patients were significantly more likely to have comorbid anxiety and depression after the multivariable adjustment including coexisting migraine.

This indicates that the bidirectional relationship between migraine and psychiatric comorbidities may further increase the risk of anxiety and depression among CH patients during a cluster bout.

Despite the strong association between CH, anxiety, and depression during active cluster bouts, anxiety and depression improved remarkably at remission in the present analysis.

A US pilot study conducted a cross-sectional comparison of the levels of anxiety and depression among ECH patients between active cluster bouts and remission periods [300].

We estimated the risk of anxiety and depression in CH and coexisting migraine during active cluster bouts based on a cross-sectional analysis.

**Conclusions**

We have quantified the risk of anxiety and depression in CH and coexisting migraine during active cluster bouts.

We have shown that coexisting migraine is a significant influencer on psychiatric comorbidities in patients with CH.

Anxiety and depression are dynamically altered between active cluster bout and remission periods, suggesting that psychiatric comorbidities may be cyclical in a similar manner to the cluster bouts observed in CH.

**Acknowledgement**

*A machine generated summary based on the work of Kim, Byung-Su; Chung, Pil-Wook; Kim, Byung-Kun; Lee, Mi Ji; Park, Jeong Wook; Chu, Min Kyung; Ahn, Jin-Young; Bae, Dae Woong; Song, Tae-Jin; Sohn, Jong-Hee; Oh, Kyungmi; Kim, Daeyoung; Kim, Jae-Moon; Kim, Soo-Kyoung; Choi, Yun-Ju; Chung, Jae Myun; Moon, Heui-Soo; Chung, Chin-Sang; Park, Kwang-Yeol; Cho, Soo-Jin. 2020 in The Journal of Headache and Pain.*

## *Demoralization Predicts Suicidality in Patients with Cluster Headache*

DOI: https://doi.org/10.1186/s10194-021-01241-7

**Abstract-Summary**

To determine the frequency of suicidal ideation and assess suicide risk in cluster headache (CH) patients compared to matched controls without CH in this observational case-control study.

CH has been linked to suicide since its early descriptions by B.T. Horton; however, there is relatively little empiric data showing the association between suicidality and CH, especially in the context of other psychological phenomena, such as depression and demoralization.

CH and control participants were recruited through community and CH patient group advertisements.

Lifetime suicidal ideation and suicide risk were assessed using the Suicidal Behavior Questionnaire-revised and the Columbia Suicide Severity Rating Scale.

More CH than control participants had lifetime active suicidal ideation (47.0% vs. 26.7%; p = 0.001), high suicide risk (38.0% vs. 18.5%; p = 0.0009), lifetime depression history (67.0%% vs. 32.6%; p < 0.00001), and demoralization (28.0% vs. 15.6%; p = 0.02).

The odds of lifetime suicidal ideation were higher in those with CH (odds [95% confidence interval]; 2.04 [1.08,3.85]), even after accounting for depression and demoralization.

In CH, suicidal ideation was associated with demoralization (6.66 [1.56,28.49]) but not depression (1.89 [0.66,5.46]).

Lifetime suicidal ideation and high suicide risk are prevalent in CH sufferers, and its likelihood is dependent on the presence of demoralization.

Extended:

Lifetime suicidal ideation and high suicide risk are prevalent in CH sufferers, significantly moreso than in sociodemographically matched control participants without CH.

The odds of passive or active SI in one's lifetime was nearly seven-fold greater in those with demoralization.

## Introduction

These recurrent intensely painful headache attacks impose a significant personal and economic burden on CH sufferers, as nearly one-fifth report losing a job due to CH and a similar number are homebound for days at a time at least once annually [10].

CH's link to suicide, the most severe consequence of depression, was first described by the American neurologist, B.T. Horton, in 1939 as he wrote, "Our patients were disabled by … pain … so severe that several had to be constantly watched for fear of suicide" [301]. In CH, however, it is unclear whether suicide or suicidal ideation (SI) is a consequence of depression or rather a perceived solution to end profound suffering in a desperate individual.

We hypothesized that SI and suicide risk would be significantly more common in CH sufferers than matched controls, even after considering sociodemographics and clinical and psychological history, and that demoralization in addition to depression would be associated with suicidality.

## Methods

Potential participants were screened through the online survey for CH, using screening questions consistent with International Classification of Headache Disorders 3rd edition (ICHD-3) diagnostic criteria for CH [1].

A person was classified in the CH group if they fulfilled the following criteria: answered "Yes" to the two questions in item (1): (1) "Have you had severe or very severe attacks of unbearable pain in the region of the eye or temple on one side?"

If the participant answered "Yes" to the prior questions, the following was asked: (4) If you have experienced feelings of helplessness, hopelessness, and/or giving up, did your state of feeling exceed a month?

Suicidality, including passive and active SI and suicide attempts, were assessed using the Suicidal Behavior Questionnaire-revised (SBQ-R) and the Columbia Suicide Severity Rating Scale (C-SSRS).

Variables associated with suicide in previous population studies (e.g. age, sex, race, marital status, education, income, and drug/alcohol abuse) were also entered in the model [302].

**Results**

While neither self-report of having depression nor report of taking an antidepressant medication were different between groups, more than two-thirds of CH sufferers had a lifetime episode of depression, more than double that of controls (67.0% vs. 32.6%; $p < 0.00001$).

From the SBQ-R, marginally more persons with CH than controls had a plan for suicide in their lifetime ($p = 0.07$), but lifetime suicide attempts did not differ between the groups.

Those found to be at high suicide risk, as evidenced by an SBQ-R score $\geq 7$, were significantly more common, 38% vs. 18.5% ($p = 0.0009$), in the CH than control group.

Demoralization was significantly more common in the chronic CH group (40.9% vs. 17.9%; $p = 0.01$), which was reflected in the significantly higher KDS scores among chronic CH sufferers.

**Discussion**

Specifically designed to study suicidality in CH, we found that persons with CH, in particular chronic CH, were significantly more likely to have had either passive or active SI in their lifetime than individuals without CH; furthermore, the likelihood of SI was best predicted by the presence of demoralization.

In controls, SI was associated with lifetime depression, but not demoralization, suggesting that demoralization may be particularly sensitive to suicidality in CH.

Future studies of suicidality in CH should in addition to assessing depression and demoralization explore these concepts of pain tolerance, attitudes toward death (fearlessness), as well as whether SI is directed inwardly toward the self or outwardly toward the disease state.

The key findings of this study that SI is increased in persons with CH and is related to both depression and demoralization highlight the importance of screening for not only suicidal ideation and intent, but also the psychological phenomenon of demoralization.

**Conclusions**

The odds of lifetime suicidal ideation were higher in those with CH than in controls, even after accounting for depression and demoralization.

In CH, suicidal ideation was associated with demoralization but not depression.

The presence of both suicidal ideation and demoralization should be screened for in patients with CH.

## Acknowledgement

*A machine generated summary based on the work of Koo, Brian B.; Bayoumi, Ahmed; Albanna, Abdalla; Abusuliman, Mohammed; Burrone, Laura; Sico, Jason J.; Schindler, Emmanuelle A. D. 2021 in The Journal of Headache and Pain.*

## Associated Factors and Clinical Implication of Cutaneous Allodynia in Patients with Cluster Headache: A Prospective Multicentre Study

DOI: https://doi.org/10.1038/s41598-019-43065-1

### Abstract-Summary

We sought to investigate the presence of CA, its associated factors, and its clinical implications in patients with cluster headache (CH).

Of 119 eligible patients, 48 and 2 (40.3% and 1.7%) had CA during and between headache attacks, respectively.

In univariable analyses, total CH duration, major depressive disorder (MDD), and generalized anxiety disorder (GAD) were associated with CA during headache attack.

They remained significantly associated with CA during headache attack in multivariable analyses.

Patients with CA during headache attack had higher headache impact (P = 0.002).

Patients with CH commonly experienced CA during headache attack, but not between headache attacks.

CA during headache attack was associated with disease duration, depression, and anxiety.

Extended:

In the present prospective study, CA during headache attack was present in 40.3% of patients with CH, whereas only 1.7% experienced CA between headache attacks.

Only two patients (1.7%) experienced mild CA between headache attacks.

The presence of CA during headache attack did not significantly influence the outcome of acute or preventive therapy in patients with CH.

Patients with CA during headache attack suffered from greater headache impact.

### Introduction

Despite some common points of pathophysiology, clinical manifestations, and treatment between migraine and CH, previous studies have shown inconsistent results with regard to the presence of CA in CH [303–308].

In a recent largest study on this issue, 35.9% of patients with CH experienced CA during a headache attack, and CA was independently associated with depression [309].

Regarding CA in CH, the present study sought to ascertain (1) the presence of CA among patients with CH in the Asian population, (2) the relation between CA and anxiety in patients with CH, (3) the association between CA severity and psychiatric comorbidities, and (4) the clinical implications of CA including headache impact and treatment response.

Using a multicentre registry of patients with CH, we investigated the presence of CA during and between headache attacks, the factors associated with CA, the relationship between CA severity and psychiatric comorbidities, and the influence of CA on headache impact and treatment response.

**Methods**

The exclusion criteria were as follows: (1) enrolment during remission period, (2) possible secondary cause, (3) no or incomplete response to allodynia questionnaire, (4) missing clinical variables, and (5) lack of follow-up visits.

In terms of the presence of CA, the study patients were dichotomously divided into a no CA (ASC score ≤2) group and a CA (ASC score ≥3) group.

We used the following clinical information in our analysis: demographic factors, social habits, headache characteristics, psychiatric comorbidity, headache impact, and treatment response.

Psychiatric comorbidity was assessed using the Korean versions of the Patient Health Questionnaire 9-item scale (PHQ-9) and the Generalized Anxiety Disorder 7-item scale (GAD-7).

Treatment-response assessment of study patients was conducted during their follow-up reservations as a part of daily clinical practice.

Because age, female sex, comorbid migraine may be associated with allodynia, the multivariate models were adjusted for these variables, regardless of whether they showed statistical significance in the univariable analyses [309, 310].

**Results**

Baseline characteristics of age, female sex, coexisting migraine history, total duration of CH illness, duration of cluster headache bout, attack duration, MDD, and GAD in patients who completed the ASC did not significantly differ from those of patients excluded due to incomplete response to the ASC.

In patients without psychiatric comorbidity, there was a clear dose–response relationship between CA during headache attack and total duration of CH illness: 6.7% after ≤1 year, 15.0% between 1 and ≤5 years, 35.7% between 5 and ≤10 years, and 53.3% after 10 years; $P = 0.013$.

The prevalences of MDD, GAD, and psychiatric comorbidity were highest in patients with severe CA during headache attack (58.3%, 83.3%, and 91.7%, respectively).

The treatment response did not differ significantly between patients with and without CA during headache attack in any of the CH treatment subgroups.

**Discussion**

In the present prospective study, CA during headache attack was present in 40.3% of patients with CH, whereas only 1.7% experienced CA between headache attacks.

In line with the Dutch study, the results of the current study indicate that CA during headache attack occurs in about 40% of patients with CH [309].

These findings indicate that the major form of CA in patients with CH is acute allodynia during headache attack.

We confirmed that CA is associated with both depression and anxiety in patients with CH, and that the frequencies of depression and anxiety increased with CA severity, partly corroborating the results of a population study of individuals who suffer migraines [310].

The presence of CA during headache attack did not significantly influence the outcome of acute or preventive therapy in patients with CH.

## Conclusions

We can confirm that a significant proportion of CH patients experience CA during headache attack, but rarely between headache attacks.

The presence of CA was associated with disease duration and psychiatric comorbidity in patients with CH.

## Acknowledgement

*A machine generated summary based on the work of Kim, Byung-Su; Park, Jeong Wook; Sohn, Jong-Hee; Lee, Mi Ji; Kim, Byung-Kun; Chu, Min Kyung; Ahn, Jin-Young; Choi, Yun-Ju; Song, Tae-Jin; Chung, Pil-Wook; Oh, Kyungmi; Lee, Kwang-Soo; Kim, Soo-Kyoung; Park, Kwang-Yeol; Chung, Jae Myun; Moon, Heui-Soo; Chung, Chin-Sang; Cho, Soo-Jin. 2019 in Scientific Reports.*


# *State and Trait Anger and Its Expression in Cluster Headache Compared with Migraine: A Cross-sectional Study*

DOI: https://doi.org/10.1007/s10072-019-03987-0

## Abstract-Summary

Individuals with migraine are more likely to hold their anger-in than controls.

Only one study evaluated anger in cluster headache (CH).

The objective is to compare anger between migraine and CH patients.

One hundred thirty-five migraine and 108 CH patients completed the State Trait Anger Expression Inventory (STAXI-2), composed of 7 subscales.

CH patients have higher median scores than migraine patients in State Anger (46 vs 44, p = 0.012).

CH patients have lower scores in Anger Control Out (44 vs 50, p = 0.016).

In subgroup analysis, CH patients during the cluster period have higher scores than chronic migraine patients in State Anger (47 vs 44, p = 0.035), while CH patients in headache-free period did not differ from migraine patients.

Migraine and CH patients differ in state anger, indicating that CH patients experienced higher intensity of anger during the time of testing.

Extended:

Individuals with migraine are more likely to hold their anger-in than those without headache [311–313].

CH patients have significant higher median scores than migraine patients (46 vs 44, p = 0.012) in State Anger and significant lower median scores in Anger Control Out subscale (50 vs 44, p = 0.016).

Possible future psychological treatments need to take into account these considerations, focusing not on the reduction or the increase of anger levels, but on the awareness of emotional status during pain [314] and on its modulation by analyzing cognitive and behavioral appraisal of pain and of other stressful events.

### Background

Individuals with migraine are more likely to hold their anger-in than those without headache [311–313].

Individuals who hold anger-in experience increased pain severity [315] and failure to express anger leads to more disability [312, 316].

Some authors found that higher anger-out at baseline predicted greater subsequent mean daily headache severity in migraine patients [317].

Contrarily to migraine and tension-type headache, in cluster headache patients, anger has not been thoroughly assessed yet.

Only one study evaluated aggressiveness differences between CH and migraine patients, indicating that CH patients (especially chronic cluster headache and active period cluster headache patients) reported higher scores in the self-aggression/ depression subscale [318].

The objective of our study is to evaluate differences between migraine and cluster headache patients in anger levels and in anger expression by using a questionnaire that evaluates multidimensional aspects of anger.

### Method

STAXI-2 questionnaire results of the groups were compared: migraine patients and cluster headache (CH) patients.

The three subgroups were selected in order to evaluate differences between cluster patients in the active period and cluster patients in the non-active period, and to compare two different primary headaches that were similar for the impairment level (such as chronic migraine and cluster headache in active period).

The Kruskal-Wallis test was used to evaluate the difference between groups (migraine vs CH) and subgroups (chronic cluster headache and cluster headache in the active period vs cluster headache in headache-free period vs chronic migraine).

The correction for multiple comparisons was not performed because the primary objective was to evaluate the differences between migraine and CH patients in State Anger and Trait Anger scales.

### Results

CH patients have significant higher median scores than migraine patients (46 vs 44, p = 0.012) in State Anger and significant lower median scores in Anger Control Out subscale (50 vs 44, p = 0.016).

CH patients have suggestive higher median scores in Anger Expression Index (58 vs 56, p = 0.059), while migraine patients have suggestive higher median scores in Anger Expression In (58 vs 56, p = 0.073).

Results showed that in migraine patients there are no significant differences in State Anger (44 [44–48] vs 44 [44–48]), and in Anger Control Out subscales (48 [42–54] vs 50 [44–54]), between patients with pharmacological therapy and patients without it.

In the CH group, there are no significant differences between patients with pharmacological therapy and patients without it in State Anger (46 [44–56] vs 44 [44–56]), and in Anger Control Out subscales (44 [36–52] vs 46 [40–54]).

## Discussion

Whereas between migraine and cluster headache patients there are differences in emotional state during pain, cluster headache patients appear to feel more anger in the cluster period than cluster headache patients do in the headache-free period and than chronic migraine patients [319].

These data could confirm the different emotional correlates to pain between migraine and cluster headache patients and support the bio-behavioral hypothesis of different behavioral responses to stress in migraine and CH patients [320].

Observations of CH patients during the attacks are consistent with the behavior of an individual fighting against pain or running away from it, actively coping with pain, and the presence of high state anger in cluster headache is in line with this hypothesis.

It is interesting to notice that cluster headache patients, especially those in active period, have lower scores than migraine patients in Anger Control Out subscale, indicating that they express their anger-out most frequently than migraine patients.

## Conclusions

These data could tell us something about the different behaviors of CH and migraine during pain and add new information about the emotional regulation involved in headache attacks.

About chronic pain (such as low back pain), evidence suggests that how anger is regulated—expression, inhibition—may have greater consequences for chronic patients' pain and functioning than their level of trait anger [321], and our data about migraine and cluster headache are in line with these results.

Possible future psychological treatments need to take into account these considerations, focusing not on the reduction or the increase of anger levels, but on the awareness of emotional status during pain [314] and on its modulation by analyzing cognitive and behavioral appraisal of pain and of other stressful events.

## Acknowledgement

*A machine generated summary based on the work of Rausa, Marialuisa; Cevoli, Sabina; Giannini, Giulia; Favoni, Valentina; Contin, Sara Anastasia; Zenesini, Corrado; Ballardini, Donatella; Cortelli, Pietro; Pierangeli, Giulia. 2019 in Neurological Sciences.*

# *Behavioral and Psychological Aspects of Cluster Headache: An Overview*

DOI: https://doi.org/10.1007/s10072-019-03831-5

**Abstract-Summary**

This paper overviews available literature addressing behavioral and psychological aspects of cluster headache.

**Introduction**

Cluster headache (CH) is a rare and extremely painful primary headache syndrome, with an estimated lifetime population prevalence of only 0.12% [158].

CH presents with a unique, distinct combination of symptoms characterized by intense unilateral pain in the orbital, supraorbital, and temporal areas, with the prototypical episode enduring 15–180 min, occurring as frequent as eight times a day, often being accompanied by restlessness or agitation [1].

This condition can be episodic (ECH), lasting as long as 7 days to a year, followed by pain-free periods up to 3 months, or chronic (CCH), persisting a year or longer nonstop or having fewer than 3 months of pain-free periods between subsequent episodes.

Having to endure such a painful, debilitating condition is certain to have pronounced psychological consequences.

We present what is currently known about the behavioral and psychological correlates of cluster headache, and explore the potential role psychology can play in the management of CH.

**Behavioral Correlates**

The self-rated quality of sleep and the level of hypocretin-1 (HCCRT-1; a neuropeptide associated with regulating sleep and arousal) is much lower in patients with CH compared to non-headache controls [79, 322].

Research consistently reveals a higher prevalence of licit and illicit drug use among individuals with CH, as compared to the general population [323].

A large-scale examination of insurance claims found that claims filed for tobacco use disorders were nearly three times greater in patients with CH when compared to that for controls [324].

Evidence points to higher use of other illicit drugs, such as cannabis and hallucinogens, among the population of individuals with CH [323].

Turning once again to insurance claims, the odds of having any type of drug dependency was recently found to be nearly three times greater, and illicit drug use two to three times greater, in patients with CH when compared to controls [324].

**Psychological Correlates**

In a large population-based cohort study that examined a health insurance database patients with CH were found to have 5.6 times greater odds of developing depression when compared to controls, similar to that of patients diagnosed with migraine [19].

Retrospective recall by 207 physicians who specialized in headache treatment from 48 different countries estimated that of the 90 patients who completed and 570 who attempted suicide, 39 and 35% had CH diagnoses, similar to rates for those diagnosed with migraine [325].

While rates of actual suicide attempts may be relatively low in this population overall, the greater observed risk when CH is present (either for CCH or CH when active) indicates that clinicians may need to be particularly vigilant during these time periods.

**Concluding Comments: The Potential Role of Psychological- and Behavioral-Based Approaches in CH Management**

We previously speculated that "just in time" training in cognitive and behavioral techniques might be of value in helping patients cope more effectively with the overwhelming and unremitting distress that arises from repeatedly having to endure the intense bouts of pain during cluster attacks [326, 327].

In our previously mentioned trial that taught patients with episodic CH multiple techniques for managing pain [328], all but one of the patients were trained intensively at varying time points during headache-free periods.

We now suggest that patients whose CH follows a somewhat predictable course delay seeking behavioral care until a month or so before the next bout of CH is likely to occur, a time when motivation for acquiring a new set of coping skills should be heightened.

The behavioral health care provider would implement a rigorous, tailored treatment program designed to directly address and dampen the heightened negative affect that occurs prior to and in anticipation of, during, and following a CH attack.

**Acknowledgement**

*A machine generated summary based on the work of Schenck, Lauren A.-M.; Andrasik, Frank. 2019 in Neurological Sciences.*

**Treatment**

Machine generated keywords: stimulation, cch, therapy, preventive, cluster, nerve, responder, cgrp, cluster headache, prophylactic, treatment cluster, attack, sumatriptan, attack frequency, oxygen

# Aids to Management of Headache Disorders in Primary Care (2nd Edition)

DOI: https://doi.org/10.1186/s10194-018-0899-2

## Abstract-Summary

The Aids to Management are a product of the Global Campaign against Headache, a worldwide programme of action conducted in official relations with the World Health Organization.

The common headache disorders (migraine, tension-type headache and medication-overuse headache) are major causes of ill health.

These Aids to Management, with the European principles of management of headache disorders in primary care as the core of their content, combine educational materials with practical management aids.

The Aids to Management may be individually downloaded and, as is the case for all products of the Global Campaign against Headache, are available without restriction for non-commercial use.

## Preface

Medical management of headache disorders does not, for the vast majority of people affected by them, require specialist skills or investigations.

Aids to management of headache disorders in primary care (2nd edition) updates the first edition, published 11 years ago [329].

It has undergone review by a wider consultation group of headache experts, including representatives of the member national societies of EHF, primary-care physicians from eight countries of Europe, and lay advocates from member organisations of the European Headache Alliance.

The European principles of management of headache disorders in primary care, laid out in 14 sections, are the core of the content.

Any of seven information leaflets may be offered to patients to improve their understanding of their headache disorders and their management.

LTB and EHF offer these aids for use without restriction for non-commercial purposes, as is the case for all products of the Global Campaign against Headache [330].

## European Principles of Management of Headache Disorders in Primary Care

Key points of information are: ■ migraine is a common disorder which, while it may be disabling, is benign; ■ it is often familial, and probably genetically inherited; ■ it cannot be cured but can be successfully treated; ■ trigger or predisposing factors are common in migraine, and should be identified and avoided or modified when possible, but not all can be; ■ a headache calendar helps good management by recording over time: ■ the symptoms and pattern of attacks (eg, menstrual relationship); ■ medication use (thus identifying overuse); ■ regular activity (eg, sport or exercise 2–3 times per week) may reduce intensity and frequency of migraine attacks.

**Instruments and Other Materials to Aid Diagnosis and Management of Headache Disorders in Primary Care**

Diagnostic criteria: A. Headache (migraine-like or tension-type-like) on $\geq 15$ days/month for >3 months, and fulfilling criteria B and C B. Occurring in a patient who has had at least five attacks fulfilling criteria B–D for 1.1 Migraine without aura and/or criteria B and C for 1.2 Migraine with aura C. On $\geq 8$ days/month for >3 months, fulfilling any of the following: 1.

Diagnostic criteria: A. At least 10 episodes of headache occurring on 1–14 days/month on average for >3 months ($\geq 12$ and <180 days/year) and fulfilling criteria B–D B. Lasting from 30 min to 7 days C. At least two of the following four characteristics: 1.

Diagnostic criteria: A. Headache occurring on $\geq 15$ days/month in a patient with a pre-existing headache disorder B. Regular overuse for >3 months of one or more drugs that can be taken for acute and/or symptomatic treatment of headache C. Not better accounted for by another ICHD-3 diagnosis.

**Patient Information Leaflets to Aid Headache Management in Primary Care (2nd Edition)**

Headache management is greatly facilitated when the patient understands his or her headache disorder and the treatment being proposed for it.

Good treatment of patients with any headache disorder therefore begins with explanations of their disorder and the purpose and means of management.

■ Explanation is a crucial element of preventative management in patients with frequent migraine or tension-type headache, who are at particular risk of escalating medication consumption.

The general principles of headache management place education and reassurance of patients first.

To assist, Lifting The Burden (LTB) has produced a series of Patient Information Leaflets (PILs).

**Translation, and the Preservation of Original Meaning, of Materials Developed to Improve Headache Management**

Coordination of the translation A translation coordinator, who oversees but does not carry out the translation, is selected according to the following criteria: ■ a headache expert; ■ bilingual in English and the target language (ideally a native speaker and a resident of the country of the target language); ■ has ability to mediate between different translators and to understand the points of view of lay and professional translators.

Coordination of the translation A translation coordinator, who oversees but does not carry out the translation, is selected according to the following criteria: ■ has technical knowledge (ie, understands the concepts underlying the questions or instrument being translated); ■ bilingual in English and the target language (ideally a native speaker and a resident of the country of the target language); ■ has ability to mediate between different translators and to understand the points of view of lay and professional translators.

**Acknowledgement**

*A machine generated summary based on the work of Steiner, T. J.; Jensen, R.; Katsarava, Z.; Linde, M.; MacGregor, E. A.; Osipova, V.; Paemeleire, K.; Olesen, J.; Peters, M.; Martelletti, P. 2019 in The Journal of Headache and Pain.*


# *Recent Advances in the Management of Cluster Headache*

DOI: https://doi.org/10.1007/s11940-020-00655-z

**Abstract-Summary**

Among the spectrum of pain conditions, cluster headache represents one of the most severe.

Targeted therapies for cluster headache are evolving thus improving the available therapeutic armamentarium.

A better understanding of the currently available therapies, as well as new and emerging options, may aide physicians to manage affected sufferers better by evolving treatment guidance.

While classic first-line medications are useful in some patients with cluster headache, they are often accompanied by significant side effects that limit their use.

A remarkable example of this is the blockage of the calcitonin gene-related peptide pathway with monoclonal antibodies, which may be a key element in the future treatment of cluster headache.

A deepening of the understanding of cluster headache mechanisms in recent years has driven the evolution of sophisticated therapeutic approaches that could allow a new era in the treatment of this difficult condition.

Extended:

This review will cover the well-established, first-line treatment options and then expand on newer targets and emerging therapies, which may represent a safer and better-tolerated option for CH management in the future.

Further studies are needed to understand the root of this relentless and extremely debilitating headache and to offer more adequate treatment strategies in the future.

**Introduction**

Cluster headache (CH) is a relatively rare primary headache disorder.

Affected patients typically report cluster headache as being the worst type of pain they have ever experienced [331, 332].

The frequency of attacks can go between one in 48 h and eight in 24 h. While the pathophysiology of cluster headache has not been entirely dissected, there are several proposed mechanisms described.

Given the severity of CH, early diagnosis and adequate management of the acute attacks, as well as prevention during the bouts, and in the chronic form, are crucial.

These include, as a first-line approach, primarily high-flow oxygen, intranasal zolmitriptan and sumatriptan, and subcutaneous sumatriptan for the acute treatment of attacks and verapamil for CH prevention [333].

### Classic Acute Attack Treatments

Oxygen is currently one of the most used acute medications for CH, with nearly 80% of patients benefitting from its use [334].

The effectiveness of high-flow oxygen in CH is remarkable; it is well tolerated with few adverse events; it is applicable repeatedly throughout the day and can also be combined with other treatments [334–336].

The possibility of a rebound headache after oxygen inhalation [337] can be mitigated by taking the treatment at the very beginning of the attack [338], by increasing the duration of inhalation or by selecting a different delivery system such as a demand valve system, which is preferred by some patients [339].

Sumatriptan 6 mg subcutaneous is an effective [340, 341] and safe option [342], which is both FDA and EMA approved and, unlike oxygen, compact and portable.

Other drawbacks include limits on daily usage [343] and a higher rate of side effects, compared to inhaled oxygen, viz.

### Classic Treatments to Prevent Attacks

Its effect in cluster headache is not entirely elucidated and may be related to the prevention of CGRP release, by inhibition of presynaptic calcium influx [344].

At a daily dose of 240–960 mg, it represents the first-line preventive treatment for most patients with cluster headache [191, 333].

Lithium at the dose of 900 mg demonstrated efficacy on chronic CH, with a longer latency period in comparison with verapamil [345] and a larger number of adverse effects, including tremor or nausea [346].

Both of these treatments seem to be beneficial for short periods, yet their prolonged use is hindered by serious side effects, such as psychosis or osteonecrosis.

GON blocks have proven effective in CH in two randomized placebo-controlled trials [347, 348].

Melatonin is a hormone that may exert an effect in cluster headache through its direct action on the suprachiasmatic nucleus of the hypothalamus [349].

It was not effective in chronic CH, although this has been investigated with variable dose regimes [102, 350].

### Emerging Treatments

CH attacks can be induced by CGRP infusion in patients with episodic cluster [351] and, with less consistency, in chronic CH patients using preventive treatment.

Of these studies, the gammaCore™ device is now CE marked in the European Union for acute and/or preventive treatment of cluster headache and has been FDA and NICE [352] approved for the treatment of both episodic and chronic CH.

The Pathway CH-2 study [353] was a randomized controlled trial involving ninety-three chronic CH patients based in the USA, treating their attacks with either active SPG stimulation or sham.

That followed the PREEMPT protocol, ten of seventeen refractory chronic CH patients treated with OBTA achieved a significant reduction in headache days [36], with mild side effects such as ptosis or a transient worsening in headaches.

**Conclusions**

A greater understanding of the basic biology of primary headaches has provided researchers with the tools to target specific pathways and design bespoke clinical studies, paving the way for novel treatments for clinical practice.

CGRP is a key element in the cluster headache pathway; new pharmacological therapies aimed at blocking it, such as monoclonal antibodies, have proven to be efficacious and well tolerated.

Emerging treatments for migraine, such as gepants or ditans, could be viable options for cluster headache patients burdened by other comorbidities and vascular risk factors.

Given the minimal amount of pharmacological interactions they present, a personalized combination of different novel therapies, targeting different elements involved in the nociceptive pathways, might well represent the future of treating cluster headache.

**Acknowledgement**

*A machine generated summary based on the work of Villar-Martínez, María Dolores; Puledda, Francesca; Goadsby, Peter J. 2020 in Current Treatment Options in Neurology.*

## *Cluster Headache: A Review and Update in Treatment*

DOI: https://doi.org/10.1007/s11910-021-01114-1

**Abstract-Summary**

The treatment of cluster headache has evolved to include a handheld neuromodulation device and a monoclonal antibody in addition to more traditional agents.

Galcanezumab is an approved treatment for episodic cluster headache.

The non-invasive vagal nerve stimulator has been shown to be effective as a treatment for episodic cluster headache.

Cluster headache is the most common trigeminal-autonomic cephalalgia, characterized by unilateral, frequent, debilitating attacks associated with ipsilateral autonomic symptoms.

Attacks have a circadian and, often, seasonal pattern with periods of remission that can last months to years in episodic patients.

Treatment in cluster headache should focus on early intervention to reduce frequency of attacks and the length of the cycle, which improves outcomes and disability.

Case 1: A 43-year-old man presents with the chief complaint of severe headaches.

He states that he hasn't "slept in over a week because of debilitating headaches."

His headaches start around the same time every night: when he lays down to go to sleep.

Similar headaches occurred last year during the month of October as well.

On further questioning, he reports that these headache attacks have been occurring almost yearly for the past 7 years.

Each year, these headaches come on as the weather is changing and occur on a nightly basis for about 3 to 4 weeks.

## Introduction

CH is the most common of the TACs yet still remains relatively rare overall, occurring in about 0.1% of the population [354].

It must be accompanied by either an ipsilateral autonomic symptom (conjunctival injection and/or lacrimation, nasal congestion, eyelid edema, forehead and facial swelling, miosis, and/or ptosis) and/or restlessness or agitation [1]. Cluster attacks tend to occur in a series of weeks to months, called cluster periods.

Most of the patients are classified as episodic, who have attacks occurring for a few weeks to months followed by periods of remission lasting months to years [355].

Chronic cluster headaches (CCH), on the other hand, are characterized by attacks occurring either without a remission period or a remission period lasting less than 3 months, for at least 1 year.

About 10–15% of the people with CH tend to have CCH rather episodic cluster headache (ECH) [1].

## Pathophysiology

Trigeminal-autonomic activation, localized to the superior salivatory nucleus, can explain the physiologic changes noted during a CH attack.

CGRP is found prominently in the trigeminovascular system, which has been shown to be activated during a cluster attack [162].

CGRP release results in the vasodilation of the arteries along with other neuropeptides, which is a direct result of activation of the trigeminal-autonomic reflex, involving the trigeminal afferent fibers and the parasympathetic nervous system, as previously mentioned [356].

Infusion of CGRP during active phase of a cluster period has also been shown to cause an attack.

## Diagnostic Work-Up

Unlike migraine, a patient with CH will typically have associated agitation.

In a study of 9 patients with treatment-resistant CH and low serum testosterone levels, hormonal supplementation with pure testosterone resulted in cessation of cluster attacks in the first 24 h in 5 of the 7 patients.

In certain reports, dedicated imaging of the pituitary gland has been recommended; however, recent data shows that the prevalence of pituitary adenomas in patients with CH is similar to those in general population and therefore do not require specific pituitary screening (unless findings on standard MRI or symptoms of pituitary disorder are elicited) [357].

One small study in 1984 showed that 60% of patients with CH had sleep apnea; however, 100% of patients with ECH had sleep apnea [278].

**Treatment**

In a study of 57 patients, in which 47 CH attacks were treated with octreotide and 46 attacks with placebo, response rates for octreotide vs. placebo were 52% vs. 36%, respectively, at 30 min (p < 0.01) [358].

A study of 69 patients showed headache relief rates of 42% and 61% at 5 mg and 10 mg doses of zolmitriptan, respectively, compared to placebo rates of 23% (p = 0.002) at 30 min.

A study of 124 patients showed that 10-mg zolmitriptan resulted in mild or no pain at 30 min in 60% of the patients, compared to 57% and 42% for 5-mg zolmitriptan and placebo, respectively (both p $\leq$ = 0.01 versus placebo).

Another study showed 11 of the 13 patients who received suboccipital nerve blocks with steroids became attack-free after 1 week compared to none out of the 11 patients in the placebo group (p = 0.0001).

**Controversies**

Case 2: A 34-year-old woman with a past medical history of episodic migraine presents with sudden increased frequency of headaches.

While CH is more common in men, approximately 20% of CH patients are women [158].

Although it is unclear from the presentation above whether this patient definitely has migraine or CH, women are often misdiagnosed without a thorough work-up.

Medication overuse headache (MOH) also remains an important, yet controversial topic in the treatment of CH.

Another review in 2008 reported that a personal or family history of migraine appeared to be strongly associated with the development of MOH in patients with CH [359].

This highlights the importance of keeping in mind the risk of MOH, which can not only worsen the patients' pain score but also their overt disability and can be avoided if proper precautions are taken, especially with patients who have other primary headache disorders such as migraine.

**Conclusion**

The attacks have a circadian and often, a seasonal pattern with periods of remission that lasts months to years in ECH patients.

Starting a patient with a bridging therapy, such as suboccipital nerve block injections with prednisone, along with an oral preventive therapy is the mainstay of treatment.

With the recent approval of galcanezumab for the treatment of ECH, we have added to the options for this patient group.

Acute therapies which have a fast onset of action such as subcutaneous sumatriptan or intranasal zolmitriptan can be used to abort CH attacks; however, a clinician must be mindful of the risk of MOH and use alternative therapies such as intranasal oxygen in conjunction.

**Acknowledgement**

*A machine generated summary based on the work of Suri, Himanshu; Ailani, Jessica. 2021 in Current Neurology and Neuroscience Reports.*


# *Cluster Headache: Present and Future Therapy*

DOI: https://doi.org/10.1007/s10072-017-2924-7

## Abstract-Summary

Cluster headache is characterized by severe, unilateral headache attacks of orbital, supraorbital or temporal pain lasting 15–180 min accompanied by ipsilateral lacrimation, rhinorrhea and other cranial autonomic manifestations.

Cluster headache attacks need fast-acting abortive agents because the pain peaks very quickly; sumatriptan injection is the gold standard acute treatment.

Monoclonal antibodies against calcitonin gene-related peptide are under investigation as prophylactic agents in both episodic and chronic cluster headache.

A number of neurostimulation procedures including occipital nerve stimulation, vagus nerve stimulation, sphenopalatine ganglion stimulation and the more invasive hypothalamic stimulation are employed in chronic intractable cluster headache.

## Introduction

According to the International Headache Society diagnostic criteria, cluster headache attacks are strictly unilateral, severe or very severe, the pain is felt in the orbital, supraorbital or temporal regions, its duration is 15–180 min [360] and the pain is accompanied by at least one of the following symptoms ipsilateral to the pain: conjunctival injection or lacrimation, nasal congestion, rhinorrhea, eyelid edema, forehead and/or facial sweating, miosis, or ptosis.

In episodic CH, attacks usually occur in periods, cluster periods, lasting 6–12 weeks followed by periods of remission of various durations [52, 361].

In chronic CH attacks occur without remission [360].

To prevent recurrent attacks during cluster periods patients need adequate prophylactic treatments while acute treatments are needed to abort single attacks.

## Acute Treatment

Patients have to treat the attack as soon as possible after onset.

Sumatriptan, a 5-HT$_{1B/D}$ agonist, is considered the gold standard to abort ongoing CH attacks both from data reported in double-blind, placebo-controlled trials and from clinical practice [340, 341].

The most effective sumatriptan formulation in CH is the injectable form [362], there are also oral and nasal-spray formulations.

The oldest treatment for CH is oral ergotamine [363]; but in one trial, intranasal application of dihydroergotamine was shown to be no superior to placebo [364].

**Preventive Treatment**

In open studies, methysergide has been demonstrated to exert some preventive effect both in episodic and chronic CH headache [365, 366].

The drug should be started at 25 mg per day and increased by 25 mg every week to minimize adverse effects, Adverse effects occur in about 40% of patients but these are rarely severe and include paresthesia of distal extremities, dizziness, cognitive symptoms, somnolence, imbalance and ataxia [367, 368].

Gabapentin at a dose of 900 mg per day produced pain free state in eight episodic and four chronic CH within 8 days in an open-label study [369].

Common dosage of oral prednisone or prednisolone is 60 mg once daily for 5–10 days or until the attacks stop; the dose should then be reduced by 5–10 mg every 4–10 days but tapering could be slower in chronic CH because relapse may occur.

**Neurostimulation**

In an another open-label study VNS (gammaCore) was used as acute treatment: it reduced attacks duration in 47% of cases: 11 vs 75 min [370] in 19 CH patients.

126 CH patients from ten open studies show an overall average efficacy of 67% reduction of headache attack frequency [371, 372].

In a 24 months open-label follow-up study 5956 CH attacks were evaluated and 45% of patients were responders (acute effectiveness in ≥50% of attacks) [373].

Sixteen years after the introduction of deep brain stimulation (DBS) of the hypothalamus as treatment of intractable chronic CH, there is only one randomized placebo-controlled trial in 11 chronic CH patients treated with this invasive procedure.

Results from more than 90 chronic CH patients treated by hypothalamic DBS have been reported and the overall proportion of responders (≥50% headache frequency reduction) is of about 66% [374].

**Acknowledgement**

*A machine generated summary based on the work of Leone, Massimo; Giustiniani, Alessandro; Cecchini, Alberto Proietti. 2017 in Neurological Sciences.*

## *Drug Treatment of Cluster Headache*

DOI: https://doi.org/10.1007/s40265-021-01658-z

**Abstract-Summary**

This review summarizes drug therapy of cluster attacks and prophylactic treatment.

The therapy for acute cluster attacks includes inhalation of 100% oxygen, subcutaneous administration of sumatriptan, and intranasal application of sumatriptan or zolmitriptan.

Best documented drugs for preventive treatment of cluster headache are verapamil and lithium, and possibly effective drugs are gabapentin, topiramate, divalproex sodium, and melatonin.

Several drug therapies are being investigated including ketamine, onabotulinumtoxinA, lysergic acid, and sodium oxybate.

## Introduction

Cluster headache is characterized by strictly unilateral attacks of severe head and facial pain.

For episodic cluster headache, bouts frequently start with one to two attacks per week, may progress to several/day over 1–2 weeks, and then taper over 1–2 weeks after occurring at the high plateau for up to several or more weeks.

It is clinically important to highlight that even patients with long-lasting chronic cluster headache show a cycling pattern and that an increase in attack frequency does not necessarily mean that medication is failing but rather that for some time add-on therapy may be necessary.

We summarize the most important data on the treatment of cluster attacks and the prevention of cluster headache with recommendations for the management of these patients.

Therapy of cluster headache consists of the medical abortion of the single attack, bridging therapy to cover the time until the prophylactic treatment takes effect, and the actual preventive therapy.

## Treatment of Cluster Attacks

In the first randomized placebo-controlled trial with 39 patients, two cluster attacks were treated in random order with 6 mg of sumatriptan subcutaneously or placebo.

The success rate of 6 mg of sumatriptan subcutaneously for pain free at 10 min was 36% and for placebo 3% [340].

Although many patients with cluster headache have vascular risk factors [375], there have been no reports of stroke or myocardial infarction in patients with cluster headache treating their attacks with subcutaneous sumatriptan.

Patients treated one attack with a sumatriptan 20-mg nasal spray and another attack with placebo.

Headache relief at 30 min was observed in 63% of patients treated with 10 mg of zolmitriptan compared with 48% treated with 5 mg of zolmitriptan and 30% treated with placebo.

## Oxygen Treatment

Inhalation of oxygen is effective in up to 60% of patients.

The recommended dosage is the inhalation of at least 12 L/min of 100% oxygen and has been tested in a randomized double-blind trial [334].

It needs to be noted that in the experience of the authors, in some patients, oxygen treatment may not end the attacks but seem to prolong them.

Oxygen inhalation seems to end the attack but comes back within 1 hour.

**Bridging or Transitional Therapy**

Prednisone in peak doses of 10–80 mg/day was used in 19 patients with cluster headache in the USA [376].

Recurrence of cluster headache occurred in most patients when the prednisone dose was reduced to below 10–20 mg daily.

Patients with episodic cluster headache within a new cluster bout lasting not longer than 30 days were randomized to 100 mg of oral prednisone for 5 days followed by tapering the dose or placebo.

Corticosteroid injections in the area of the ipsilateral greater occipital nerve were investigated in a double-blind placebo-controlled trial in 16 patients with episodic headache and seven patients with chronic cluster headache [347].

Another randomized, double-blind, placebo-controlled trial enrolled patients with more than two cluster headache attacks per day [348].

Patients who were treated with cortivazol also had fewer cluster attacks in the first 15 days after injections than controls.

**Prevention of Cluster Headache**

The first randomized placebo-controlled trial with 30 patients investigated the efficacy of verapamil compared with placebo in the prophylaxis of episodic cluster headache.

A second open study investigated verapamil in 84 patients with cluster headache [377].

Another open study of 36 consecutive patients including 26 with episodic cluster headache and ten with chronic cluster headache reported a reduction in cluster attacks of more than 50% in 7/33 patients.

A prospective study from Spain with 26 patients, 12 with episodic cluster headache and 14 with chronic cluster headache used a maximum dose of topiramate of 200 mg.

In a small Italian study in eight patients with episodic cluster headache and four patients with chronic cluster headache, all of whom were refractory to traditional prophylactics, a dose of 1000 mg of gabapentin resulted in a significant reduction in the length of the cluster period [378].

**Future Therapy of Cluster Headache**

In a study in 2016, 13 patients with chronic headache and 16 with episodic cluster headache were treated with low doses of intravenous ketamine at 2-week intervals [379].

In patients with episodic cluster headache, this resulted in a suspension of cluster attacks for a period of between 3 and 18 months.

Half of the patients with chronic cluster headache also responded to ketamine.

A ketamine-magnesium combination was studied in an open trial in patients with chronic cluster headache who were resistant to at least three preventive treatments [380].

An ongoing trial in Denmark is a proof-of-concept study for the evaluation of the effect of a ketamine intranasal spray in the treatment of chronic cluster headache (EudraCT2019-001260-29).

Patients with episodic and chronic cluster headache were enrolled in a randomized, double-blind, placebo-controlled phase II trial.

OnabotulinumtoxinA was investigated in an open trial in patients with chronic cluster headache [381].

## Conclusions

Cluster headache is extremely distressing owing to the high intensity of pain attacks and significantly affects the quality of life of affected patients [382].

In a real-life study in Denmark, of 399 patients with cluster headache, only 30 treated their attacks with subcutaneous sumatriptan.

There is a considerable need to develop new fast-acting therapies for the treatment of cluster attacks.

Even more problematic is the prophylactic therapy of cluster headache.

These substances are not approved for the prophylaxis of cluster headache.

It would be desirable if there were effective and well-tolerated new therapies for the prophylaxis of cluster headache.

## Acknowledgement

*A machine generated summary based on the work of Diener, Hans Christoph; May, Arne. 2021 in Drugs.*

## *Pharmacotherapy for Cluster Headache*

DOI: https://doi.org/10.1007/s40263-019-00696-2

## Abstract-Summary

Cluster headache is characterised by attacks of excruciating unilateral headache or facial pain lasting 15 min to 3 h and is seen as one of the most intense forms of pain.

Cluster headache attacks are accompanied by ipsilateral autonomic symptoms such as ptosis, miosis, redness or flushing of the face, nasal congestion, rhinorrhoea, peri-orbital swelling and/or restlessness or agitation.

Cluster headache treatment entails fast-acting abortive treatment, transitional treatment and preventive treatment.

The primary goal of prophylactic and transitional treatment is to achieve attack freedom, although this is not always possible.

Subcutaneous sumatriptan and high-flow oxygen are the most proven abortive treatments for cluster headache attacks, but other treatment options such as intranasal triptans may be effective.

Verapamil and lithium are the preventive drugs of first choice and the most widely used in first-line preventive treatment.

Since the evidence level is low, we also recommend considering one of several neuromodulatory options in patients with refractory chronic cluster headache.

A new addition to the preventive treatment options in episodic cluster headache is galcanezumab, although the long-term effects remain unknown.

Since effective preventive treatment can take several weeks to titrate, transitional treatment can be of great importance in the treatment of cluster headache.

Extended:

Cluster headache is considered the most severe primary headache disorder and is characterised by attacks of excruciating unilateral headache or facial pain lasting 15 min to 3 h [1].

The primary goal of prophylactic therapy is attack freedom.

Since the evidence level is low, we recommend also considering one of several neuromodulatory options.

**Introduction**

Cluster headache is considered the most severe primary headache disorder and is characterised by attacks of excruciating unilateral headache or facial pain lasting 15 min to 3 h [1].

In eCH, the attacks occur in 'bouts' (clusters) that last from weeks to months and alternate with remission periods of months to years [60].

Cluster headache exhibits a remarkable circadian pattern, with attacks often occurring at the same time of the day.

Cluster headache treatment entails both fast-acting abortive treatment to effectively abort an ongoing attack and preventive treatment.

This article provides an overview of currently available pharmacological treatment for cluster headache.

Since this is an overview of pharmacological treatment options for cluster headache, invasive and non-invasive neurostimulation treatment options are not discussed.

**Pathophysiology**

The exact pathophysiology of cluster headache remains unknown.

Several structures have been found to contribute to cluster headache attacks: the trigeminovascular system, the parasympathetic nerve fibres and the hypothalamus [355].

Early imaging studies indeed showed hypothalamic activation in cluster headache attacks [121, 383–385].

How this hypothalamic activation contributes to the generation of cluster headache attacks remains unclear, but the hypothalamus is currently regarded as the 'attack generator'.

Although cluster headache is a primary headache, cases of atypical cluster headache and even 'classic' cluster headache secondary to underlying structural pathology have been described.

A case review describing 63 cases of symptomatic cluster headache revealed that a significant proportion of secondary cases were associated with structural changes in the pituitary region and with arterial dissection [386].

## Cluster Headache Treatment

The only double-blind randomised placebo-controlled trial studying verapamil (1:1 treatment allocation, verapamil 360 mg vs. placebo) showed a significant decrease in daily attack frequency (0.66 ± 0.88 vs. 1.65 ± 1.01, respectively; p < 0.001) and daily analgesic use (0.5 ± 0.87 vs. 1.2 ± 1.03, respectively; p < 0.004) in 30 patients with eCH [387].

In an early open-label trial, sodium valproate (600–2000 mg) was effective in the treatment of cluster headache in 11 of 15 patients: nine patients achieved complete remission and two showed a partial effect [388].

This therapeutic intervention for the treatment of chronic local neuropathic pain has existed since the 1960s, with effectiveness in cluster headaches being reported as early as 1985 in 12 patients with eCH and eight patients with cCH [389].

## Conclusion and Clinical Recommendation

Treatment of cluster headache entails a combination of fast-acting abortive treatment, transitional treatment and preventive treatment.

Very few pharmacological treatment options have a high level of evidence.

When treating patients with cluster headache, it is important to first start abortive treatment.

Prophylactic therapy is necessary for patients with cCH or for patients with eCH in an active cluster episode.

In patients with eCH, the type of prophylactic treatment depends on bout length, because titrating to an adequate dosage of prophylactic drug can take weeks.

When patients are in a sustained period of attack freedom, prophylactic therapy can be tapered.

Since effective preventive treatment can take several weeks to titrate, transitional treatment can be of great importance in the treatment of cluster headache.

Cluster headache therapy needs to be highly individualised, especially in patients with cCH since attack freedom cannot always be achieved.

## Acknowledgement

*A machine generated summary based on the work of Brandt, Roemer B.; Doesborg, Patty G. G.; Haan, Joost; Ferrari, Michel D.; Fronczek, Rolf. 2020 in CNS Drugs.*


## *Anti-CGRP in Cluster Headache Therapy*

DOI: https://doi.org/10.1007/s10072-019-03786-7

## Abstract-Summary

The pathophysiology of cluster headache comprises mechanisms both in the peripheral and central nervous system, involving the trigeminovascular system, the trigemino-parasympathetic reflex, and central modulating systems.

Drugs against this neuropeptide have been developed for the treatment of different headache disorders.

Monoclonal antibodies vs CGRP as galcanezumab and fremanezumab have been tested in cluster headache, with promising results for the episodic form.

Considering the relevance of central mechanisms in CH, drugs interfering with the CGRP pathway in the central nervous system can enlarge the therapeutic armamentarium against this highly disabling condition.

Extended:

Considering that cluster headache is not just peripheral vasodilation of cranial arteries, the possibility to employ central acting molecules interfering with the CGRP pathway open highways for future treatment of CH.

## Cluster Headache

Cluster headache (CH) is a primary headache characterized by strictly unilateral pain, of severe intensity, associated with autonomic phenomena in the ipsilateral face (conjunctival injection, lacrimation, nasal congestion, rhinorrhea, forehead and facial sweating, miosis, ptosis, and/or eyelid edema) and psychological-behavioral manifestations (agitation, restlessness) [60].

About 1 out of 7 CH patients has been afflicted by headaches for at least a year without a sustained remission [158], and thus suffers from what is defined as "chronic cluster headache" [60].

Despite its rarity, CH is deemed to be the most painful headache condition, and patients are afflicted by a significant burden.

A survey in the USA observed that CH had caused a lost job in almost 20% of patients, while another 8% were out of work or on disability secondary to their headaches, while 11% stated they were literally bed-bound for 31 days or more per year because of headaches [10].

## Calcitonin Gene–Related Peptide

CGRP is expressed in nearly a quarter of trigeminal ganglionic sensory neurons, and particularly in 1/3 of the neurons innervating the cerebral and meningeal vasculature [390].

CGRP could also exert an action inside the trigeminal ganglion: in vitro observations support the hypothesis that the neuropeptide can be released at this level by sensory neurons, inducing the activation of satellite glial cells via CGRP receptor with the increase of iNOS expression and the release of NO [391].

In the human sphenopalatine ganglion, Csati and others observed thin CGRP-containing fibers, probably originating from the trigeminal ganglion as C-fibers, and the two CGRP receptor components together in the satellite glial cells [392], establishing a possible peripheral link between the sensory afferents and the autonomic efferents.

Walker and others found expression of both CTR and RAMP1 in some neurons of the trigeminal ganglion and in the spinal trigeminal complex, potentially also implicating the $AMY_1$ receptor in the CGRP signaling [393].

## CGRP in Cluster Headache

Goadsby and colleagues observed a raise in blood levels of CGRP and VIP during acute spontaneous attacks of CH measured from the ipsilateral external jugular vein.

During nitroglycerine-induced attacks, plasma CGRP levels rose [394, 395], and reversed to the baseline both after spontaneous and sumatriptan-induced remission.

Intravenous CGRP induced CH attacks in 8 of 9 episodic CH patients in the active phase while placebo provoked headache only in 1.

None of the episodic CH patients in remission developed headache after both CGRP and placebo infusion.

Vasodilators in general, such as alcohol, nitroglycerine, and CGRP itself, are able to induce CH attacks, but only during cluster periods or in chronic patients [351].

The observation that the CGRP concentration in the jugular vein is increased at the peak of severity of NO-induced CH attacks, but not before or at the onset of the headache [395], might indicate that CGRP is involved in the ramp up of the attack, but is not essential for its initiation; otherwise, this observation may be due to a delay needed by CGRP to reach the venous circulation [396].

**Anti-CGRP in Cluster Headache**

The efficacy of two different monoclonal antibodies against CGRP, galcanezumab and fremanezumab, has been recently investigated in the prophylaxis of CH.

Results from a placebo-controlled study of galcanezumab in patients with episodic CH have been reported.

The mean reduction in weekly CH attack frequency across weeks 1–3 was −8.7 for galcanezumab compared to −5.2 for placebo (treatment groups difference in mean change, −3.5 [95% CI −6.7, −0.2]; p = 0.036).

The proportion of CH patients showing ≥50% reduction in weekly CH attack frequency at week 3 was 76% for galcanezumab compared to 57% for placebo (p = 0.04).

Two trials exploring anti-CGRP monoclonal antibodies efficacy for the prevention of chronic CH, galcanezumab NCT02438826 and fremanezumab NCT02964338, stopped recruitment because futility analysis revealed that the primary endpoint was unlikely to be met.

**Conclusions**

Monoclonal antibodies against CGRP have the potential to improve CH and initial data from randomized clinical trials support this view.

The blood brain barrier (BBB) avoids antibodies to reach the brain, so monoclonal antibodies against CGRP exert their therapeutic effects outside the brain, in the extracerebral arteries and the trigeminal ganglion and fibers.

**Acknowledgement**

*A machine generated summary based on the work of Giani, Luca; Proietti Cecchini, Alberto; Leone, Massimo. 2019 in Neurological Sciences.*

# *Cluster Headache Pathophysiology—Insights from Current and Emerging Treatments*

DOI: https://doi.org/10.1038/s41582-021-00477-w

**Abstract-Summary**

Preventive medications were borrowed from non-headache indications, so management of cluster headache is challenging.

As our understanding of cluster headache pathophysiology has evolved on the basis of key bench and neuroimaging studies, crucial neuropeptides and brain structures have been identified as emerging treatment targets.

In this Review, we provide an overview of what is known about the pathophysiology of cluster headache and discuss the existing treatment options and their mechanisms of action.

We also consider emerging treatment options, including calcitonin gene-related peptide antibodies, non-invasive vagus nerve stimulation, sphenopalatine ganglion stimulation and somatostatin receptor agonists, discuss how evidence from trials of these emerging treatments provides insights into the pathophysiology of cluster headache and highlight areas for future research.

Extended:

In this Review, we provide an overview of cluster headache, including the key clinical features, epidemiology and current understanding of pathophysiology based on bench and neuroimaging studies.

We explore the results of the clinical studies in the context of understanding cluster headache pathophysiology, and conclude by identifying areas of research for the future.

**Introduction**

Treatment options for cluster headache have been limited, but key clinical studies from the past 5 years have provided promising new treatment options.

In this Review, we provide an overview of cluster headache, including the key clinical features, epidemiology and current understanding of pathophysiology based on bench and neuroimaging studies.

We explore the results of the clinical studies in the context of understanding cluster headache pathophysiology, and conclude by identifying areas of research for the future.

**Clinical Characteristics**

Patients with cluster headache experience repeated, severe attacks of unilateral pain in the trigeminal nerve distribution that can last from 15 min to 3 h [1].

Cluster headache attacks are often experienced in clusters or 'bouts' that occur at particular times of the year with a circannual periodicity.

Multiple bouts can occur throughout the year, and if the time between bouts is >3 months without preventive medication, patients are classified as having episodic cluster headache.

Bouts can also be continuous; if this is the case or if the time between bouts is <3 months, patients are classified as having chronic cluster headache [1].

**Pathophysiology**

Given the trigeminal [397] and cervical [398] afferent innervation distribution, the clinical presentation of cluster headache strongly suggests that activation of second-order trigeminocervical neurons is responsible for the pain.

Are the key neuropeptides and neurotransmitters involved in the trigeminovascular system, trigeminal autonomic reflex and retinohypothalamic tract that are thought to have a role in the pathogenesis of cluster headache.

Activation of the trigeminal autonomic reflex can be secondary to activation of the trigeminovascular system, and peripheral activations of the afferent and efferent arms of the trigeminal autonomic reflex alone are insufficient to trigger cluster headache attacks.

Although uncertain, the hypothalamus is likely to have a central role in the activation of these mechanisms; this hypothesis is supported by clinical findings of neuroendocrine changes in patients with cluster headache, the association between cluster bouts and photoperiods, and functional neuroimaging that shows hypothalamus activation during acute attacks.

**Established Treatments**

The use of corticosteroids for the treatment of cluster headache was first reported in 1952, but in this study, 100 mg of cortisone (equivalent to 20 mg prednisolone) was effective in only 4 of 21 patients [399].

This effect was reflected in a clinical study in which external jugular vein plasma levels of CGRP (a biomarker of trigeminal activation) and urine levels of a metabolite of melatonin (a biomarker of hypothalamic function) were compared before and after methylprednisolone treatment in patients with episodic cluster headache and controls with multiple sclerosis [400].

In a subsequent open-label study that involved 34 patients with chronic cluster headache, verapamil at doses of 160–480 mg/day decreased attack frequency and severity in 79% of patients [401].

One double-blind pilot study suggested that treatment with melatonin helps prevent attacks in patients with episodic cluster headache when compared with placebo [102].

**Emerging Treatment Options**

Of the CGRP antibody fremanezumab, in which the primary end point was assessed at a later time point than with galcanezumab, treatment was not effective in patients with episodic cluster headache [402].

Double-blind, randomized studies have shown that nVNS effectively aborts cluster headache attacks within 15 min, but only in patients with episodic cluster headache and not in those with chronic cluster headache [403–405].

In one study, low-frequency stimulation induced cluster headache attacks in three of six patients with cluster headache, either during the 3 min of stimulation or within the 30 min after stimulation [406].

In a more extensive double-blind, randomized, sham-controlled, crossover study, 21 patients with cluster headache underwent 30 min of low-frequency or sham stimulation, and the low-frequency stimulation induced more cranial autonomic symptoms than sham stimulation.

### Invasive Treatment

In small studies of patients with medically refractory cluster headache, DBS of the ipsilateral posterior hypothalamus reduced the severity and frequency of attacks [219, 374, 407].

In a study of eight patients with cluster headache [408], ONS was well tolerated, and the adverse effect profile was less severe than that of DBS.

Further open-label studies of the use of ONS in the treatment of chronic cluster headache have shown that it can reduce attack frequency in 66.7–70% of patients [372, 409–411].

ONS could be a treatment option for medically refractory chronic cluster headache, provided that patients are selected carefully to ensure all other avenues have been explored.

### Episodic vs Chronic Cluster Headache

The results of clinical trials of CGRP monoclonal antibodies and nVNS have highlighted the fact that episodic cluster headache and chronic cluster headache respond differently.

Differences between episodic and chronic cluster headache are also apparent from triggering studies in humans.

Intravenous nitroglycerin infusion to induce cluster headache attacks has revealed phenotypic differences between the subtypes of cluster headache: patients with episodic cluster headache in bout or chronic cluster headache developed attacks in response to nitroglycerin but the time until attack onset was shorter in those with episodic cluster headache than in those with chronic cluster headache [412].

Further studies to identify the differences in the pathophysiology of episodic and chronic cluster headache are crucial for improvement in treatment options, as the therapeutic approaches used to date clearly target only some aspects of the complex pathogenesis of cluster headache.

### Conclusion

Great strides have been made in the treatment of cluster headache in the past decade.

Not all patients respond to the novel and targeted treatments, indicating that the targets of existing therapeutic approaches do not fully explain the pathogenesis of cluster headache.

The underlying cause of cluster headache chronicity needs to be identified — to this end, patients who develop cluster headache secondary to episodic cluster headache should be compared with patients with de novo chronic cluster headache.

These studies are important, because as long as our understanding of cluster headache remains incomplete, our treatments are unlikely to be sufficient to control this debilitating condition.

### Acknowledgement

*A machine generated summary based on the work of Wei, Diana Y.; Goadsby, Peter J. 2021 in Nature Reviews Neurology.*

## *Oxygen Treatment for Cluster Headache Attacks at Different Flow Rates: A Double-Blind, Randomized, Crossover Study*

DOI: https://doi.org/10.1186/s10194-018-0917-4

### Abstract-Summary

Oxygen at flow rates of both 7 L/min and 12 L/min was shown to be effective.

In a double-blind, randomized, crossover study, oxygen naïve cluster headache patients, treated attacks with oxygen at 7 and 12 L/min.

The primary outcome measure was the percentage of attacks after which patients (treating at least 2 attacks/day) were painfree after 15 min, in the first two days of the study.

Secondary outcome measures were percentage of successfully treated attacks, percentage of attacks after which patients were painfree, drop in VAS score and patient preference in all treatment periods (14 days).

We could only include 5 patients, treating 27 attacks on the first two days of the study, for our primary outcome, which did not show a significant difference (p = 0.180).

Patients tended to prefer 12 L/min (p = 0.005).

Contradicting this result, more patients were painfree using 7 L/min (p = 0.039).

The exploratory analysis showed an odds ratio of being painfree using 12 L/min of 0.73 (95% CI 0.52–1.02) compared to 7 L/min (p = 0.061) as scored on a 5-point scale.

Slightly more patients noticed, no or not much, relief on 7 L/min, and found 12 L/min to be effective in all their attacks.

There is lack of evidence to support differences in the effect of oxygen at a flow rate of 12 L/min compared to 7 L/min.

More patients were painfree using 7 L/min, but our other outcome measures did not confirm a difference in effect between flow rates.

Extended:

Oxygen at both 7 L/min and 12 L/min was shown to be effective [334, 413].

We could only include 5 patients for analysis of our primary outcome measure.

Contradicting this result, a higher percentage of attacks after which patients were painfree, as scored on a 5-point scale, was found in the 7 L/min group.

On all other outcome measures, group 3 and 4 were equal to the other groups.

It remains unclear which outcome measure is the most appropriate for a trial on the treatment of cluster headache.

## Background

A study by Kudrow (1981) (N = 52) demonstrated that 75% of patients treated with oxygen at a flow rate of 7 L/min have adequate or complete relief, in at least 7 out of 10 attacks [413].

In a small study by Fogan (1985) (N = 19) oxygen at a flow rate of 6 L/min was shown to be more effective than room air [335].

The usual oxygen flow rate applied has remained 7 L/min until the study by Cohen (2009) (N = 76) showed that treatment with oxygen at a flow rate of 12 L/min was effective as well [334].

We compared treatment of CH attacks with 100% oxygen via a non-rebreather mask at different flow rates, 7 L/min vs. 12 L/min.

We hypothesized that oxygen at a higher flow rate (12 L/min) might be more effective for the treatment of cluster headache attacks.

## Methods

During the treatment period patients were asked to fill in a diary, in which they described, for each attack, the time until the start of oxygen treatment, pain scores before and following treatment, how long the oxygen treatment lasted, and any side effects using valve A or B. Following the 14-day study period or at the end of the cluster period, patients were asked to fill in a final questionnaire.

The secondary endpoints were, percentage of attacks treated successfully (defined as drop in VAS score of over 50%), percentage of attacks after which patients were painfree, absolute drop in VAS-score, and the patient preference to the flow rates of 7 or 12 L/min in all treatment periods.

If patients dropped out before using both treatments, or if all attacks using one flow rate had to be excluded, they were not included in the primary and secondary endpoints.

## Results

These patients treated a total of 680 attacks, of which 76 attacks had to be excluded, leaving 604 attacks for the analysis.

Five patients had an average attack duration of longer than 180 min and 3 patients had less than one attack in 2 days.

Only 5 patients met the inclusion criteria for our primary outcome measure; two treated attacks on each of the first 2 days.

These patients treated a total of 27 attacks on the first 2 days.

Patient's preference at the end of the study, expressed on a scale of 0–10, showed a median score of 3.5 (favouring 12 L/min).

Contradicting this result, a higher percentage of attacks after which patients were painfree, as scored on a 5-point scale, was found in the 7 L/min group.

No significant differences were found between randomization groups on success or painfree percentages and patient preference.

## Discussion

We could not confirm this trend in our other outcome measures and contradicting these results, patients tended to favour 12 L/min.

These results, combined with our other outcome measures, suggest that although more patients were painfree using 7 L/min, this is insufficient to state that 7 L/min is the more effective treatment.

This could be interpreted in a way that there seems to be a subgroup of patients, who absolutely favours 12 L/min, while in the rest of the population there does not seem to be a difference between both treatment groups.

As our study did not show any difference in the occurrence of side effects between groups, we can state that there is no consistent difference in treatment effect and safety between oxygen at a flow rate of 7 and 12 L/min.

As these were nearly equally distributed between flow rates and treatment results were not significantly different in these patients, we have no reason to assume selective drop-out.

## Conclusion

Patients preferred the treatment with oxygen at a flow rate of 12 L/min compared to 7 L/min.

The preference for 12 L/min might be explained by the fact that there were more patients in which treatment with 12 L/min was effective in all attacks, and less patients in which treatment was ineffective.

These results suggest, that although more patients were painfree using 7 L/min, this is insufficient to state that 7 L/min is the more effective treatment.

As no difference in side effects were found, the usage of oxygen at a flow rate of 12 L/min is at least equally safe as 7 L/min and could be used in all patients.

## Acknowledgement

*A machine generated summary based on the work of Dirkx, Thijs H. T.; Haane, Danielle Y. P.; Koehler, Peter J. 2018 in The Journal of Headache and Pain.*

# *Safety and Efficacy of Percutaneous Pulsed Radiofrequency Treatment at the C1–C2 Level in Chronic Cluster Headache: A Retrospective Analysis of 21 Cases*

DOI: https://doi.org/10.1007/s13760-019-01203-6

## Abstract-Summary

We performed a study of the safety and efficacy of percutaneous pulsed radiofrequency (PRF) treatment directed at C1 and C2 levels as performed at our local pain clinic in refractory chronic cluster headache (CCH) patients.

Data were collected through retrospective analysis of patients' files and include demographic variables, onset and duration of the headache, mean attack frequency, and prior pharmacological treatment.

Safety and reduction of attack frequency in the first 3 months after a first PRF treatment was the primary outcome parameter of this study.

Ten patients (47.6%) reported no meaningful effect, four patients (19%) reported a meaningful reduction of <50%, and seven patients (33.3%) reported a reduction in headache burden of at least 50% in the 3 months following treatment.

Two patients reported occurrence or increase in frequency of contralateral cluster attacks.

Upper cervical PRF treatment appears to be a safe procedure that could prove effective in the treatment of patients with refractory CCH and warrants a prospective study.

**Introduction**

Patients with primary headaches not only report pain from the anterior part of the head innervated by the trigeminal nerve, but also from the back of the head and neck innervated by the upper cervical roots [414].

No studies have reported on radiofrequency ablation or pulsed radiofrequency (PRF) treatment directed at upper cervical neural structures.

There has been some interest in using the PRF technique for cluster headache patients and a few case series of PRF interventions directed at the pterygopalatine ganglion have been published (the largest series reported the results in 16 patients) [415–418].

Studies on PRF treatment directed at the trigeminal ganglion are lacking, but limited retrospective data on radiofrequency ablation of this structure are available [419].

We present the results from a study that we conducted on the safety and effectiveness of percutaneous PRF treatment directed at the C1 and C2 levels in chronic cluster headache (CCH) patients at our pain clinic.

**Methods**

Informed consent was not required for this retrospective clinical study.

A retrospective chart review of patients' medical records was performed of all cluster headache patients who underwent the procedure at the Pain Clinic of the Ghent University Hospital between January 2010 and August 2017.

The entry point for C1 is at the junction of the upper 2/3 and lower 1/3 of the bony pillar of C1.

The position of the needle is checked in the antero-posterior axis while identifying the lateral margin of the atlanto-axial joint.

The needle is advanced to the lateral border of the atlanto-axial joint.

The entry point for C2 lies at the junction of the upper 1/3 and lower 2/3 of the bony pillar of C2.

A 22G 50 mm RF needle is inserted and advanced using tunnel vision until contact with bone at the target point.

## Results

All patients had tried at least two prophylactic drugs prior to PRF treatment; all had been on an adequate dose of verapamil, 19 out of 21 on lithium, 19 on topiramate, 11 on gabapentin, 10 on methysergide (which is currently no longer available in Belgium), 10 on melatonin, and 9 on valproate.

Ten patients (47.6%) reported no meaningful effect after PRF treatment, four patients (19%) reported a meaningful reduction in headache burden of <50% and seven patients (33.3%) reported a reduction in headache burden of more than 50% in the 3 months following treatment.

Changes in prophylactic cluster treatment occurred in seven patients in the first 3 months of follow-up and of these three patients reported a reduction in headache burden of more than 50%.

One other patient with strictly unilateral attacks at baseline and a complete resolution of cluster attacks after ipsilateral PRF treatment reported recurrence of contralateral cluster attacks 11 months after the procedure.

## Discussion

A global improvement of at least 50% reported by a third of this group with difficult to treat CCH patients is promising and could be clinically meaningful if confirmed in further prospective (and preferably controlled) studies.

Comparison to our results should be done with caution, since the patient characteristics in this study could be significantly different from our population, as it included CCH patients regardless of medication history and no information was provided on previous standard of care prophylactic treatments.

The stimulation of C1 in patients with chronic occipital pain evoked periorbital and frontal pain in the subgroup of six migraine patients only, suggesting that C1 has a particular link with migraine; there were no cluster patients included in this study, but a similar phenomenon cannot be excluded [398].

Since solid data from a prospective study are lacking, we can only speculate on the potential place of PRF treatment at the high cervical level in the interventional treatment algorithm of CCH.

## Acknowledgement

*A machine generated summary based on the work of Kelderman, Tim; Vanschoenbeek, Giel; Crombez, Erwin; Paemeleire, Koen. 2019 in Acta Neurologica Belgica.*

# *A Retrospective Observation on 105 Patients with Chronic Cluster Headache Receiving Indomethacin*

DOI: https://doi.org/10.1007/s10072-021-05114-4

## Abstract-Summary

Indomethacin (IMC) as a prophylactic treatment is considered to be ineffective in cluster headache (CH).

We described clinical features of IMC responders in a retrospective cohort of chronic cluster headache (CCH).

We included all patients fulfilling CCH criteria (ICHD-3-beta).

We recorded all the prescriptions of IMC as a prophylactic treatment.

The study consisted of 324 CCH, 121 female (37%) and 203 males (63%) with an average age at onset of 33.93 (±14.71) years.

Thirty-four patients (32%) were non-responders.

Responding status was undefined for 41 patients (39%).

Twelve patients (11%) had a complete response.

This study shows the interest of IMC in CCH patients.

We recommend an IMC test as a third-line treatment in CCH.

**Introduction**

Cluster headache (CH) is a primary headache, classified into 2 subforms: episodic (ECH) and chronic (CCH).

To its anti-inflammatory properties, IMC may provoke vasoconstriction, decrease cerebro-spinal fluid pressure, decrease blood flow velocity, and inhibit neuronal trigemino-vascular responses and lower levels of CGRP and VIP in the jugular veins.

IMC could prevent CH's attacks by inhibiting the trigemino-vascular response and the vasodilatation.

Despite lack of systematic evaluation for CH prophylaxis, IMC is largely considered to be ineffective in patients with CH.

There were many case reports/series of CH in the literature where IMC was effective [420, 421].

The headache center in La Timone hospital (Marseille) follows a large number of CCH patients, and some of them have been treated with IMC as prophylactic treatment.

The objective of this study was to describe the clinical features of chronic cluster headache responding to IMC.

**Patients and Methods**

The response to IMC was defined by a 50% or higher reduction in attack frequency as it was done in other studies in CH [387].

For each patient, the physician filled a questionnaire reporting clinical, paraclinical, and therapeutic data during the first consultation.

For patients who had an IMC prescription during the follow-up, we also noted clinical data they presented at that time.

The failure to follow up was defined by the absence of consultation for more than one year, or if it was mentioned that the patient decided to stop the follow-up.

All prophylactic CCH treatments the patients received, before and during their follow-up, were documented.

Because IMC is not given to all CCH patient, we tried to identify which patients received this treatment by comparing the clinical characteristics of treated patients (at the time of prescription) with those of untreated patient (at the time of the first consultation).

## Results

105 patients (32%) received IMC as a prophylactic treatment.

The responders (30 patients) comprised 18 women (60%) and 12 men (40%); they had on average 44.89 years (±12.88) at IMC prescription.

Only 3 patients (10%) had an IMC prescription in the past (as a prophylactic or attack treatment).

We compared patients receiving IMC and those who did not receive it (control group).

The IMC group received in total, at the last follow-up, more prophylactic treatments (6.75 ± 3.12) than the control group (3.30 ± 2.7).

On the 105 treated patients we could describe 5 main reasons why IMC was chosen as a prophylactic treatment: as a diagnostic test (26%), because of the lack of other therapeutics left (47%), because of the knowledge of previous effectiveness of IMC (6%), because of the presence of an interictal dull pain (20%), because the patients should receive NSAID for other reasons (6%).

## Discussion

Regarding the scientific literature about CH and IMC, Prakash and others [421], in a review, reported 13 articles [422–425] describing 24 CH patients responding to IMC and added 4 new cases.

An oral presentation by Lisotto in 2015 reported one new case of a CCH patient responding absolutely to IMC [426].

Only 13 CCH patients responding to IMC were reported in literature in 2019.

In this situation, the fact that we showed in our IMC group that 29% patients were responders and 11% had a complete initial response (11%), could affirm the role of IMC as a therapeutic option for the management of CCH.

Prakash and others, according to the observation of 28 cases of CH responding to IMC, affirm its efficiency in CH at high dose (≥300 mg daily) and would need a delay between 1 and 2 weeks [421].

This retrospective observational cohort study helps to understand the interest of IMC in the management of CCH patients.

## Conclusion

Chronic cluster headache as an IMC-resistant headache disorder is not true anymore.

Chronic cluster headache can respond to IMC even at lower doses than previously reported.

We recommend that all patients with CCH should have a trial of IMC before CH neurosurgery.

## Acknowledgement

*A machine generated summary based on the work of Monta, Anaé; Redon, Sylvain; Fabre, Cyprien; Donnet, Anne. 2021 in Neurological Sciences.*

## *Galcanezumab Effectiveness on Comorbid Cluster Headache and Chronic Migraine: A Prospective Case Series*

DOI: https://doi.org/10.1007/s10072-021-05624-1

### Abstract-Summary

Cluster headache (CH) and migraine are recurrent painful primary cephalalgies, typically with different clinical appearance and some shared features, such as unilateral pain, common triggers and response to triptans and/or monoclonal antibodies against the calcitonin gene-related peptide (CGRP) pathway.

Very few case series have been conducted so far investigating anti-CGRP treatments in patients with comorbid CH and migraine, and no cases have been reported which assess both CH and chronic migraine outcomes.

Taking into account the role of CGRP in migraine and CH pathophysiology, a usually well-tolerated treatment with CGRP blockade could be a rationale-based option to treat patients with coexisting chronic migraine and cluster headache.

Additional studies are needed to assess the role of anti-CGRP drugs in episodic and chronic CH treatment, as well as to establish correct timing and patient prerequisites to begin therapy.

### Introduction

In most patients, attacks occur for weeks or months, separated by pain-free remission periods (episodic CH), whereas in approximately 10–15% of patients, pain attacks occur without remission periods or with remissions lasting <3 months (chronic CH) [427].

Although poorly investigated, migraine has been reported to coexist in a subgroup (10–16.7%) of CH patients [428].

Although clinical trials on galcanezumab in chronic CH and fremanezumab in both episodic and chronic CH were prematurely discontinued due to futility [429], galcanezumab was found to ameliorate episodic CH, and the drug has been authorized in the USA as a preventive CH treatment.

We describe, in four patients comorbid for migraine and CH, the tolerability and effectiveness profile of galcanezumab (240 mg loading dose followed by 120 mg monthly) in these two conditions.

### Case Series

A 48-year-old woman reported episodes of unilateral orbital-periorbital and temporal pain localization with ipsilaterally associated autonomic symptoms, such as rhinorrhea and eyelid edema, which occurred up to 3 times per day (30/month) and lasted approximatively 60 min if untreated, which started 15 days before the visit.

The patient also reported headache episodes of throbbing quality, moderate intensity, with unilateral temporal localization, associated with nausea, vomiting, phonophobia and photophobia, lasting more than 4 h. Since 2002, these attacks occurred with a frequency of 18–20 days/month, leading to a diagnosis of chronic migraine.

A 27-year-old man referred to the Headache Centre for a 5-year history of chronic migraine (28–30 days/month) without aura, with headache attacks lasting 6–10 h if untreated, characterized by unilateral temporal localization, throbbing quality and moderate to severe intensity, associated to phonophobia, photophobia, nausea and vomiting.

## General

The HIT-6 questionnaire, associated with quality-of-life (QoL) measures and headache severity [430], is commonly used to measure the overall impact of headache on the patient's life, and, unlike the MIDAS questionnaire, it can be applied to a variety of headache disorders, including cluster headache [431].

In our four patients, the mean total HIT-6 score was reduced from 68 at baseline to 51 at month 3, indicating an overall pain reduction and improvement in QoL. No patient reported serious adverse events, while irritation at the site of the subcutaneous injection was described only in a few cases as a mild reaction.

## Discussion

A case series of five cluster headache patients treated with erenumab (70 mg then 140 mg) because of concomitant episodic migraine showed improvement in intensity and number of CH attacks and an amelioration in migraine days in all patients after 3 months of treatment with the higher dose [432].

Previous case series [432, 433] identified a specific time-response pattern which entailed either a rapid reduction in CH attacks in the first month of treatment with galcanezumab or after at least 3 months of treatment with monthly erenumab 140 mg administration.

Our case series did not show a similar [433] rapid response to galcanezumab, as at least 3 months of treatment seemed to be necessary to observe a clinical response to therapy in CH.

This is the first open-label case series specifically reporting the effectiveness and tolerability of galcanezumab in patients with coexisting CH and chronic migraine.

## Conclusions

Chronic migraine and cluster headache are primary cephalalgias with a severe impact on quality of life, usually requiring the combination of numerous acute and preventive treatments.

According to the recognized role of the CGRP pathway in migraine and CH, a well-tolerated treatment based on CGRP blockade could be a rational-based option to treat naïve and drug-resistant patients with episodic and chronic migraine with coexisting CH, limiting potential harmful preventive co-therapies and reducing the need for acute medications.

Additional studies that rigorously select patients in strict adherence with guidelines, avoiding uneven groups, are necessary to further assess the role of anti-CGRP drugs in episodic and chronic CH treatment.

**Acknowledgement**

*A machine generated summary based on the work of Iannone, Luigi Francesco; Fattori, Davide; Geppetti, Pierangelo; De Cesaris, Francesco. 2021 in Neurological Sciences.*

## *Different Doses of Galcanezumab Versus Placebo in Patients with Migraine and Cluster Headache: A Meta-analysis of Randomized Controlled Trials*

DOI: https://doi.org/10.1186/s10194-020-1085-x

**Abstract-Summary**

It has been tested for the preventive treatment of migraine and episodic cluster headache by multiple randomized clinical trials (RCTs) and have been found to reduce headache frequency.

120 mg group has the same treatment efficacy with 240 mg group (50% response: RR = 1.06; 95% CI, 0.92 to 1.22; P = 0.425; 75% response: RR = 1.07; 95% CI, 0.94 to 1.23; P = 0.301; 100% response; RR = 1.06; 95% CI, 0.81 to 1.37; P = 0.682; MHD: RR = −0.08; 95% CI, −0.55 to −0.40; P = 0.748) while related to a lower risk for adverse events for the treatment of migraine (120 mg RR = 1.06; 95% CI, 0.99 to 1.14; P = 0.084; 240 mg: RR = 1.17; 95% CI, 1.09 to 1.25; P < 0.001).

300 mg per month galcanezumab is effective for the prevention of episodic cluster headache measured by at least 50% reduction of cluster headache frequency at week 3 (RR = 1.36; 95% CI, 1.00–1.84; P = 0.048).

Use of galcanezumab is related to a significantly reduced monthly headache frequency compared with placebo for the treatment of migraine and episodic cluster headache, 120 mg has the same treatment efficacy with 240 mg group while related to a lower risk for adverse effects for the treatment of migraine.

300 mg per month galcanezumab is effective for the prevention of episodic cluster headache with no significantly increased adverse events.

Extended:

Use of galcanezumab for the treatment of primary headaches have a promising clinical application, it is related to a significantly reduced monthly headache frequency for the treatment of migraine and episodic cluster headache.

Major limitation of this study is the lack of the clinical outcome of long-term use, thus, further studies are required to evaluate efficacy and safety in a long-term setting.

**Background**

Increased serum CGRP level is observed after migraine and cluster headache attack in both human and animal models [434, 435].

CGRP will, induce potent vasodilatory effects on cerebral arteries [436], modulate the sensitivity of nociceptive trigeminal neurons [437] and subsequently trigger migraine and cluster headache attacks.

CGRP is considered a promising target for treatment of migraine and cluster headache.

Previous clinical trials have supported the use of CGRP monoclonal antibodies as a preventive treatment for migraine and episodic cluster headache [438–444].

Systemic reviews have confirmed the effectiveness and safety of CGRP monoclonal antibodies for the treatment of migraine and cluster headache [445, 446].

## Methods

All of the studies included in this meta-analysis (1) were all randomized clinical trials (RCTs); (2) enrolled participants with migraine or cluster headache (3) used galcanezumab as intervention; (4) enrolled over 100 participants.

The extracted data include (1) literature information (title, author, publication time, sample size, etc); (2) characteristic of the object of the study (age, BMI, smoking status, headache attack status before study); (3) content of the expose or interfere (experiment doses in different groups); (4) outcome data including migraine headache days (MHD), 50%, 75%, 100% response rate, which was defined as a reduction of the frequency of headache attacks by at least given percentage, treatment-emergent adverse events (TEAE), serious adverse events (SAE) and number of patients discontinue.

Weighted mean differences (WMD) and relative risk (RR) with their 95% confidence intervals (CIs) were used to evaluate the effect of galcanezumab on migraine or cluster headache.

## Results

7 studies were found to be directly related to our study, but one ongoing clinical trial on chronic cluster headache (NCT02438826) was excluded because the trial did not reach its primary endpoint.

Three of the seven studies are at high risk of attrition bias [439, 442, 444] which can be explained by a relatively high discontinue rate related to prolonged experiment period [439, 444] and high proportion of discontinue in placebo group due to lack of efficacy [442].

One study is at high risk of selection bias [444].

We conducted a sensitivity test to evaluate potential bias of the studies involved in our meta-analysis.

Of the seven included studies, all the studies were at low risk of publication bias.

## Discussion

Our study is the first meta-analysis of the clinical use of galcanezumab in the treatment of migraine and cluster headache.

For the does-response relationship, our data suggest that 120 mg galcanezumab per month is superior for treatment of migraine than 240 mg per month and 300 mg galcanezumab is effective for the treatment of episodic cluster headache with no significantly increased risk for adverse events.

We also demonstrated that 300 mg galcanezumab is effective against episodic cluster headache when measured by response rate and have no significantly increased risk for causing adverse events.

One ongoing clinical trial of galcanezumab for the preventive treatment of chronic cluster headache was excluded from of study due to it didn't reach its primary endpoint.

Further studies are needed to reveal the overall outcome and potential interaction of combining galcanezumab with traditional therapies or direct CGRP receptor antagonists for the treatment of migraine and cluster headache.

**Conclusion**

Use of galcanezumab for the treatment of primary headaches have a promising clinical application, it is related to a significantly reduced monthly headache frequency for the treatment of migraine and episodic cluster headache.

As for the dose-response relationship, 120 mg has the same treatment efficacy with 240 mg group while related to a lower risk for adverse effects for the treatment of migraine.

300 mg per month galcanezumab is effective against episodic cluster headache that was proved by one randomized clinical trial and the use of 300 mg galcanezumab is not related to an increased risk for adverse events.

**Acknowledgement**

*A machine generated summary based on the work of Yang, Yanbo; Wang, Zilan; Gao, Bixi; Xuan, He; Zhu, Yun; Chen, Zhouqing; Wang, Zhong. 2020 in The Journal of Headache and Pain.*

## *Great Occipital Nerve Long-Acting Steroid Injections in Cluster Headache Therapy: An Observational Prospective Study*

DOI: https://doi.org/10.1007/s00415-021-10884-0

**Abstract-Summary**

Injections targeting the occipital nerve are used to reduce headache attacks and abort cluster bouts in cluster headache patients.

The aim of this study was to verify the effectiveness and safety of greater occipital nerve long-acting steroid injections in the management of episodic and chronic cluster headache.

We conducted a prospective observational cohort study on episodic (ECH) and chronic cluster headache patients (CCH).

ECH were included in the study at the beginning of a cluster period.

We registered the frequency and intensity of attacks three days before and 3, 7 and 30 days after the treatment, the latency of cluster relapse, adverse events, scores evaluating anxiety (Zung scale), depression (Beck's Depression Scale) and quality of life (Disability Assessment Schedule II, 12-Item Self-Administered Version).

We observed a complete response in 47.8% (22/46) of episodic and 33.3% (4/12) of chronic patients.

A partial response (reduction of at least 50% of attacks) was obtained in further 10.8% (5/46) of episodic and in 33.3% (4/12) of chronic patients at 1 month.

Median pain-free period was of 3 months for CCH responders.

We suggest three greater occipital nerve injections of 60 mg methylprednisolone on alternate days as useful therapy in episodic and chronic cluster headache.

This leads to a long pain-free period in chronic forms.

Extended:

The aim of our study was to verify the effectiveness and safety of GON long-acting steroid injections alone in the management of ECH and CCH patients.

We observed a complete response in near half of ECH and in a third of CCH for at least of 1 month after the last injection.

## Introduction

Medical treatment of CH includes acute, transitional and preventive therapy.

Acute treatment aims to abort the pain of each attack, while preventive therapy modulates attack frequency, intensity and cluster duration.

Transitional therapy should provide almost immediate relief to decrease pain until preventive therapy becomes effective or until the cluster period ends spontaneously [447].

We hypothesized that repeated injections of long-acting steroid could be useful in CH treatment.

The aim of our study was to verify the effectiveness and safety of GON long-acting steroid injections alone in the management of ECH and CCH patients.

## Materials and Methods

Inclusion criteria were: subjects over the age of 18; diagnosis of ECH and CCH according to the criteria of "The international classification of headache disorders" ICHD Edition 3-beta [1]; ECH in active cluster within the first week from cluster onset and CCH during the exacerbation phase; if taking preventive therapies, these should have not been modified in the previous 3 months.

Exclusion criteria were: patients with another type of headache; patients with non-active cluster headache; patients with contraindications to methylprednisolone; patients taking anticoagulants or with coagulation disorders; patients using oral steroid therapy; patients with preventive therapies introduced or modified in the previous 3 months; patients unable to sign the informed consent.

Secondary outcomes were to evaluate the number of partial responders, i.e., those with an improvement of at least 50% in the frequency of attacks after one month from treatment compared to previous frequency, the reduction of the intensity of pain, the evaluation of recurrence of cluster attacks at one-year of follow-up, the improvement of anxiety, depression and quality of life.

## Results

Sixty CH patients were enrolled: 47 ECH and 13 CCH.

Oral preventive therapy was ongoing in 10 out of 13 CCH patients (76.9%) and in 18 out of 47 ECH patients (38.3%).

Among the remaining 58 patients, 26 (44.8%) were attack free after 1 month from the third injection.

A proportion of 23 patients of the whole sample (38.3%) reported mild adverse events: 21 complained of neck stiffness and 2 of mild pain on the site of injection.

Complete responders underwent a 1-year follow-up: 50% of ECH were still pain-free at 1-year of follow-up, while 50% had recurrence of cluster attacks with a mean latency of 8 months (242 days, SD ± 130.49).

All CCH patients relapsed with a median pain-free period of 3 months (94 days, SD ± 7.85).

## Discussion

Our study shows the effectiveness and safety of GON long-acting steroid injections alone as a transitional therapy in a large sample of CH patients.

We found a high efficacy in stopping the cluster period: 45% of patients (48% of ECH and 33% of CCH) were attack free for at least one month after the third injection.

Most protocols provide a combination of steroid plus anesthetic injection or a simple anesthetic block, however, only a few studies can boast an adequate randomized, placebo-controlled design.

Drawing inspiration from the experience of Leroux, we selected methylprednisolone which is a low-cost and easily available medication and whose use is supported by most previous studies on GON injections.

Our study demonstrates for the first time that previous response to oral steroid therapy does not correlate with that of steroid injection therapy.

## Conclusions

Repeated greater occipital nerve injections of 60 mg methylprednisolone, performed on alternate days, is an effective therapy in CH.

This protocol seems particularly useful in the treatment of CCH, leading to a 3-month pain-free period in responder patients.

Adverse effects are mild and support its use as first choice compared to oral therapies.

## Acknowledgement

*A machine generated summary based on the work of Merli, Elena; Asioli, Gian Maria; Favoni, Valentina; Zenesini, Corrado; Mascarella, Davide; Sartori, Alex; Cortelli, Pietro; Cevoli, Sabina; Pierangeli, Giulia. 2021 in Journal of Neurology.*

# Non-invasive Vagus Nerve Stimulation for Treatment of Cluster Headache: Early UK Clinical Experience

DOI: https://doi.org/10.1186/s10194-018-0936-1

## Abstract-Summary

Evidence supports the use of non-invasive vagus nerve stimulation (nVNS; gammaCore®) as a promising therapeutic option for patients with cluster headache (CH).

We conducted this audit of real-world data from patients with CH, the majority of whom were treatment refractory, to explore early UK clinical experience with nVNS used acutely, preventively, or both.

We retrospectively analysed data from 30 patients with CH (29 chronic, 1 episodic) who submitted individual funding requests for nVNS to the National Health Service.

All patients had responded to adjunctive nVNS therapy during an evaluation period (typical duration, 3–6 months).

The mean (SD) CH attack frequency decreased from 26.6 (17.1) attacks/wk.

Significant decreases in attack frequency, severity, and duration were observed in these patients with CH who did not respond to or were intolerant of multiple preventive and/or acute treatments.

These real-world findings complement evidence from clinical trials demonstrating the efficacy and safety of nVNS in CH.

Extended:

We retrospectively analysed data from patients with CH who previously had an inadequate response and/or intolerable side effects with ≥3 current or previous CH treatments and were offered nVNS therapy for use during an evaluation period.

These findings represent the practical use of this treatment and complement results from clinical trials demonstrating the efficacy and safety of nVNS therapy in patients with CH.

## Background

A non-invasive vagus nerve stimulation (nVNS) device (gammaCore®) has demonstrated safety and efficacy for prevention and acute treatment of CH attacks in clinical trials [403, 404, 448].

The use of novel treatments in practice can provide data to complement those from clinical trials by documenting qualitative details that are not typically captured during such trials, enabling a real-world view of patient- and health care–centric management.

To add further insight to the data on nVNS from randomised clinical trials, we conducted this retrospective analysis of data from patients in the United Kingdom with CH who were at various stages in the process of applying for individual funding requests (IFRs) for nVNS from the National Health Service.

The process is reserved for patients with rare conditions that have not responded to available therapies and who are considered exceptional individuals with regard to the treatment of their CH.

**Methods**

Patients who reported a clinically meaningful decrease in the frequency, severity, or duration of their attacks after ≥3 months of evaluation were considered for inclusion in the IFR process.

Clinical centres provided data on CH attacks and treatments before the nVNS evaluation period, which were obtained from patient diaries and/or medical records, as well as the following data from patient interviews, treatment diaries, and physician notes documented during the nVNS evaluation period (from May 2012 through March 2016): CH type, patient demographics/other characteristics; CH attack frequency, duration, and severity (rated on a 0–10 scale, higher numbers indicating greater severity); number and timing of stimulations administered; concomitant use of preventive and/or abortive treatments; adverse events (AEs); and subjective feedback on nVNS.

Within-patient changes from baseline (i.e., during treatment with the standard of care [SoC] regimen alone) to the end (or latest available point) of the nVNS evaluation period in attack frequency, duration, and severity were assessed via paired t tests.

**Results**

Sixteen patients (53%) used nVNS exclusively as preventive therapy, 1 (3%, a patient with episodic CH) used it exclusively as acute treatment, and 13 (43%) used it as both preventive and acute therapy.

Patients used a mean (range) of 0.8 (0–2) preventive treatments before the initiation of nVNS therapy and 0.7 (0–2) preventive treatments afterward.

The mean (range) number of acute treatments used was 1.8 (1–4) before the initiation of nVNS therapy and 1.1 (0–2) afterward.

Twenty-two patients used triptan injection or nasal spray as acute treatment before the initiation of nVNS therapy.

Twenty-nine patients reported use of high-flow oxygen; 27 (93%) used it as acute treatment before the initiation of nVNS therapy.

After treatment with nVNS was initiated, 9 patients (33%) stopped and 17 (63%) decreased high-flow oxygen use; use of this treatment was unchanged in the remaining patient.

**Discussion**

In previous clinical trials, nVNS demonstrated efficacy as preventive therapy in patients with chronic CH [448] and as acute treatment in patients with episodic CH [403, 404], but not as acute treatment in patients with chronic CH [403, 404, 448].

Patients in this analysis, who predominantly had chronic CH (29/30), reported significant decreases in attack duration and severity, indicating a benefit from nVNS as an acute treatment in chronic CH in this practical setting when the acute use was added to daily preventive use.

Results from the initial open-label exploratory study of nVNS therapy in CH suggested that several patients with chronic CH had a stable favourable response to nVNS as acute treatment [370].

Such dosing individualisation, which is common with pharmacologic treatments, could explain why patients with chronic CH benefited from acute nVNS treatment in the current study but not in the acute clinical trials, which did not allow for daily preventive use.

Further study is needed to determine whether acute treatment regimens in patients with chronic CH might benefit from increased nVNS dosing.

## Conclusions

Treatment with nVNS led to significant decreases in attack frequency, severity, and duration in patients with CH who previously did not benefit from or could not tolerate multiple preventive and/or acute treatments.

These findings represent the practical use of this treatment and complement results from clinical trials demonstrating the efficacy and safety of nVNS therapy in patients with CH.

## Acknowledgement

*A machine generated summary based on the work of Marin, Juana; Giffin, Nicola; Consiglio, Elizabeth; McClure, Candace; Liebler, Eric; Davies, Brendan. 2018 in The Journal of Headache and Pain.*


# *Peripheral Nerve Stimulation for Chronic Pain: A Systematic Review of Effectiveness and Safety*

DOI: https://doi.org/10.1007/s40122-021-00306-4

## Abstract-Summary

Peripheral nerve stimulation (PNS) was the first application of neuromodulation.

This systematic review was written to assess the current status of high-quality evidence supporting the use of PNS for pain conditions treated by interventional pain physicians.

The available literature on PNS, limited to conditions treated by interventional pain physicians, was reviewed and the quality assessed.

One RCT was of high quality and four were of moderate quality; all four case series were of moderate quality.

Three of the RCTs and all four case series evaluated peripheral nerve neuropathic pain.

Based upon these studies, there is level II evidence supporting the use of PNS to treat refractory peripheral nerve injury.

One moderate-quality RCT evaluated tibial nerve stimulation for pelvic pain, providing level III evidence for this indication.

One moderate-quality RCT evaluated surgically placed cylindrical leads for cluster headaches, providing level III evidence for this indication.

The evidence suggests that approximately two-thirds of patients with peripheral neuropathic pain will have at least 50% sustained pain relief.

No studies dealt with joint-related osteoarthritic pain.

Extended:

This systematic review will assess the literature on PNS for nerve entrapment, joint pain, or axial or radicular pain up until June 2021.

## Introduction

Following the publication of a comprehensive text on peripheral nerve entrapments [449], the role of peripheral nerves as a source of pain and as an avenue of treatment has become more widely recognized.

Neuromodulation of peripheral nerves to treat pain is an area of great intellectual activity.

Stimulation of mixed nerves at 100 Hz can selectively activate the largest sensory afferents; however, stimulation of mixed nerves at a low frequency such as 12 Hz can equally stimulate muscle efferent fibers, leading to remote selective targeting.

The role of the current review is to assess the current status of the evidence supporting the use of neuromodulation of peripheral nerves to treat subacute or chronic pain, including treatment of cranial/facial pain, nerve entrapment/injury, joint degeneration, or axial or radicular pain.

This systematic review will assess the literature on PNS for nerve entrapment, joint pain, or axial or radicular pain up until June 2021.

## Methods

The methodology utilized in this systematic review followed the review process derived from evidence-based systematic reviews and meta-analysis of randomized trials and observational studies [450–465].

This review differs in that it includes databases not previously utilized and non-randomized studies, and excludes both occipital and peripheral nerve field stimulation.

Utilizing Cochrane review criteria of risk of bias, studies meeting the inclusion criteria with at least 8 of 12 criteria were considered high quality and 5–7 criteria were considered moderate quality.

Based on ASIPP criteria for randomized trials and non-randomized studies, the studies meeting the inclusion criteria scoring of 32–48 were considered high-quality trials, studies with scores between 21 and 31 were considered moderate quality, and studies scoring 20 or less were considered low quality and were excluded.

## Data Analysis

Table 6 illustrates the characteristics of the eight RCTs and 12 observational studies considered for inclusion.

Table 8, The ASIPP IPM–QRB Analysis, shows the ASIPP bias and quality analysis for the eight RCTs.

Table 9, The ASIPP IPM–QRBNR Analysis for non-randomized studies, shows ASIPP's bias and quality analysis for the 11 non-randomized studies.

Of the eight RCTs and 11 observational studies considered for inclusion, three RCTs [466–468] and eight observational studies [469–476] were considered low quality on the appropriate ASIPP analysis and were excluded.

Table 10 shows the study characteristics of the five randomized trials and four case series evaluating PNS which were included for consideration.

## Results

Of the RCTs evaluating the treatment of peripheral nerve pain, Wilson and others found 60% relief at 16 weeks [477].

Eisenberg and others [478], looking at peripheral nerve injury, also provided long-term follow-up, from 3 to 16 years, with 78% of patients having at least 50% relief.

Of the three RCTs evaluating relief of peripheral nerve neuropathic pain at a minimum of 3 months, two showed greater than 50% relief at the end point.

A recent review of surgically implanted leads placed on peripheral nerves for treatment of CRPS over a 30-year time frame, documenting the experience at the Cleveland Clinic from 1990 to 2017, showed a mean 25% relief at 12 months [479].

One high-quality RCT and two moderate-quality RCTs documented the efficacy of PNS in treating refractory peripheral nerve neuropathic pain.

Four moderate-quality case series reports corroborate the findings of the RCTS and provide documentation of long-term, multiple-year relief.

## Complications

The early cuff and paddle leads, which required open surgical dissection for proper placement, had a high incidence of scarring and concomitant nerve damage, limiting adoption of PNS [480].

Chmiela and others reported the complications seen in their 27-year history of surgically placed PNS leads for CRPS [479].

Of these, five were explanted for infection, one for lead erosion, and four for resolution of pain.

Seventeen patients required revision, nine for lead migration, five for device malfunction, five for lead or anchor erosion, and four for infection.

Eldabe and others, in a review of complications of spinal cord and peripheral stimulation, found lead migration to be the primary concern [481].

Current stimulator systems, in which leads do not cross joints, markedly reduce the risk of lead fracture.

Of their 22 study-related events, 21 were skin irritation or redness from the bandage or pain due to implantation or stimulation.

## Discussion

PNS has been an area of interest since 1967, when Wall and Sweet, applying the gate theory of pain, first stimulated peripheral nerves [482].

Deer and others [483] in 2016 published an RCT evaluating percutaneously implanted stimulators for peripheral nerve pain, with a mean reduction of pain of 27% at 3 months.

Gilmore and others [484], in the only high-quality study reviewed, published an RCT in 2020 looking at pain in amputees, providing ultrasound-guided placement of percutaneous leads with stimulation for 8 weeks, at which time the leads were removed.

Their findings highlight the extent of the need for high-quality studies confirming the role of PNS in treating joint or back pain.

Finch and others [480] performed a high-quality double-blind analysis of the characteristics of PNS relief looking at the time necessary for PNS to provide relief (wash-in) and for pain to return after the stimulator was turned off (wash-out).

**Limitations**

Despite having been used for over 50 years, PNS has a paucity of high-quality literature supporting its use.

Of the literature reviewed, only one study was of high quality.

Some indications which are currently generating much clinical interest, such as the treatment of joint pain from osteoarthritis, have limited literature supporting their use.

**Conclusion**

PNS was the first application of neuromodulation.

While the vast majority of the reviewed studies were of small samples, collectively they reveal significant improvement in pain utilizing PNS for treatment of neuropathic pain conditions.

The best studied application is refractory neuropathic pain involving a peripheral nerve, an indication which has level II evidence.

Cluster headaches and pelvic pain treated with tibial nerve stimulation have level III evidence.

Further research on the efficacy of therapy and on the mode of action will help expand the applications of PNS.

**Acknowledgement**

*A machine generated summary based on the work of Helm, Standiford; Shirsat, Nikita; Calodney, Aaron; Abd-Elsayed, Alaa; Kloth, David; Soin, Amol; Shah, Shalini; Trescot, Andrea. 2021 in Pain and Therapy.*

## *High Dosage of Methylprednisolone in Cluster Headache*

DOI: https://doi.org/10.1007/s10072-018-3383-5

**[Section 1]**

After 30 days, 6/32 patients remained pain-free (3 ECH, 3 CCH), 10 had a recurrence of attacks with a reduced frequency than the pre-treatment condition (7 ECH, 3 CCH), and 2 had a clinical worsening (1 ECH, 1 CCH).

It concerned a patient with chronic CH and long history of disease, in continuous 2-year treatment with oral steroids and verapamil at high dosages (10–50 mg/day and 720–960 mg daily, respectively), which developed a respiratory failure for which he was transferred to a sub-intensive unit and subjected to CPAP for a few days.

Our data show that steroid treatment with high doses iv MP, administered over several days, is highly effective in interrupting the cluster period in episodic patients and in reducing the "burden" of the disease in chronic patients.

**Acknowledgement**

*A machine generated summary based on the work of D'Arrigo, Giacomo; Di Fiore, Paola; Galli, Alberto; Frediani, Fabio. 2018 in Neurological Sciences.*


# *The Sensitivity to Change of the Cluster Headache Quality of Life Scale Assessed Before and After Deep Brain Stimulation of the Ventral Tegmental Area*

DOI: https://doi.org/10.1186/s10194-021-01251-5

**Abstract-Summary**

Since specific measures to assess the quality of life (QoL) in TACs are lacking, we recently developed and validated the cluster headache quality of life scale (CH-QoL).

Specifically we aimed to (i) assess the sensitivity of CH-QoL to change before and following deep brain stimulation of the ventral tegmental area (VTA-DBS), (ii) evaluate the relationship of changes on CH-QoL with changes in other generic measures of quality of life, as well as indices of mood and pain.

The CH-QoL total score was significantly reduced after compared to before VTA-DBS.

Changes in the CH-QoL total score correlated significantly and negatively with changes in HAL, the SF-36, and positively and significantly with depression and the evaluative domain on the McGill Pain Questionnaire.

Our findings demonstrate that changes after VTA-DBS in CH-QoL total scores are associated with the reduction of frequency, duration, and severity of headache attacks after surgery.

Post VTA-DBS improvement in CH-QoL scores is associated with an amelioration in quality of life assessed with generic measures, a reduction of depressive symptoms, and evaluative pain experience after VTA-DBS.

These results support the sensitivity to change of the CH-QoL and further demonstrate the validity and applicability of CH-QoL as a disease specific measure of quality of life for CH.

Extended:

The CH-QoL total score was significantly reduced after (M = 70.3, SD = 21.6) compared to before VTA-DBS (M = 77.6, SD = 14.5), t(9) −2.0, p = 0.03, d = −0.6), indicating better health-related quality of life reported by the patients after VTA-DBS.

As for most patients with cluster headache, standard medical treatment would entail medication, future studies could also further evaluate the sensitivity to change of CH-QoL by examining its responsiveness to change following effective medical treatment.

## Introduction

Quality of life (QoL) scales have increasingly emerged as an essential clinical outcome measure for assessing the impact of a disorder, the symptoms, and its medical or surgical treatment on patients' well-being and daily life.

These measures might not be specifically sensitive for CH and might, for example, fail to discriminate between CH patients and migraineurs, highlighting the need for a specific scale to assess QoL in CH [485].

It was shown that the cluster headache quality of life scale (CH-QoL) has essential psychometric properties, including good construct validity, convergent validity, internal consistency and test retest reliability [63].

The aim of the present study was to evaluate the sensitivity to change of the CH-QoL. Specifically, the aims were (i) to assess the sensitivity of CH-QoL to change before and after VTA-DBS intervention, (ii) to assess the association of change on CH-QoL with change in other generic standardized measures of quality of life, as well as indices of mood and pain in CH.

## Methods

Headache load (HAL) is a composite score to simultaneously measure frequency, severity and duration of cluster headache episodes.

On both Depression and Anxiety subscales scores range from 0 to 21, with higher scores indicating more severe depression or anxiety.

The Headache Impact Test (HIT-6) [486] is a six-item questionnaire used to measure the adverse impact of headaches on role and social functioning, cognitive functioning, vitality, psychological distress, and pain severity.

The total possible score ranges from 0 to 78, with higher scores indicating worse pain.

Pearson correlational analyses were performed to explore the relationship between the change scores in the CH-QoL scale (before and after VTA-DBS) and change scores in measures of the SF-36, mood, and pain.

Standardized response mean (SRM) was calculated for the CH-QoL total score and the four subdomains: Cohen's d and SRM are standardized indices of power to detect a true change, and larger values indicate higher sensitivity to change [487, 488].

## Results

The CH-QoL total score was significantly reduced after (M = 70.3, SD = 21.6) compared to before VTA-DBS (M = 77.6, SD = 14.5), t(9) −2.0, p = 0.03, d = −0.6), indicating better health-related quality of life reported by the patients after VTA-DBS.

We found significant positive correlations between the CH-QoL total score and ratings of mood on the BDI r = 0.63, p < 0.05, indicating that lower CH-QoL score (better QoL) is associated with a reduction of depressive symptoms after VTA-DBS.

There were significant positive correlations between the CH-QoL total score and the evaluative domain on the McGill Pain Questionnaire r = 0.73, p < 0.05, and a correlation approaching significance with HIT6 r = 0.58, p = 0.06, indicating that lower/improved CH-QoL scores are associated with a reduction of pain evaluation and the impact of pain after VTA-DBS.

## Discussion

The change scores of the CH-QoL total score and the reduction of headache load were significantly related, indicating that the reduction of the frequency, duration and severity of headache attacks after VTA-DBS are reflected by the pre versus post-operative change scores of the CH-QoL. Second, the associations of change scores of the CH-QoL total score with change scores of the generic QoL measure the SF-36, indices of mood (BDI), pain (HIT-6 and McGill), and pain-related behaviors (Pain Behaviour Checklist-Help Seeking behaviours) were in the expected direction; all reflecting an association between the improvement of disease-specific and generic QoL, mood, pain and pain-related behaviours following VTA-DBS surgery.

While change on the 'restrictions of ADL' subscale was significant and the other three subscales of the CH-QoL also reflected improved functioning following VTA-DBS, these other features of CH-QoL such as 'mood and interpersonal relations' and 'lack of vitality' 'pain and anxiety' may require a longer time post-DBS to adequately and significantly reflect change following reduction of headache load, since interpersonal relations and vitality unlike daily activities may be aspects of quality of life that require a longer period for a move towards readjustment and 'normalization'.

## Conclusions

The lack of a gold standard to assess QoL in CH is currently limited to using a combination of generic tests not explicitly devised to assess CH patients.

Our study indicates that CH-QoL responds similarly to other validated generic scales, supporting CH-QoL's validity and sensitivity to detect CH patients' clinical changes following surgical treatment.

The small number of patients and the lack of testing for other medical therapies limit the generalizability of our results on CH-QoL's sensitivity to change.

## Acknowledgement

*A machine generated summary based on the work of Cappon, Davide; Ryterska, Agata; Akram, Harith; Lagrata, Susie; Cheema, Sanjay; Hyam, Jonathan; Zrinzo, Ludvic; Matharu, Manjit; Jahanshahi, Marjan. 2021 in The Journal of Headache and Pain.*

## *Regional Cerebral Blood Flow as Predictor of Response to Occipital Nerve Block in Cluster Headache*

DOI: https://doi.org/10.1186/s10194-021-01304-9

### Abstract-Summary

Greater occipital nerve blockades can transiently suppress attacks in approximately 50% of patients, however, its mechanism of action remains uncertain, and there are no reliable predictors of treatment response.

To address this, we investigated the effect of occipital nerve blockade on regional cerebral blood flow (rCBF), an index of brain activity, and differences between treatment responders and non-responders.

21 male, treatment-naive patients were recruited while in a cluster headache bout.

During a pain-free phase between headaches, patients underwent pseudo-continuous arterial spin labelled MRI assessments to provide quantitative indices of rCBF.

Following treatment, patients demonstrated relative rCBF reductions in posterior temporal gyrus, cerebellum and caudate, and rCBF increases in occipital cortex.

Responders demonstrated relative rCBF increases, compared to non-responders, in medial prefrontal cortex and lateral occipital cortex at baseline, but relative reductions in cingulate and middle temporal cortices.

rCBF was increased in patients compared to healthy controls in cerebellum and hippocampus, but reduced in orbitofrontal cortex, insula and middle temporal gyrus.

We provide new mechanistic insights regarding the aetiology of cluster headache, the mechanisms of action of occipital nerve blockades and potential predictors of treatment response.

Extended:

Greater occipital nerve blockade (GONB) is a relatively successful therapy for suppressing CH attacks with minimal side effects [489].

Forthcoming studies including a larger number of patients and healthy controls may replicate these findings and shed further light into perfusion patters that may reliably act as predictors of GONB response in CH patients.

Our findings provide further characterisation of underlying brain mechanisms in CH that extend beyond the traditional midbrain hubs widely discussed in the literature.

### Introduction

Functional magnetic resonance imaging (fMRI) and in particular blood-oxygen-level dependent (BOLD) fMRI, can describe differences in activity and connectivity between CH patients and healthy controls [154], both in the resting state and during headache attacks [490, 491], pointing towards the hypothalamus as a key area involved in triggering headache attacks during bouts, as well as in marking the beginning and end of bouts in episodic CH patients, causing the circadian nature of CH symptoms.

We hypothesised that prefrontal rCBF at baseline could relate to the capacity of treatment response, ultimately contributing to differential responses to GONB; therefore we anticipated that prefrontal CBF at baseline would differ between CH patients and healthy controls, as well as between those who respond positively to GONB (i.e. responders) and treatment non-responders.

We explored i) rCBF changes in CH patients following their first GONB treatment to further understand the mechanisms of action of GONB, ii) differences in rCBF across CH patients at baseline during interictal phase in relation to response to GONB treatment, and iii) brain perfusion differences between CH patients at baseline and healthy controls.

## Materials and Methods

For all patients, the study required three visits to the imaging centre; (i) a neuropsychological screening and a mock scanning session to familiarise patients to the scanner environment; (ii) a baseline MRI scanning session (including structural T2-weighted images and pCASL measurements) followed by GONB treatment; (iii) a third session, taking place between 7 and 21 days following treatment to examine treatment effects once the effects of the injection were allowed to emerge.

Despite the fact that all patients were scanned during an interictal phase in a pain-free state, CBF maps from episodic CH and chronic CH patients were compared at baseline via an independent sample t-test, to assess the appropriateness of their inclusion in subsequent modelling as a single sample.

Patients age, duration of CH (measured in number of years from the first CH attack to the moment of first visit) and global CBF signal were also included as additional nuisance covariates.

## Results

Eight patients were designated as non-responders; within this group, two patients reported a reduction in weekly attacks lower than 50%, no changes were reported by two patients and remaining subjects reported an increased number of attacks after treatment.

Repeated-measures ANOVA indicated a main effect of Treatment (i.e. pre vs post GONB); patients presented local decreases in rCBF after treatment across three main clusters in the left hemisphere, including posterior temporal gyrus, cerebellum and caudate, in comparison to the post GONB session.

Our hypothesis-led analysis (i.e. SVC) to test for prefrontal cortical CBF differences between responders and non-responders indicated that patients who responded to GONB treatment had greater rCBF at baseline in left medial PFC (mPFC), compared to patients who did not experience a substantial improvement after treatment (pFWE = 0.015, t-score = 5.56, 115 voxels).

## Discussion

We compared patients' rCBF maps at baseline with matched healthy controls, in order to provide further meaningful information on the pathophysiology of CH.

Perfusion decreases in primary visual cortex after GONB, as well as in comparison to healthy controls have been previously reported [492]; the authors speculated that these differences could be due to the existence of visual aura in CH patients.

We also identified greater rCBF in the dorsal hippocampus in CH patients compared to healthy controls.

GMV reductions in CH patients compared to healthy controls have been reported [136], that develop and change with time and disease stage, suggesting that the hippocampus could be involved in pain memory, and its activation is related to pain expectancy and harm avoidance [493].

We observed decreased rCBF in the rostral anterior insula in the CH patients group compared to healthy controls at baseline.

Qiu and others [494] found decreased FC between the hypothalamus and the salience network, of which the anterior insula is a key component, in pain-free CH patients in bout compared to healthy controls.

**Conclusions**

Our results indicate that the pathophysiology of CH includes, but is not limited to, brain areas typically linked to pain perception; while changes in brain perfusion after GONB point out as possible main targets areas innervated by the trigeminal nerve (i.e. cerebellum, striatum, visual cortex), we propose that there is a heavy psychological component that might be driving treatment responses through poor anxiety and stress response regulation, attentional bias towards pain, and ruminating thoughts; our results point to differences in areas previously associated with these psychological states at baseline.

Future research may elucidate whether response to GONB may be improved by combining it with therapies focused on controlling negative thoughts towards pain promoting cognitive flexibility.

Further investigation of GONB responses including placebo-controlled designs might disentangle differential responses to treatment.

**Acknowledgement**

*A machine generated summary based on the work of Medina, Sonia; Bakar, Norazah Abu; O'Daly, Owen; Miller, Sarah; Makovac, Elena; Renton, Tara; Williams, Steve C. R.; Matharu, Manjit; Howard, Matthew A. 2021 in The Journal of Headache and Pain.*

## *Sphenopalatine Ganglion Stimulation for Cluster Headache, Results from a Large, Open-Label European Registry*

DOI: https://doi.org/10.1186/s10194-017-0828-9

**Abstract-Summary**

This study examines outcomes of a cohort of mainly chronic CH patients treated with sphenopalatine ganglion (SPG) stimulation.

Ninety-seven CH patients (88 chronic, 9 episodic) underwent trans-oral insertion of a microstimulator targeting the SPG.

Frequency, use of preventive and acute medications, headache impact (HIT-6) and quality of life measures (SF-36v2) were monitored at clinic visits.

Eighty-five patients (78 chronic, 7 episodic) remained implanted and were evaluated for effectiveness at 12 months.

68% of all patients were responders, 55% of chronic patients were frequency responders and 32% of all patients were acute responders.

67% of patients using acute treatments were able to reduce the use of these by 52% and 74% of chronic patients were able to stop, reduce or remain off all preventive medications.

59% of all patients were HIT-6 responders, 67% were SF-36 responders.

This open-label registry corroborates that SPG stimulation is an effective therapy for CH patients providing therapeutic benefits and improvements in use of medication as well as headache impact and quality of life.

Extended:

Stimulation duration and timing may play a role and future studies should investigate this and possible predictive factors.

## Background

CH exists as episodic CH (eCH), where attacks occur in clusters lasting weeks-months separated by attack-free intervals >1 month, and chronic CH (cCH) with no periods of remission lasting >1 month for >1 year.

Preventive therapies are taken daily during the cluster period, or in cCH continuously, and consist of verapamil or lithium [495].

With up to eight attacks/day use of acute medications may exceed recommendations, and often doses of preventive medications higher than recommended are necessary, increasing the risk of side-effects [496].

The aim of this study is to evaluate the effectiveness of SPG stimulation through 12 months in an open label setting, in a large population including cCH and a limited number of eCH patients.

As opposed to the previously mentioned forms of neurostimulation, ONS and DBS, SPG stimulation elicits both an acute and preventive effect which this study was specifically designed to capture.

## Methods

Exclusion criteria included changes in preventive medication in the month prior to enrollment and patients who have bony facial deformities, inappropriate surgical anatomy or have had facial surgery that would prevent the proper placement of the Pulsante Microstimulator.

Average attack frequency, laterality and acute and preventive medication use were collected retrospectively at each clinic visit, with patients asked to recall their attack frequency and acute medication usage over the prior 4 week period.

Per protocol analyses included percent change in attack frequency, percent of attacks achieving effective therapy, the number of patients achieving acute and/or frequency effect, changes in acute and preventive medication, characterization of

HIT-6 headache disability and SF-36v2 quality of life and patient evaluation of therapy using the patient experience questionnaire.

Analysis of the acute response included all attacks where SPG stimulation was applied and for which the patient entered diary responses through the 12 month study visit.

## Results

The remaining 85 patients (78 chronic, 7 episodic) continued through the study to 12 months and are included in the present 12 month evaluation of effectiveness (average time from microstimulator insertion to 12 month study visit: $368 \pm 42$ days (range 245–475)).

For these cCH patients experiencing no attacks, the preventive effect manifested $150 \pm 102$ (range 8–390) days after microstimulator insertion.

32% (27/85) of patients were acute responders achieving effective therapy in at least 50% of their attacks.

Patients using SPG stimulation experience both acute and frequency effects, and therapeutic response was therefore defined as experiencing either acute and/or frequency response.

In the chronic patients, 65% (51/78) were considered responders per protocol (achieving effective therapy in at least 50% of attacks or experiencing a 50% reduction in attack frequency or both).

## Discussion

In this prospective study of 85 eCH and cCH patients treated with an implantable neurostimulator, we have demonstrated the effectiveness of SPG stimulation for attack frequency reductions and acute pain relief.

The data presented here is very similar to previously published results of SPG stimulation [373, 497, 498] with one exception: The proportion of acute uses of the stimulator achieving effective therapy was lower than previously reported (39% vs. 65%).

This difference may be attributed to acute non-responders choosing the SPG stimulator over other acute treatments, despite it not being effective in them.

SPG stimulation provides acute relief in some, a preventive effect in others, or both.

At current, no positive or negative predictors for efficacy of SPG stimulation have been identified therefore patients with no immediate acute effect should keep stimulating as a preventive effect may manifest at a later point.

## Acknowledgement

*A machine generated summary based on the work of Barloese, Mads; Petersen, Anja; Stude, Philipp; Jürgens, Tim; Jensen, Rigmor Højland; May, Arne. 2018 in The Journal of Headache and Pain.*

# *Gamma Knife Radiosurgery for the Treatment of Cluster Headache: A Systematic Review*

DOI: https://doi.org/10.1007/s10143-021-01725-9

**Abstract-Summary**

Cluster headache (CH) is a severe trigeminal autonomic cephalalgia that, when refractory to medical treatment, can be treated with Gamma Knife radiosurgery (GKRS).

The outcomes of studies investigating GKRS for CH in the literature are inconsistent, and the ideal target and treatment parameters remain unclear.

The aim of this systematic review is to evaluate the safety and the efficacy, both short and long term, of GKRS for the treatment of drug-resistant CH.

A systematic review of the literature was performed to identify all clinical articles discussing GKRS for the treatment of CH.

The literature review revealed 5 studies describing outcomes of GKRS for the treatment of CH for a total of 52 patients (48 included in the outcome analysis).

Trigeminal sensory disturbances were observed in 28 patients (58%) and deafferentation pain in 3 patients (6%).

GKRS targeted on the trigeminal nerve or sphenopalatine ganglion is associated to a frequent risk of trigeminal disturbances and possibly deafferentation pain.

Extended:

Cluster headache (CH) is a primary headache disorder characterized by unilateral excruciating headaches lasting 15 to 180 min, accompanied by agitation and cranial autonomic features [499, 500].

For studies that did not quantify pain reduction, a significant outcome was left up to the discretion of the respective study's authors.

Future controlled studies with larger groups of patients are necessary to draw definitive conclusions regarding the efficacy and safety of GKRS in patients with CH.

**Introduction**

Ablative surgical procedures targeted on the trigeminal nerve (TN), which were used in the past for the treatment of CH, have been largely abandoned due to risk of causing bothersome facial sensory disturbances and deafferentation pain.

The introduction of effective and non-destructive neuromodulation techniques, such as deep brain stimulation of the posterior hypothalamus or occipital nerve stimulation, has also caused these ablative procedures to fall out of favor [219, 407].

Gamma Knife radiosurgery (GKRS) has been explored as a less invasive ablative treatment option for reducing pain in patients with drug-resistant CH.

We have systematically reviewed the medical literature related to GKRS for the treatment of drug-resistant CH in order to aid neurosurgeons in understanding the limitations, actual risks, and efficacy of this procedure.

**Methods**

Peer-reviewed articles for this systematic review were selected based on the following criteria: (1) neuroablation was performed with the Gamma Knife (Elekta AB Instruments, Stockholm, Sweden), (2) GKRS was performed for the treatment of drug-resistant CH, (3) the study included post-treatment outcomes data, (4) the study was written in English, and (5) GKRS was performed as the upfront radiosurgical treatment for CH.

Duplicate articles and articles with overlapping patient populations were accounted for to avoid redundancy.

Thirty articles were then selected, among which 25 were excluded from the analysis.

For studies that did not quantify pain reduction, a significant outcome was left up to the discretion of the respective study's authors.

**Results**

Of the 48 patients who were included in the outcome analysis, initial pain reduction following GKRS was reported in 60–100% of patients, with an aggregate initial meaningful pain reduction in 37 patients (77%) patients.

Meaningful pain reduction at the last follow-up assessment was reported in 20 (42%) patients.

Three patients were treated with repeat GKRS for recurrent CH, and all of them had pain reduction at the last follow-up assessments.

Meaningful pain reduction at the last follow-up assessment was observed in 14 out of 24 patients treated with upfront GKRS targeted on the TN, 5 out of 13 treated with GKRS targeted on both the TN and SPG, and in the single patient treated with GKRS targeted on the SPG alone.

TN dysfunction of varying grade was observed in 28 (58%) CH patients following GKRS.

**Discussion**

Further confirming this hypothesis, this group later reported a single patient with CH and trigeminal neuralgia who developed deafferentation pain and contralateral CH following an initially effective GKRS-mediated ablation of the TN and the SPG [501].

In that study, six patients had transient pain reduction and five developed trigeminal disturbances.

Ten patients had considerable pain reduction after a mean follow-up period of 34 months, and 8 patients developed trigeminal sensory disturbances, including one case of deafferentation pain.

The main issue with GKRS targeted on the TN and SPG appears to be the high rate of post-procedural trigeminal sensory disturbances and deafferentation pain, although there are differences among studies.

In the study of Donnet and others, the three patients with a successful outcome did not develop trigeminal disturbances, but these disturbances did occur in all the seven patients who did not have pain reduction after GKRS [502].

### Limitations

There is considerable variability in methods for reporting pain reduction across studies.

All studies were observational open-label patient series and therefore subject to bias from the placebo effect.

Controlled studies should be carried out in patients with drug-refractory chronic CH.

### Conclusions

The available clinical evidence supports the short-term efficacy of GKRS targeted to the TN and/or SPG in reducing pain of CH patients.

The procedure was demonstrated to cause excessive trigeminal sensory disturbances and deafferentation pain in some patients.

The possibility of safely repeating the radiosurgical procedure to prolong pain reduction time cannot be recommended due to the lack reported patients undergoing repeat GKRS for this indication.

The decision whether to use GKRS in patients with CH should be made based on those considerations.

Future controlled studies with larger groups of patients are necessary to draw definitive conclusions regarding the efficacy and safety of GKRS in patients with CH.

### Acknowledgement

*A machine generated summary based on the work of Franzini, Andrea; Clerici, Elena; Navarria, Pierina; Picozzi, Piero. 2022 in Neurosurgical Review.*

## *Other Trigeminal Autonomic Cephalalgias*

Machine generated keywords: hemicrania, indomethacin, sunct, tac, continua, hemicrania continua, hemicrania continuum, neuralgiform headache, neuralgiform, unilateral neuralgiform, autonomic, paroxysmal hemicrania, trigeminal autonomic, paroxysmal, galcanezumab

## *Treatment of SUNCT/SUNA, Paroxysmal Hemicrania, and Hemicrania Continua: An Update Including Single-Arm Meta-analyses*

DOI: https://doi.org/10.1007/s11940-020-00649-x

### Abstract-Summary

This review presents a critical appraisal of the treatment strategies for short-lasting unilateral neuralgiform headache attacks (SUNHA), paroxysmal hemicrania (PH), and hemicrania continua (HC).

We present estimated pooled analyses of the most common treatments and emphasize recent promising findings.

Pooled analyses reveal that lamotrigine for SUNHA and indomethacin for PH and HC are the preventative treatments of choice.

Second-line choices include topiramate, gabapentin, and carbamazepine for SUNHA; verapamil for PH; and cyclooxygenase-2 inhibitors and gabapentin for HC.

Parenteral lidocaine is highly effective as a transitional treatment for SUNHA.

Lamotrigine as a prophylactic and parenteral lidocaine as transitional treatment remain the therapies of choice for SUNHA.

Extended:

We hand-searched the reference lists of reviews on TACs.

Parenteral lidocaine is useful when a transitional treatment is required.

## Introduction

Short-lasting unilateral neuralgiform headache attacks (SUNHA), paroxysmal hemicrania (PH), and hemicrania continua (HC) are all classified as trigeminal autonomic cephalalgias (TACs) by the International Classification of Headache Disorders [1].

TACs are mainly characterized by unilateral trigeminal distribution pain that occurs in association with ipsilateral cranial autonomic features [503].

SUNHA and PH are characterized by short-lasting intense headache attacks, with their main difference being in attack duration and frequency as well as the response to therapy.

PH and HC are characterized by absolute responsiveness to indomethacin.

## Methods

We constructed a literature base from their reference list, combined with an updated literature search.

Treatments with two or more reports of at least five patients were included in pooled single-arm meta-analyses.

The literature search for SUNHA yielded 147 records.

Six reports of five cohorts [504–509] (n = 154) with five or more patients were included in the pooled analyses.

The literature search for PH yielded 40 records.

Thirteen studies [213, 510–521] (n = 189) with five or more patients were included in pooled analyses.

The literature search for HC yielded 48 records.

Ten studies [512, 515, 520–527] with a total of 131 patients were included in the pooled analyses.

## Pathophysiology and Indomethacin Response

The most widely accepted pathophysiological construct is that an abnormality in the posterior hypothalamus leads to an activation of the trigeminal autonomic reflex—the phenomenon in which trigeminal nociceptive stimulation may elicit cranial parasympathetic outflow [528].

The pain is likely mediated by activation of the trigeminovascular nociceptive afferents from the peripheral cranium leading to the trigeminal nucleus caudalis (TNC) [529].

This reflex connection mediates the parasympathetic outflow via the sphenopalatine ganglion (SPG) and the facial nerve, explaining the autonomic symptoms [162].

Indomethacin appears to inhibit the production of nitric oxide, distinguishing it from other non-steroidal anti-inflammatory drugs (NSAID), and thereby inhibit neurogenic-induced vasodilatation activating nociceptive trigeminovascular nerve fibers [530].

It is therefore believed that indomethacin may antagonize the nitric oxide pathway occurring in the parasympathetic outflow ganglia and SPG, and through this mechanism exert its effect on headache syndromes characterized by activation of the trigeminal autonomic reflex [531].

### Short-Lasting Unilateral Neuralgiform Headache Attacks

In the largest available study, comprising 102 SUNHA patients [509], a total of 18/29 SUNCT patients and 5/16 SUNA patients reported effect of the drug.

In the largest available dataset, gabapentin was effective in 11/29 SUNCT patients and in 7/18 SUNA patients [509].

In the largest study, carbamazepine was effective 20/63 patients [509].

Pooled analyses of lidocaine in 38 patients [505, 509] showed a responder proportion of 0.91 (95% CI 0.79 to 0.99).

In one case series, using lidocaine and methylprednisolone greater occipital nerve block (GONB), improvement was seen in 6/12 SUNCT patients and 3/4 SUNA patients [509].

Implantation of occipital nerve stimulators (ONS) has been performed in a study of 31 patients in which the mean daily attack frequency was reduced by 69% at median follow-up of 45 months [532].

### Paroxysmal Hemicrania

Reports of patients with clinical symptoms consistent with PH where indomethacin is not effective [516, 533].

In the largest prospective study of 31 PH patients, 30 could tolerate indomethacin and all had an effect [213].

A retrospective study of likely PH cases found a consistent response to indomethacin in 30/40 patients [516].

Adverse events are the same as for commonly used NSAIDs, and approximately 25% of PH patient on indomethacin seems to develop gastrointestinal side effects [515].

In the first study, 4/6 PH patient reported a treatment benefit.

In the second study, treatment response was observed in 6/8 patients and the mean monthly headache frequency was reduced by 75% at 6 months follow-up.

In a larger series of different chronic headaches that had failed GONB, response to MCNB was seen in 1/4 PH patients [534].

## Hemicrania Continua

Most patients with HC has unremitting pain, but up to 20% of cases have pain-free periods from 1 day to several months [524].

In a case series of 14 patients, 6 responded completely to COX-2 [527].

Another case series of four patients found complete response to celecoxib in all [535].

A case report of two patients from 2019 suggests that topiramate may have an indomethacin-sparing effect [536].

In a retrospective series of seven HC patients, non-invasive vagus nerve stimulation provided reduction in severity of continuous pain in all patients, and reduction in exacerbation intensity in two patients [518].

A series of seven HC patients found reduction in pain intensity with superior orbital nerve blockades (SONB) with lidocaine [521], but no pain relief for any of the patients with GONB.

Radiofrequency ablation of the superior orbital nerve has been effective in a case series of three patients [537].

## Conclusion

SUNHA, PH, and HC are rare headache syndromes that can be difficult to diagnose and treat correctly.

PH and HC can usually be readily treated with indomethacin when tolerated, but some patients will require other treatments.

Non-invasive vagus nerve stimulation is emerging as a promising and readily accessible prophylactic for both PH and HC.

A subset of PH and HC patients may benefit from ONS or invasive SPG procedures.

## Acknowledgement

*A machine generated summary based on the work of Stubberud, Anker; Tronvik, Erling; Matharu, Manjit. 2020 in Current Treatment Options in Neurology.*


# *Do Paroxysmal Hemicrania and Hemicrania Continua Represent Different Headaches? A Retrospective Study*

DOI: https://doi.org/10.1007/s10072-019-03980-7


## Abstract-Summary

Hemicrania continua and paroxysmal hemicrania are considered different headaches belonging to a group of trigeminal autonomic cephalalgias.

The patients with hemicrania continua and paroxysmal hemicrania were compared for severity, location, character, and mean effective indomethacin dose.

The natural history of headache was looked into to see the evolution of hemicrania continua and paroxysmal hemicrania from episodic and chronic pains, respectively.

The mean age of patients with paroxysmal hemicrania was 34.42 years, and hemicrania continua was 37 years.

Paroxysmal hemicrania had higher pain severity.

Five patients transformed from paroxysmal hemicrania to hemicrania continua, and 3 patients transformed from hemicrania continua to paroxysmal hemicrania.

Paroxysmal hemicrania and hemicrania continua were similar on majority of pain characteristics and autonomic features.

The paroxysmal hemicrania and hemicrania continua are not exclusive headaches and can transform into each other.

Extended:

The mean age of patients with PH was 34.42 years and those with HC was 37 years.

## Background

Hemicrania continua (HC) and paroxysmal hemicrania (PH) are considered different headache types belonging to a group of trigeminal autonomic cephalalgias [60, 538].

HC and PH clearly differ from each other by the duration of pain.

Some experts believe that the pain and autonomic symptoms in PH are more severe as compared with HC [213, 539, 540].

The brain areas that brighten up due to pain on functional MRI in patients with HC and PH are posterior hypothalamus and ventrolateral midbrain [224].

The differences in the characteristics/severity of pain and autonomic features between HC and PH have never been compared.

We conducted this study to compare the severity, character, distribution, and other characteristics of pain, autonomic symptoms, and mean effective indomethacin dose in patients with HC and PH.

We propose a null hypothesis that HC and PH will have significant difference in characteristics of pain and autonomic features.

## Methods

We reviewed the clinical data of patients with the diagnosis of HC and PH that visited the out-patient department between July 2015 and March 2017.

In 2015, we generated the patient's performance for documentation of pain characteristics, autonomic features, and other clinical characteristics of patients with new daily persistent headache (NDPH), chronic migraine, chronic tension type headache, and hemicrania continua.

Since 2015, we have been using the same performance for routine evaluation and documentation of clinical features of patients with TACs.

All consecutive patients with HC and PH were evaluated and documented in the patient's performa.

We identified patients of HC with preceding history of paroxysmal unilateral headaches.

We identified patients of PH with preceding continuous unilateral headaches and reviewed the clinical details and treatment history of their continuous headaches.

**Statistical Methods**

The categorical variables were compared by using the chi-square test.

The continuous variables were compared by independent t test.

The Kruskal-Wallis test or Mann-Whitney U test was used to compare the non-parametric data.

**Results**

We included 35 patients with HC and 27 patients with PH.

None of the patients with PH had background continuous interictal pain.

Patients with PH and HC were comparable in age, male:female ratio, majority of pain characteristics, number of autonomic symptoms, severity of autonomic symptoms, and median effective dose of indomethacin to relieve headache.

Majority of patients with HC and PH had frontal-periorbital location of headache.

One patient transformed from paroxysmal attacks of pain into continuous pain of HC directly without any time gap, whereas four patients had spontaneous resolution of their paroxysmal attacks for 6 to 18 months prior to the new onset of HC.

One patient transformed directly into PH, whereas 2 patients had resolution of this continuous headache for 18 months and 3 years, respectively, prior to the appearance of the pain of PH.

**Discussion**

HC and PH appear to be different headaches based only on the duration of headache.

We could not find any significant difference in most of the headache characteristics and the number/severity of autonomic features between HC and PH.

Despite higher severity of pain in PH, we did not find any significant difference in the severity of autonomic features in our patients with PH.

Three patients with PH had preceding continuous ipsilateral headaches with autonomic features similar to HC.

Despite the fact that we quantified autonomic features and other pain characteristics in order to be more objective in comparing the two groups, we could not define definite end points so as to call two headaches similar or different.

We believe that our study will convince people to agree that there are more similarities than differences between HC and PH.

**Conclusion**

Except for the episodic nature and higher pain severity in PH, most other pain characteristics and autonomic features in PH are similar to HC.

Our study raises an important question that whether HC and PH represent the episodic and chronic variants of same headache type.

A prospective long-term study that determines the natural history of HC and PH and also compares the clinical characteristics, therapeutic response to indomethacin and functional imaging between HC and PH may give some answers.

**Acknowledgement**

*A machine generated summary based on the work of Paliwal, Vimal Kumar; Uniyal, Ravi; Aneez, A; Singh, Laxmi Shankar. 2019 in Neurological Sciences.*

## *Therapeutical Approaches to Paroxysmal Hemicrania, Hemicrania Continua and Short Lasting Unilateral Neuralgiform Headache Attacks: A Critical Appraisal*

DOI: https://doi.org/10.1186/s10194-017-0777-3

### Abstract-Summary

The aim of this review is to summarize all articles dealing with treatments for HC, PH, SUNCT and SUNA, comparing them in terms of effectiveness and safety.

Indomethacin is the best treatment both for HC and PH.

For the acute treatment of HC, piroxicam and celecoxib have shown good results, whilst for the prolonged treatment celecoxib, topiramate and gabapentin are good options besides indomethacin.

For PH the best drug besides indomethacin is piroxicam, both for acute and prolonged treatment.

For SUNCT and SUNA the most effective treatments are intravenous or subcutaneous lidocaine for the acute treatment of active phases and lamotrigine for the their prevention.

Other effective therapeutic options are intravenous steroids for acute treatment and topiramate for prolonged treatment.

Besides a great number of treatments tried, HC, PH, SUNCT and SUNA management remains difficult, according with their unknown pathogenesis and their rarity, which strongly limits the studies upon these conditions.

Extended:

The aim of this study is to rank all therapeutic options available in literature for HC, PH, SUNCT and SUNA treatment and to compare, when possible, their effectiveness and safety.

Indomethacin is the most used treatment (168 patients), followed by verapamil (30 patients), sumatriptan (24 patients) and oxygen (18 patients).

For SUNCT and SUNA 95 articles were excluded: 60 were reviews, 20 of them didn't deal with SUNCT or SUNA therapy or reported it unsatisfactorily, 11 reported symptomatic cases and 4 didn't full-filled all diagnostic criteria.

### Background

The International Classification of Headache Disorders 3rd Edition beta version (ICHD-III-beta) recognizes 4 TACs: cluster headache (CH), hemicrania continua (HC), paroxysmal hemicrania (PH) and short-lasting unilateral neuralgiform headache attacks (SUNCT and SUNA) [60].

TACs rather than CH are uncommon and neglected syndromes: the annual prevalence of PH and short lasting unilateral neuralgiform headache attacks is about 0.5/1000 in the general population and is still unknown for HC [541], this facilitate their misdiagnosis, which often delays the correct treatment [542].

There aren't studies clearly ranking treatments to manage TACs, nor one comparing them in terms of effectiveness and/or safety.

The aim of this study is to rank all therapeutic options available in literature for HC, PH, SUNCT and SUNA treatment and to compare, when possible, their effectiveness and safety.

## Methods

A MEDLINE search using the electronic data-base pubmed has been performed to check all articles dealing with the treatment of primary HC, PH, SUNCT and SUNA form the 1st of January 1989 (the first complete year in which the first International Headache Society classification was available) onwards.

For PH, 195 articles were excluded: 67 reported and summarized only the results of different works, 90 didn't consider PH therapy or described it unsatisfactorily, 29 referred to symptomatic PH and 9 didn't fulfill all ICHD-III diagnostic criteria, making a diagnosis of "probable PH".

For every article, each patient was analyzed and only those treatments correctly stated in terms of regimen and response were considered.

Drug mean dosage and therapeutic standards for non-pharmacological treatments were considered and summarized, even if not statistically analyzed.

## Results

Indomethacin has a significantly higher odds of responders than celecoxib ($p < 0.001$), piroxicam ($p < 0.001$) and GONB ($p < 0.001$), but a similar proportion of responders than SONB, which reduced painful symptoms in each patient ($p = 0.541$).

Considering other treatments rather than indomethacin, piroxicam and celecoxib haven't shown a significantly different odds of responders ($p = 0.837$) and complete responders ($p = 0.219$).

Indomethacin has a significantly higher odds of responders than all other treatments except for OnabotA ($p = 0.723$) and SONB ($p = 0.541$); moreover, it has a significantly higher odds of pain-free patients compared to the other types of treatment (all $p < 0.001$).

Considering pain-free patients, indomethacin has a lower odds than lamotrigine, topiramate, gabapentin, GONB, VTA DBS and ONS (all p-values $< 0.001$).

## Discussion

It should also be considered that SONB has been tested only in a smaller number of patients than indomethacin and currently the experience on the use of these techniques is scarce, both for long-term availability (mean follow-up time = 93 days-data not show) and AEs profile.

The prolonged use of drugs which were effective exacerbation control is a common practice and drugs like indomethacin, piroxicam and celecoxib are frequently used in HC patients outside active phases, even for many months: in our sample the duration of indomethacin assumption ranged between 5 and 1440 days, whereas from 18 to 540 for celecoxib.

Piroxicam seems to be the most effective treatment other than indomethacin, even if the possibility of having GI AEs remains [543] and, like indomethacin, its use should be avoided for long periods of time.

## Conclusion

PH, HC, SUNCT and SUNA represent a hard challenge for clinicians who work in headache or pain fields.

Their infrequence makes difficult to study the pathogenesis of these conditions, as well as design well-done RCPCT for new drugs.

From the review of the available literature indomethacin emerges as the best treatment for HC and PH, while other drugs like celecoxib, topiramate and gabapentin may be useful.

## Acknowledgement

*A machine generated summary based on the work of Baraldi, Carlo; Pellesi, Lanfranco; Guerzoni, Simona; Cainazzo, Maria Michela; Pini, Luigi Alberto. 2017 in The Journal of Headache and Pain.*

# *Hemicrania Continua: A Clinical Perspective on Diagnosis and Management*

DOI: https://doi.org/10.1007/s11910-018-0899-2

## Abstract-Summary

Hemicrania Continua (HC) is a daily and persistent form of headache that is characterized by side-locked pain which is continuous, varies in severity and can be associated with conjunctival injection, lacrimation, nasal congestion, rhinorrhea, eyelid edema, forehead or facial sweating and miosis and/or ptosis.

A similar pathway activation is seen in other Trigeminal autonomic cephalalgias (TAC) which solidifies HC as a TAC.

While we also discuss promising treatments in our review, more evidence is needed before making them a standard of therapy for HC.

Extended:

Hemicrania Continua (HC) is an indomethacin-responsive primary headache disorder.

## Introduction

Secondary HC is a clinical phenomenon that has been widely reported in the literature and refers to patients who have HC like headache secondary to underlying pathology.

Prakash and others 2009 states patients who present with either HC evolving from a remitting form or HC with fading effects of indomethacin may indicate a secondary pathology [544].

Cases have been reported of patients with indomethacin induced headaches during HC treatment.

In Cittadini's and others 2010 cohort study of 39 patients diagnosed with HC patients, one patient with a history of migraines experienced a bilateral headache on higher doses of indomethacin [524, 545].

Eleven HC patients in this study were treated with indomethacin for 6 months (unless patients developed side effects or tolerance) before undergoing an indomethacin taper and switch to Melatonin [546].

**Conclusion**

Recent advancements in neurological treatment options have investigators and clinicians determined to find the best method to therapeutically manage patients with HC.

In order to expand our treatment options for HC, further research is first needed to better understand the pathophysiology and neurological structures involved in this headache disorder.

**Acknowledgement**

*A machine generated summary based on the work of Mehta, Amit; Chilakamarri, Priyanka; Zubair, Adeel; Kuruvilla, Deena E. 2018 in Current Neurology and Neuroscience Reports.*

# *Hemicrania Continua Associated with an Unruptured Anterior Communicating Artery Aneurysm: First Case Report*

DOI: https://doi.org/10.1186/s10194-021-01219-5

**Discussion**

This is the first case report of hemicrania continua in association with an anterior communicating artery aneurysm.

Hemicrania continua predominantly affects females and it is typically a moderately severe unilateral continuous headache which may be associated with intermittent jabs and jolts as is the case with this patient [547, 548].

Hemicrania continua has been reported in association with a variety of intracranial pathologies especially traumatic brain injury, sinusitis, primary and secondary brain tumours, internal carotid artery dissection, dental, orbital and temporomandibular joint problems [549, 550].

There is however only one case report of hemicrania continua in relation to an intracranial aneurysm, and this was of the internal carotid artery [551].

This case report nevertheless emphasises the importance of investigating patients with hemicrania continua for associated intracranial causes.

**[Section 2]**

I present this 51-year-old woman who presented with a 24-month history of a gradual onset right sided headache which was continuous from the start.

The headache was associated with watering of the right eye, and occasionally blockage of the right nostril.

She has a history of hypertension and was on Ramipril; a temporary withdrawal did not resolve the headache.

The clinical diagnosis of hemicrania continua was made and her headaches resolved promptly on Indomethacin but only at a dose of 50 mg three times a day.

**Acknowledgement**

*A machine generated summary based on the work of Imam, Ibrahim. 2021 in The Journal of Headache and Pain.*

## First Case of Hemicrania Continua Responsive to Galcanezumab

DOI: https://doi.org/10.1007/s10072-021-05476-9

### Introduction

Pain and associated symptoms in some primary headaches, such as migraine and trigeminal autonomic cephalalgias (TACs), are due to the activation of the trigemino-vascular system.

Calcitonin gene-related peptide (CGRP) is key in this process as exemplified by the fact that monoclonal CGRP antibodies (CGRP-mABs) are efficacious against migraine [552].

Galcanezumab has shown efficacy in episodic cluster headache patients [442, 553].

### Case Report

Six years earlier, she began with continuous headache, strictly located in her left anterior hemicranium and accompanied by ipsilateral conjunctival injection and eyelid edema.

We tried twice indomethacin, plus omeprazole, but she could not tolerate it, even at very low doses of 25 mg/tid due to gastric discomfort, nausea, dizziness, and unsteadiness, though she felt headache improvement with this drug.

On "November 23rd" and for the whole first month of treatment, she felt a dramatic improvement: background pain disappeared and she just complained of hint of pain episodes every few days, which ceased spontaneously.

In the next two months, she has remained asymptomatic, both for pain and autonomic symptoms, for the first three weeks after the injection, but noticed, only between 5 and 7 days before the next monthly dose of galcanezumab, reappearance of her previous background hemicranial pain together with ipsilateral autonomic symtpoms, though usually mild and allowing her a normal life.

### Discussion

This experience shows that CGRP-mABs, and galcanezumab in particular, can be efficacious in patients with HC.

This case fulfills criteria for unremitting HC, except for an absolute response to indomethacin as she could not tolerate it, though she noticed headache improvement even with low indomethacin doses.

Many medications have been tested in cases with indomethacin intolerance, but, concurring with our experience, their efficacy is limited and anecdotal.

The efficacy of galcanezumab and other CGRP-mABs in migraine [552] and episodic cluster headache [442, 553] is well demonstrated, but results in chronic cluster headache are still controversial [429, 553], and there are no data on the remaining TACs.

**Conclusion**

This experience shows that CGRP antibodies, and galcanezumab in particular, can be efficacious in patients with HC.

With the limitation of having treated just one case in mind, this case supports a key role of CGRP in the pathophysiology of TACs and calls for a clinical trial with CGRP antibodies in HC.

**Acknowledgement**

*A machine generated summary based on the work of González-Quintanilla, Vicente; Pérez-Pereda, Sara; Fontanillas, Noelia; Pascual, Julio. 2021 in Neurological Sciences.*

## Increase in CGRP Levels in a Case of Hemicrania Continua Normalizes After a Successful Response to Galcanezumab

DOI: https://doi.org/10.1007/s10072-022-06063-2

**Dear Editor,**

Our aim here was to analyse the behaviour of blood CGRP levels in our patient with hemicrania continua with a successful response to galcanezumab to try to correlate her clinical response with a theoretical objective marker of the activation of the trigeminovascular system.

CGRP levels were assessed from blood morning samples of this hemicrania continua woman aged 68 immediately before and then 15 days and 3 months after the initiation of galcanezumab.

With the limitation of having examined just one patient, we show for the first time a very clear increase in serum CGRP levels in a case of hemicrania continua as compared to control women without the headache and the progressive normalization of these increased CGRP levels after successful treatment with galcanezumab, which confirms the value of the peripheral levels of this neuropeptide as a biomarker of the activation of the trigeminovascular system [554].

**Acknowledgement**

*A machine generated summary based on the work of Gárate, Gabriel; Pereda, Sara Pérez; González-Quintanilla, Vicente; Madera, Jorge; Pascual, Julio. 2022 in Neurological Sciences.*

# *SUNCT and SUNA: An Update and Review*

DOI: https://doi.org/10.1007/s11916-018-0707-3

## Abstract-Summary

The purpose of this review is to provide an update on the clinical features, diagnosis, pathogenesis, epidemiology, and treatment of the rare primary headache disorders short-lasting unilateral neuralgiform headache attacks with conjunctival injection and tearing (SUNCT) and short-lasting unilateral neuralgiform headache attacks with autonomic symptoms (SUNA).

Recent case reports of secondary SUNCT and SUNA due to medullary infarcts support the theory that the trigeminohypothalamic pathway is involved in the pathophysiology of SUNHA.

We will discuss the pathophysiology of both the pain and the autonomic symptoms experienced in SUNCT and SUNA attacks as well the medical, procedural, and surgical options for treatment with emphasis on recent advances.

## Clinical Case

A 46-year-old otherwise healthy man presented with new onset facial pain triggered by nose blowing.

1.5 years later, the patient developed the episodes again with a frequency of >100 attacks/day lasting up to 10 s in duration.

The following medications either provided him with short-term pain relief, reduced pain, or reduced severity or frequency of attacks: lidocaine, extracranial nerve blocks, sphenopalatine ganglion (SPG) block, and fosphenytoin intravenously.

The images on MRI suggested that the patient likely had compression of the trigeminal nerve by a venous structure as well as an arterial structure.

Following microvascular decompression of these vessels, the patient was able to wean off of all of his medications and has remained pain free.

## Introduction, Clinical Features, and Diagnosis

The ICHD 3-beta classifies SUNCT and SUNA as part of the trigeminal autonomic cephalgias (TACs) [60].

SUNCT and SUNA are distinguished from trigeminal neuralgia (TN) by their associated autonomic features—conjunctival injection and tearing being characteristic for SUNCT and either one or none of the autonomic symptoms of conjunctival injection or tearing for SUNA [555, 556].

Autonomic features can aid in the diagnosis but even tearing has been noted in trigeminal neuralgia [555].

Unlike SUNCT and SUNA, trigeminal neuralgia has a refractory period during which time it is near impossible to trigger another episode.

The absence of a refractory period in SUNHA may be due to its pathophysiology which includes a central source of pain and disinhibitor of the trigeminal nucleus caudalis which is thought to come from the posterior hypothalamus and will be discussed further below [499, 555, 557, 558].

**Pathophysiology**

In rat studies cited by Leone, a trigeminohypothalamic tract has been identified where the trigeminal nucleus caudalis can stimulate the posterior hypothalamus.

It is also thought that the posterior hypothalamus can modulate activity of the trigeminal nucleus caudalis which has been demonstrated in cluster headache research.

Goadsby's work on cluster headache suggests secondary activation of areas of the cortex once the trigeminocervical complex has been activated, leading to the severe pain associated with this headache disorder [159].

Miller published a study involving 11 patients with SUNCT and SUNA who had either failed or been denied occipital nerve stimulation and underwent DBS to the ventral tegmental area (VTA) ipsilateral to the side of the attacks, and showed 78% improvement in median attack frequency and 50% improvement in attack severity [559].

The actual pathophysiologic data linking the ventral tegmental area to the pain involved in SUNCT and SUNA is limited, and the posterior hypothalamus has been speculated to be involved in cluster headache by fMRI and PET studies [560].

**Secondary SUNCT and SUNA**

Although considered a primary headache disorder, cases of secondary SUNCT and SUNA have been reported.

There have also been two recent case reports of ischemic injuries resulting in secondary SUNCT.

Report, a 64-year-old man suffered a left ischemic dorsolateral medullary infarct and 13 days later and headaches described as SUNCT.

These case reports clearly demonstrate SUNCT syndrome due to a secondary cause.

**Epidemiology**

SUNCT and SUNA have comparable symptomology to TN, but their epidemiology does differ in some respects.

The age of onset of these conditions may differ with trigeminal neuralgia average age of onset between 50 and 60 and SUNCT/SUNA being reported from childhood through advanced age [555].

One recent case report of a familial SUNCT syndrome has been reported [561].

**Current Medical Therapy and Recent Advances**

A critical appraisal from Baraldi and others in The Journal of Headache and Pain 2017 effectively analyzed both acute and prophylactic (or prolonged) treatments for SUNCT and SUNA by looking at published treatments dating back to 1989.

Of the four medications used to treat acute attacks (lidocaine, prednisone, methylprednisolone, and phenytoin), lidocaine (both intravenous and subcutaneous) had the highest odds of responders and those that were pain free after administration.

Lamotrigine is not only the most commonly administered prolonged treatment, but when compared to other therapies, it has a higher odds of responders compared to topiramate (although their complete responders were similar).

Although not typically occurring in children, a recent case report describes the success of onobotulinum toxin A in the treatment of acute-onset idiopathic SUNCT in a 12-year-old boy [562].

Reportedly, it had only been used once before in a 55-year-old man with chronic SUNCT who was being treated with multiple other medical therapies [562, 563].

## Other Therapy and Recent Advances

A study from Japan identified 2 patients out of 800 with trigeminal neuralgiform pain who had concomitant autonomic symptoms and underwent microvascular decompression.

Occipital nerve stimulation (ONS) is considered a potential option for SUNCT and SUNA patients with medically refractory symptoms.

In a literature review performed by Baraldi and others, 7 patients who had occipital nerve stimulation not only had pain reduction, they were complete responders, meaning pain free, after the procedure [564].

All nine patients in Baraldi's review who underwent DBS of the VTA were complete responders; notably, all nine also experienced side effects related to the procedure that were not detailed in the review [564].

In a case series of 11 patients in the UK with medically refractory SUNHA that had either failed ONS or had been denied access to this procedure, DBS to the ipsilateral VTA was performed.

## Controversy

He also questions why patients initially diagnosed with trigeminal neuralgia can have evolution of their symptoms such that they then fit a diagnosis of SUNHA and then can even de-volve back to the symptomatology of solely trigeminal neuralgia.

Classical cases of trigeminal neuralgia have compression of the superior cerebellar artery as the etiology, and as discussed above, secondary SUNHA can share this common mechanism and treatment with vascular decompression [60, 557, 565, 566].

Lambru and Matharu point out that the spectrum of SUNCT, SUNA, and trigeminal neuralgia may cause misdiagnosis of patients as not all patients with SUNHA present with pain in the V1 division, and as so their practitioner may not ask about autonomic symptoms associated with their condition, which is an important part of the history in order to make an accurate diagnosis [558].

## Conclusion

While primary in nature they can also have potential secondary etiologies which if identified can lead to a different course of treatment.

While medical therapies have not significantly changed in recent years, surgical and procedural interventions have been more frequently reported in the literature with positive results.

These results, however, do not come without risk, some of which can be significant.

Further research directed at the potential hormonal involvement in this condition may expand the number of therapies available.

**Acknowledgement**

*A machine generated summary based on the work of Arca, Karissa N.; Halker Singh, Rashmi B. 2018 in Current Pain and Headache Reports.*

## Trigeminal Autonomic Cephalalgias Presenting in a Multidisciplinary Tertiary Orofacial Pain Clinic

DOI: https://doi.org/10.1186/s10194-019-1019-7

### Abstract-Summary

To assess the headache disorders presenting in a tertiary multidisciplinary orofacial pain clinic, after dental causes have been excluded.

The most common trigeminal autonomic cephalalgia diagnosis was hemicrania continua (n = 13, 9%), which is higher than the reported prevalence in neurology and headache clinics.

This study demonstrates the importance of a multidisciplinary approach to diagnosing complex orofacial pain patients and the importance of awareness of primary headache disorders, in particular trigeminal autonomic cephalalgias, thereby reducing unnecessary diagnostic delays or procedures.

Extended:

The most common cranial autonomic symptom, within the whole group with possible TAC, was lacrimation (n = 35), followed by nasal congestion (n = 27) and conjunctival injection (n = 23).

### Introduction

The pain CH patients experience can be easily and often misdiagnosed as dental pulp pain.

58% had a dental procedure ipsilateral to the side where CH developed and in 24 out of 54 (44%) oral surgery was performed afterwards in order to resolve this pain.

With regards to patients with CH, Bahra and Goadsby documented that dentists and ear, nose and throat (ENT) surgeons were most commonly consulted prior to neurologists (45% of 511 subjects) and that 52% had an invasive procedure performed for pain [266].

The application of the ICHD-II criteria to 502 patients who presented with Temporo-Mandibular Dysfunction (TMD) and orofacial pain in a Temporo-Mandibular Joint and Orofacial Pain Clinic found, surprisingly, one single case of CH with no other TACs reported, and being tension-type headache the most frequent entity, diagnosed in 246 patients [567].

### Methods

Clinic letters from the initial consultation and subsequent follow up reviews of the 142 patients, who were seen in the tertiary Multidisciplinary Orofacial Pain clinic between January 2015 until January 2018 were reviewed as a clinical audit.

In this clinic, all patients are first reviewed by an experienced Orofacial Surgeon (TR) to exclude a dental cause for their facial pain.

The Multidisciplinary Orofacial Pain clinic has approximately 300 new patients a year, approximately 12% of patients present with a dental cause for primary complaint, of which the most common is painful post-traumatic trigeminal neuropathic (48%) and TMD is second most common (23%).

Of the patients with a possible TAC diagnosis, the pain localisation, cranial autonomic symptoms and result of the indomethacin test (if applicable) were recorded.

A positive test was deemed to be at least a 50% reduction in pain intensity and/or 50% in frequency or duration of the worsenings present with the indomethacin and not with the placebo.

## Results

A TAC was suspected in 62 patients (44%) based on the history of unilateral pain in the trigeminal distribution and the presence of ipsilateral cranial autonomic symptoms, as per ICHD-III beta criteria.

A previous suspected diagnosis was only reported in 17 patients, including trigeminal neuralgia (n = 6), migraine (n = 8), SUNCT (n = 1) and painful trigeminal neuropathy (n = 2).

Time to diagnosis for the whole cohort was 5.6 years, in patients with a confirmed TAC (HC, PH, CH and SUNCT/SUNA) was 7 years.

Time to diagnosis in patients with HC, the most common diagnosis among TACs, was 8.7 years.

Among patients with possible TAC (including all patients with suspected HC who underwent the indomethacin test), different dental procedures were recorded.

Twenty-six out of 62 patients (42%) had a previous pain background, migraine being the most common.

## Discussion

HC has been considered a rare condition and a recent study by Hryvenko and colleagues reviewed 1617 new patients seen in their TMD and Orofacial Pain Clinic, and only found 6 (0.4%) patients with HC, with 5 patients with nearly complete response with oral indomethacin (150–225 mg/day) and one patient had to remain on 75 mg/day due to intolerable side effects, and therefore had partial pain relief [568].

We have found a higher prevalence of HC in our cohort of 142 patients from our tertiary Multidisciplinary Orofacial Pain clinic.

Our findings suggest HC patients present to orofacial pain services due to the distribution and characteristics of the pain, and we encourage orofacial pain services to consider this diagnosis perhaps more often than may have been the case.

## Conclusion

TACs are an important group of primary headache disorders dentists and oral surgeons should be aware of as many patients with unilateral side-locked primary headaches present to the dental services.

HC is underdiagnosed and this may be due to the presentation to other speciali-ties rather than to neurology and headache services.

We have found the most effective way to ensure patients are diagnosed correctly and managed optimally is a multidisciplinary service with dentists, oral surgeons and headache specialists.

**Acknowledgement**

*A machine generated summary based on the work of Wei, D. Y.; Moreno-Ajona, D.; Renton, T.; Goadsby, P. J. 2019 in The Journal of Headache and Pain.*

# CT-Guided Thermocoagulation of the Pterygopalatine Ganglion for Refractory Trigeminal Autonomic Cephalalgia

DOI: https://doi.org/10.1007/s40122-022-00406-9

**Abstract-Summary**

Trigeminal autonomic cephalalgia (TAC) is a type of one-sided cerebral painful headache, with attacks regularly accompanied by autonomic responses, such as tearing, runny nose, panic, nausea and vomiting on the affected side.

We report the case of thermocoagulation treatment of the pterygopalatine gan-glion in an uncommon TAC under local anesthesia.

A rare case of TAC was treated with computed tomography (CT)-guided thermo-coagulation within the pterygopalatine ganglion.

In the case reported here, we performed CT-guided thermocoagulation of the pterygopalatine ganglion at 90 °C for 180 s for treatment of a trigeminal autonomic headache.

This is the first report of using thermocoagulation at 90 °C to treat the pterygo-palatine ganglion.

Computed tomography-guided thermocoagulation of the pterygopalatine gan-glion at 90 °C for 180 s for treatment of trigeminal autonomic headache is a safe and economical treatment option.

Extended:

We report a case of standard radiofrequency treatment of the pterygopalatine ganglion (SPG) in a uncommon TAC performed under local anesthesia, a strategy that has fewer side effects and is more cost-effective than other treatments for such patients.

These results indicate that CT-guided SPG standard radiofrequency treatment can be expected to be an effective treatment for TACs.

**Introduction**

Trigeminal autonomic cephalalgias (TACs) are a group of primary headaches char-acterized by paroxysmal, fluctuating unilateral headaches distributed along the trigeminal nerve, with pain often located in the orbital, forehead and temporal regions, accompanied by clinical manifestations, such as ipsilateral autonomic dysfunction including, for example, lacrimation and bulbar conjunctival congestion.

TACS are grouped into four distinct primary headache types: cluster headache, paroxysmal migraine, persistent migraine and unilateral transient persistent neuralgia-like headache with conjunctival congestion and tearing [1].

TAC appeared for the first time as an independent headache type in the 2013 International Classification of Headache, version 3β [569].

We report a case of standard radiofrequency treatment of the pterygopalatine ganglion (SPG) in a uncommon TAC performed under local anesthesia, a strategy that has fewer side effects and is more cost-effective than other treatments for such patients.

## Case Presentation

The patient, a 44-year-old women, was admitted to the hospital with "recurrent attacks of left-sided cephalofacial pain for more than 29 years, aggravated for 1 month".

There had been an onset of pain on the left side of the head and face that had worsened 1 month previously, affecting sleep, with attacks ranging in frequency from one to several times a day, with each attack lasting between 3 and 4 h. The pain could be relieved by forceful defecation and vomiting.

On the third night, she reported a sudden worsening of pain, with an NRS score of 9–10 for pain and slight relief of symptoms after forceful defecation and vomiting.

On postoperative day 1, she reported significant improvement in the paroxysmal head and facial pain, and there was no swelling of the left side of the face, no nausea and vomiting; the NRS score was 2.

## Discussion

Of these, the sensory nerve originates from the pterygopalatine nerve of the maxillary branch of the trigeminal nerve and is located above the SPG; the parasympathetic nerve originates from the Iambda nerve of the facial nerve and is located posterior to the SPG; and the sympathetic nerve originates from the Iambda deep nerve of the superior cervical plexus and is located posteriorly below the pterygopalatine SPG.

The associations of these nerve branches also explains the pain attack with nausea and vomiting and strong bowel movement in this patient, and can be used as a basis for electrical stimulation to determine whether the radiofrequency needle is close to the SPG.

When performing radiofrequency ablation of the pterygopalatine ganglion in the pterygopalatine fossa, high- and low-frequency electrophysiological tests should be performed first to prevent damage to the V2 branch of the trigeminal nerve in the external orifice of the foramen magnum from causing numbness in the innervation area of this branch.

## Conclusion

There are very few treatment options for TACs.

After giving the patient several stellate nerve blocks with less than satisfactory results, we obtained the patient's consent to go forward with CT-guided radiofrequency treatment of the SPG.

These results indicate that CT-guided SPG standard radiofrequency treatment can be expected to be an effective treatment for TACs.

**Acknowledgement**

*A machine generated summary based on the work of Ma, Ying; Xu, Shuangshuang; Liu, Xiaolan; Xia, Zhangtian; Zhao, Wei; Huang, Bing. 2022 in Pain and Therapy.*

## *Treatment of Disabling Headache with Greater Occipital Nerve Injections in a Large Population of Childhood and Adolescent Patients: A Service Evaluation*

DOI: https://doi.org/10.1186/s10194-018-0835-5

**Abstract-Summary**

Evidenced-based options for the treatment of primary headache disorders with preventive medication is limited and clinical outcomes are often unsatisfactory.

Greater occipital nerve injections represent a rapid and well-tolerated therapeutic option, which is widely used in clinical practice in adults, and has previously shown a good outcome in a pediatric population.

This service evaluation reviewed greater occipital nerve injections performed unilaterally with 30 mg 1% lidocaine and 40 mg methylprednisolone, to treat disabling headache disorders in children and adolescents.

Of the population, 79% had chronic migraine, 14% new daily persistent headache, 4% a trigeminal autonomic cephalalgia, 3% secondary headache and one patient had chronic tension-type headache.

Improvement was seen in 68% of patients with chronic migraine, 67% with a trigeminal autonomic cephalalgia and 59% with new daily persistent headache.

This large single centre service evaluation confirms that unilateral injection of the greater occipital nerve is a safe, rapid-onset and effective treatment strategy in disabling headache disorders in children, with a range of diagnoses and severity of the condition, and with minimal side effects.

Extended:

Greater occipital nerve (GON) injections have shown to provide a quick onset of therapeutic response, which is also sustained [570], while avoiding the common side effects of classic migraine preventives or more invasive treatments [571].

Greater occipital nerve injections are a safe, effective and useful strategy for disabling primary headache disorders in children.

Improvement was seen in 68% of the chronic migraine population (n = 85) and 59% (n = 13) in the NDPH subgroup.

A binary logistic regression analysis was performed in order to determine the effect of several predictor variables on the dichotomous primary outcome measure of improvement.

Research should focus on performing large randomized controlled studies in paediatric subjects to establish how objectively effective this approach may be.

## Background

Headache disorders with high frequency of attacks in children and adolescents can be extremely disabling.

Infiltration of the area around the greater occipital nerve with a mixture of local anesthetic and corticosteroids is a well-established therapy for primary headache prevention in adults [347, 572] that has been recently reported in children to have excellent results [573].

The mechanism of action is linked to the anatomical overlap between spinal afferents providing sensory innervation from the C2 occipital region and trigeminal afferents at the trigeminocervical complex, a complex brain area involved in the pathophysiology of primary headache disorders [574].

Our objective was to determine the efficacy and safety of greater occipital nerve injections in a large population of paediatric headache patients.

## Methods

A retrospective chart review was performed on all letters and clinical correspondence for patients who received a greater occipital nerve injection between 2009 and 2016.

For each patient who received a GON injection, information on age (measured as a continuous variable), gender, headache diagnosis, date of first visit, time from first visit to injection, site of injection, past and current medication, effects of injection and eventual follow-up treatment was collected using a standardized pro forma.

The clinician palpated over the greater occipital nerves and injected the side that was most tender.

The primary outcome of 'improvement' from the injection was defined as either a significant, more than one third, decrease in headache frequency or intensity or by a documented headache improvement in the clinical notes.

A binary logistic regression analysis was performed in order to determine the effect of several predictor variables on the dichotomous primary outcome measure of improvement.

## Results

Of these, 159 patients with follow-up, 79% (n = 126) had chronic migraine, 15% (n = 24) with aura, 14% (n = 22) new daily persistent headache (NDPH), 4% (n = 6) a trigeminal autonomic cephalalgia (TAC), 3% (n = 4) a form of secondary headache and one patient had chronic tension-type headache.

Of patients who had subsequent injections n = 15 were headache free and n = 67 had a general benefit after treatment.

A binary logistic regression model was created in order to examine the effect of age, gender, medication overuse, headache diagnosis and frequency, years of disease, number of past preventives used and presence of side effects, on the primary outcome measure of improvement for the first GON injection.

No specific variable was responsible for significantly predicting a positive outcome, although a diagnosis of migraine and a trigeminal autonomic cephalalgia increased the odds of having an improvement from the injection by 4 and 3 times, respectively.

**Discussion**

Our study found no significant difference with regards to response to treatment in different headache phenotypes, even if we observed an increased likelihood of response in migraineurs and patients with TACs.

Conditions normally associated with a more severe clinical picture, such as an increased number of headache preventive medications used in the past and a diagnosis of medication overuse, not only did not predict a poorer response to treatment but on the contrary were linked with a higher likelihood of improvement.

It is therefore possible to infer that greater occipital nerve injections are a valid therapeutic approach even in refractory headache patients who would normally be bound to fail normal preventives [575]; patients should also be informed that side effects are not to be considered as a marker of poor outcome.

It is worth noting this is a relatively invasive procedure and the proportion of patients showing a placebo response in headache studies is well established [576].

**Conclusions**

Greater occipital nerve injections are a safe, effective and useful strategy for disabling primary headache disorders in children.

Presence of side effects and refractory headache does not predict poor treatment outcome.

In the clinical approach to the treatment of chronic primary headache disorders in a paediatric setting, GON injections should be considered as first line management alongside the classic medications, which are often more side-effect prone.

**Acknowledgement**

*A machine generated summary based on the work of Puledda, Francesca; Goadsby, Peter J.; Prabhakar, Prab. 2018 in The Journal of Headache and Pain.*

# References

1. Headache Classification Committee of the International Headache Society (IHS). The International Classification of Headache Disorders, 3rd edition. Cephalalgia. 2018;38:1–211. https://doi.org/10.1177/0333102417738202. Diagnostic Criteria by IHS. This is the brand new edition of the International Classification of Headache Disorders. Next to describing >200 headache disorders, it contains up-to-date references and commentaries on all headache types, including cluster headache.
2. Kudrow L. The cyclic relationship of natural illumination to cluster period frequency. Cephalalgia. 1987;7:76–8. https://doi.org/10.1177/03331024870070S623.

3. Wilbrink LA, Teernstra OPM, Haan J, van Zwet EW, Evers SMAA, Spincemaille GH, et al. Occipital nerve stimulation in medically intractable, chronic cluster headache. The ICON study: rationale and protocol of a randomised trial. Cephalalgia. 2013;33:1238–47. https://doi.org/10.1177/0333102413490351.

4. Torelli P, Beghi E, Manzoni GC. Cluster headache prevalence in the Italian general population. Neurology. 2005;64:469–74.

5. Ekbom K, Svensson DA, Pedersen NL, Waldenlind E. Lifetime prevalence and concordance risk of cluster headache in the Swedish twin population. Neurology. 2006;67:798–803.

6. Donnet A, Lanteri-Minet M, Guegan-Massardier E, Mick G, Fabre N, Géraud G, et al. Chronic cluster headache: a French clinical descriptive study. J Neurol Neurosurg Psychiatry. 2007;78:1354–8.

7. Manzoni GC, Taga A, Russo M, Torelli P. Age of onset of episodic and chronic cluster headache – a review of a large case series from a single headache centre. J Headache Pain. 2016;17:4–9.

8. Steinberg A, Fourier C, Ran C, Waldenlind E, Sjo C, Belin AC. Cluster headache – clinical pattern and a new severity scale in a Swedish cohort. Cephalalgia. 2018;38:1286–95. https://doi.org/10.1177/0333102417731773.

9. Diamond S, Urban G. Cluster headache. Pain Manag. 2006;1:474–91.

10. Rozen TD, Fishman RS. Cluster headache in the United States of America: demographics, clinical characteristics, triggers, suicidality, and personal burden. Headache. 2012;52:99–113.

11. Gaul C, Christmann N, Schröder D, Weber R, Shanib H, Diener HC, et al. Differences in clinical characteristics and frequency of accompanying migraine features in episodic and chronic cluster headache. Cephalalgia. 2012;32:571–7.

12. Dong Z, Di H, Dai W, Pan M, Li Z, Liang J, et al. Clinical profile of cluster headaches in China - a clinic-based study. J Headache Pain. 2013;14:1–10.

13. Imai N, Yagi N, Kuroda R, Konishi T, Serizawa M, Kobari M. Clinical profile of cluster headaches in Japan: low prevalence of chronic cluster headache, and uncoupling of sense and behaviour of restlessness. Cephalalgia. 2011;31:628–33.

14. Lin KH, Wang PJ, Fuh JL, Lu SR, Chung CT, Tsou HK, et al. Cluster headache in the Taiwanese - a clinic-based study. Cephalalgia. 2004;24:631–8.

15. Bhargava A, Pujar GS, Banakar BF, Shubhakaran K, Kasundra G, Bhushan B. Study of cluster headache: a hospital-based study. J Neurosci Rural Pract. 2014;5:369–73.

16. Moon HS, Park JW, Lee KS, Chung CS, Kim BK, Kim JM, et al. Clinical features of cluster headache patients in Korea. J Korean Med Sci. 2017;32:502–6.

17. Schürks M, Kurth T, De Jesus J, Jonjic M, Rosskopf D, Diener HC. Cluster headache: clinical presentation, lifestyle features, and medical treatment. Headache. 2006;46:1246–54.

18. Robbins MS, Bronheim R, Lipton RB, Grosberg BM, Vollbracht S, Sheftell FD, et al. Depression and anxiety in episodic and chronic cluster headache: a pilot study. Headache. 2012;52:600–11.

19. Liang JF, Chen YT, Fuh JL, Li SY, Liu CJ, Chen TJ, et al. Cluster headache is associated with an increased risk of depression: a nationwide population-based cohort study. Cephalalgia. 2013;33:182–9.

20. Absinta M, Rocca MA, Colombo B, Falini A, Comi G, Filippi M. Selective decreased grey matter volume of the pain-matrix network in cluster headache. Cephalalgia. 2012;32:109–15.

21. Yang F-C, Chou K-H, Fuh J-L, Huang C-C, Lirng J-F, Lin Y-Y, et al. Altered gray matter volume in the frontal pain modulation network in patients with cluster headache. Pain. 2013;154:801–7.

22. Naegel S, Holle D, Desmarattes N, Theysohn N, Diener H-C, Katsarava Z, et al. Cortical plasticity in episodic and chronic cluster headache. NeuroImage Clin. 2014;6:415–23.

23. May A, Bahra A, Büchel C, Frackowiak RS, Goadsby PJ. Hypothalamic activation in cluster headache attacks. Lancet (London, England). 1998;352:275–8.

24. Morelli N, Pesaresi I, Cafforio G, Maluccio MR, Gori S, Di Salle F, et al. Functional magnetic resonance imaging in episodic cluster headache. J Headache Pain. 2009;10:11–4.

25. Leone M, Proietti CA. Long-term use of daily sumatriptan injections in severe drug-resistant chronic cluster headache. Neurology. 2016;86:194–5.
26. Blau JN, Engel HO. Individualizing treatment with verapamil for cluster headache patients. Headache. 2004;44:1013–8. https://doi.org/10.1111/j.1526-4610.2004.04196.x.
27. Huang W, Lo M, Wang S, Tsai J, Wu H. Topiramate in prevention of cluster headache in the Taiwanese. Neurol India. 2010;58:284–7. http://www.neurologyindia.com/article.asp?issn=0028-3886
28. Koverech A, Cicione C, Lionetto L, Maestri M, Passariello F, Sabbatini E, Capi M, De Marco CM, Guglielmetti M, Negro A, Di Menna L, Simmaco M, Nicoletti F, Martelletti P. Migraine and cluster headache show impaired neurosteroids patterns. J Headache Pain. 2019;20(1):61. https://doi.org/10.1186/s10194-019-1005-0.
29. Vollesen AL, Benemei S, Cortese F, Labastida-Ramírez A, Marchese F, Pellesi L, Romoli M, Ashina M, Lampl C. School of advanced studies of the European Headache Federation (EHF-SAS). Migraine and cluster headache—the common link. J Headache Pain. 2018;19(1):89. https://doi.org/10.1186/s10194-018-0909-4.
30. Barloese M. Current understanding of the chronobiology of cluster headache and the role of sleep in its management. Nat Sci Sleep. 2021;13:153–62. https://doi.org/10.2147/NSS.S278088. (eCollection 2021)
31. Kim BS, Chung PW, Kim BK, Lee MJ, Park JW, Chu MK, Ahn JY, Bae DW, Song TJ, Sohn JH, Oh K, Kim D, Kim JM, Kim SK, Choi YJ, Chung JM, Moon HS, Chung CS, Park KY, Cho SJ. The impact of remission and coexisting migraine on anxiety and depression in cluster headache. J Headache Pain. 2020;21(1):58. https://doi.org/10.1186/s10194-020-01120-7.
32. Steiner TJ, Jensen R, Katsarava Z, et al. Aids to management of headache disorders in primary care (2nd edition). J Headache Pain. 2019;20:57.
33. de Andrés F, Lionetto L, Curto M, Capi M, Cipolla F, Negro A, Martelletti P. Acute, transitional and long-term cluster headache treatment: pharmacokinetic issues. Expert Opin Drug Metab Toxicol. 2016;12(9):1011–20. https://doi.org/10.1080/17425255.2016.1201067.
34. Martelletti P, Curto M. Headache: cluster headache treatment—RCTs versus real-world evidence. Nat Rev Neurol. 2016;12(10):557–8. https://doi.org/10.1038/nrneurol.2016.134.
35. Martelletti P, Jensen RH, Antal A, Arcioni R, Brighina F, de Tommaso M, et al. Neuromodulation of chronic headaches: position statement from the European Headache Federation. J Headache Pain. 2013;14:86. https://doi.org/10.1186/1129-2377-14-86.
36. Lampl C, Rudolph M, Bräutigam E. OnabotulinumtoxinA in the treatment of refractory chronic cluster headache. J Headache Pain. 2018;19(1):45. https://doi.org/10.1186/s10194-018-0874-y.
37. https://www.ema.europa.eu/en/documents/smop/questions-answers-refusal-change-marketing-authorisation-emgality-galcanezumab_en.pdf. Viewed 2 May 2021.
38. Argyriou AA, Vikelis M, Mantovani E, Litsardopoulos P, Tamburin S. Recently available and emerging therapeutic strategies for the acute and prophylactic management of cluster headache: a systematic review and expert opinion. Expert Rev Neurother. 2021;21(2):235–48. https://doi.org/10.1080/14737175.2021.1857240.
39. Mudugal D, Monteith TS. Drug profile: galcanezumab for prevention of cluster headache. Expert Rev Neurother. 2021;21(2):145–55. https://doi.org/10.1080/14737175.2021.1852931.
40. Ossipov MH, Raffa RB, Pergolizzi JV. Galcanezumab: a humanized monoclonal antibody for the prevention of migraine and cluster headache. Drugs Today (Barc). 2020;56(1):5–19. https://doi.org/10.1358/dot.2020.56.1.3069863.
41. Alexandre J, Humbert X, Sassier M, Milliez P, Coquerel A, Fedrizzi S. High-dose verapamil in episodic and chronic cluster headaches and cardiac adverse events: is it as safe as we think? Drug Saf Case Rep. 2015;2(1):13. https://doi.org/10.1007/s40800-015-0015-3.
42. Negro A, Sciattella P, Spuntarelli V, Martelletti P, Mennini FS. Direct and indirect costs of cluster headache: a prospective analysis in a tertiary level headache centre. J Headache Pain. 2020;21(1):44. https://doi.org/10.1186/s10194-020-01115-4.

43. Cruz S, Lemos C, Monteiro JM. Familial aggregation of cluster headache. Arq Neuropsiquiatr. 2013;71(11):866–70.

44. Leone M, Rigamonti A, Bussone G. Cluster headache sine headache: two new cases in one family. Cephalalgia. 2002;22(1):12–4.

45. Bordini CA, et al. Cluster headache: report of seven cases in three families. Funct Neurol. 1997;12(5):277–82.

46. D'Amico D, et al. Familial cluster headache: report of three families. Headache. 1996;36(1):41–3.

47. Russell MB, Andersson PG. Clinical intra- and interfamilial variability of cluster headache. Eur J Neurol. 1995;1(3):253–7.

48. Leone M, et al. Increased familial risk of cluster headache. Neurology. 2001;56(9):1233–6.

49. Vikelis M, Rapoport AM. Cluster headache in Greece: an observational clinical and demographic study of 302 patients. J Headache Pain. 2016;17(1):88.

50. Naber WC, Fronczek R, Haan J, Doesborg P, Colwell CS, Ferrari MD, et al. The biological clock in cluster headache: a review and hypothesis. Cephalalgia. 2019;39(14):1855–66.

51. Rossi P, Little P, De La Torre ER, Palmaro A. If you want to understand what it really means to live with cluster headache, imagine... fostering empathy through European patients' own stories of their experiences. Funct Neurol. 2018;33(1):57–9. Highlights importance of understanding patients' with cluster headache experiences.

52. Kudrow L. Cluster headache: mechanisms and management. Oxford: Oxford University Press; 1980.

53. Manzoni GC, Terzano MG, Bono G, Micieli G, Martucci N, Nappi G. Cluster headache – clinical findings in 180 patients. Cephalalgia. 1983;3:21–30.

54. Ekbom K, Svensson DA, Träff H, Waldenlind E. Age at onset and sex ratio in cluster headache: observations over three decades. Cephalalgia. 2002;22:94–100.

55. Sjaastad O, Bakketeig LS. Cluster headache prevalence. Vågå study of headache epidemiology. Cephalalgia. 2003;23:528–33.

56. Sutherland JM, Eadie MJ. Cluster headache. Res Clin Stud Headache. 1972;3:92–125.

57. Manzoni GC. Cluster headache and lifestyle: remarks on a population of 374 male patients. Cephalalgia. 1999;19:88–94.

58. Manzoni GC, Stovner LJ. Epidemiology of headache. In: Headache NG, Moskowitz MA, editors. Handbook of clinical neurology, vol. 97. Amsterdam: Elsevier; 2010. p. 3–22.

59. Manzoni GC, Micieli G, Granella F, Tassorelli C, Zanferrari C, Cavallini A. Cluster headache – course over ten years in 189 patients. Cephalalgia. 1991;11:169–74.

60. Headache Classification Committee of the International Headache Society (IHS). The International Classification of Headache Disorders (beta version). Cephalalgia. 2013;33(9):629–808.

61. Manzoni GC, Maffezzoni M, Lambru G, Lana S, Latte L, Torelli P. Late-onset cluster headache: some considerations about 73 cases. Neurol Sci. 2012;33(Suppl 1):S157–9.

62. D'Amico D, et al. Mapping assessments instruments for headache disorders against the ICF biopsychosocial model of health and disability. Int J Environ Res Public Health. 2021;18(1):246.

63. Bakar NA, et al. The development and validation of the cluster headache quality of life scale (CHQ). J Headache Pain. 2016;17(1):79.

64. Klan T, et al. Determination of psychosocial factors in cluster headache–construction and psychometric properties of the cluster headache scales (CHS). Cephalalgia. 2020;40(11):1240–9.

65. May A, et al. Cluster headache. Nat Rev Dis Prim. 2018;4(1):1–17.

66. D'Amico D, et al. Disability, quality of life, and socioeconomic burden of cluster headache: a critical review of current evidence and future perspectives. Headache. 2020;60(4):809–18.

67. Jensen RM, Lyngberg A, Jensen RH. Burden of cluster headache. Cephalalgia. 2007;27(6):535–41. https://doi.org/10.1111/j.1468-2982.2007.01330.x.

68. Choi YJ, Kim BK, Chung PW, et al. Impact of cluster headache on employment status and job burden: a prospective cross-sectional multicenter study. J Headache Pain. 2018;19(1):78. https://doi.org/10.1186/s10194-018-0911-x.

69. Sjöstrand C, Russell MB, Ekbom K, Waldenlind E. Familial cluster headache: demographic patterns in affected and nonaffected. Headache. 2010;50(3):374–82. https://doi.org/10.1111/j.1526-4610.2009.01426.x.
70. Gaul C, et al. Treatment costs and indirect costs of cluster headache: a health economics analysis. Cephalalgia. 2011;31(16):1664–72.
71. Buse DC, Manack AN, Fanning KM, Serrano D, Reed ML, Turkel CC, et al. Chronic migraine prevalence, disability, and sociodemographic factors: results from the American Migraine Prevalence and Prevention study. Headache. 2012;52(10):1456–70.
72. D'Amico D, Sansone E, Grazzi L, Giovannetti AM, Leonardi M, Schiavolin S, et al. Multimorbidity in patients with chronic migraine and medication overuse headache. Acta Neurol Scand. 2018;138(6):515–22.
73. Sinnige J, Korevaar JC, Westert GP, Spreeuwenberg P, Schellevis FG, Braspenning JC. Multimorbidity patterns in a primary care population aged 55 years and over. Fam Pract. 2015;32(5):505–13.
74. Vetrano DL, Calderón-Larrañaga A, Marengoni A, Onder G, Bauer JM, Cesari M, et al. An international perspective on chronic multimorbidity: approaching the elephant in the room. J Gerontol A Biol Sci Med Sci. 2018;73(10):1350–6.
75. Lateef T, He J-P, Nelson K, Calkins ME, Gur R, Gur R, et al. Physical–mental comorbidity of pediatric migraine in the Philadelphia neurodevelopmental cohort. J Pediatr. 2019;205:210–7.
76. Steiner TJ, Stovner LJ, Vos T, Jensen R, Katsarava Z. Migraine is first cause of disability in under 50s: will health politicians now take notice? J Headache Pain. 2018;19(1):17. https://doi.org/10.1186/s10194-018-0846-2.
77. Stovner LJ, Nichols E, Steiner TJ, et al. Global, regional, and national burden of migraine and tension-type headache, 1990–2016: a systematic analysis for the Global Burden of Disease Study 2016. Lancet Neurol. 2018;17:954–76.
78. Marx P, Antal P, Bolgar B, Bagdy G, Deakin B, Juhasz G. Comorbidities in the diseasome are more apparent than real: what Bayesian filtering reveals about the comorbidities of depression. PLoS Comput Biol. 2017;13(6):e1005487.
79. Barloese MC. Neurobiology and sleep disorders in cluster headache. J Headache Pain. 2015;16:562. https://doi.org/10.1186/s10194-015-0562-0.
80. Seo JG, Park SP. Validation of the patient health Questionnaire-9 (PHQ-9) and PHQ-2 in patients with migraine. J Headache Pain. 2015;16:65. https://doi.org/10.1186/s10194-015-0552-2.
81. Seo JG, Park SP. Validation of the generalized anxiety Disorder-7 (GAD-7) and GAD-2 in patients with migraine. J Headache Pain. 2015;16:97. https://doi.org/10.1186/s10194-015-0583-8.
82. Warttig SL, Forshaw MJ, South J, et al. New, normative, English-sample data for the short form perceived stress scale (PSS-4). J Health Psychol. 2013;18:1617–28. https://doi.org/10.1177/1359105313508346.
83. Lee EH, Chung BY, Suh CH, et al. Korean versions of the perceived stress scale (PSS-14, 10 and 4): psychometric evaluation in patients with chronic disease. Scand J Caring Sci. 2015;29:183–92. https://doi.org/10.1111/scs.12131.
84. Steiner TJ, Stovner LJ, Katsarava Z, Lainez JM, Lampl C, Lantéri-Minet M, et al. The impact of headache in Europe: principal results of the Eurolight project. J Headache Pain. 2014;15(1):31.
85. Stovner LJ, Andrée C. Impact of headache in Europe: a review for the Eurolight project. J Headache Pain. 2008;9(3):139.
86. Lampl C, Thomas H, Stovner LJ, et al. Interictal burden attributable to episodic headache: findings from the Eurolight project. J Headache Pain. 2016;17:9.
87. Taga A, Russo M, Manzoni GC, Torelli P. Cluster headache with accompanying migraine-like features: a possible clinical phenotype. Headache. 2017;57:290–7.
88. Manzoni GC, et al. Cluster headache—clinical findings in 180 patients. Cephalalgia. 1983;3:21–30.

89. Bacchelli E, et al. A genome-wide analysis in cluster headache points to neprilysin and PACAP receptor gene variants. J Headache Pain. 2016;17:114.

90. Sprenger T, et al. Altered metabolism in frontal brain circuits in cluster headache. Cephalalgia. 2007;27:1033–42.

91. Chou K-H, et al. Altered white matter microstructural connectivity in cluster headaches: a longitudinal diffusion tensor imaging study. Cephalalgia. 2014;34:1040–52.

92. Qiu E, Tian L, Wang Y, Ma L, Yu S. Abnormal coactivation of the hypothalamus and salience network in patients with cluster headache. Neurology. 2015;84:1402–8.

93. Barloese M, et al. Sleep and chronobiology in cluster headache. Cephalalgia. 2015;35:969–78.

94. Louter MA, et al. Cluster headache and depression. Neurology. 2016;87:1899–906.

95. Liang J-F, et al. Cluster headache is associated with an increased risk of depression: a nation-wide population-based cohort study. Cephalalgia. 2013;33:182–9.

96. Bahra A, May A, Goadsby PJ. Cluster headache: a prospective clinical study with diagnostic implications. Neurology. 2002;58:354–61.

97. Chervin RD, et al. Sleep disordered breathing in patients with cluster headache. Neurology. 2000;54:2302–6.

98. Barloese MCJ, Jennum PJ, Lund NT, Jensen RH. Sleep in cluster headache—beyond a temporal rapid eye movement relationship? Eur J Neurol. 2015;22:656–e640.

99. Monstad I, et al. Preemptive oral treatment with sumatriptan during a cluster period. Headache. 1995;35:607–13.

100. Zebenholzer K, Wober C, Vigl M, Wessely P. Eletriptan for the short-term prophylaxis of cluster headache. Headache. 2004;44:361–4.

101. Mulder LJ, Spierings EL. Naratriptan in the preventive treatment of cluster headache. Cephalalgia. 2002;22:815–7.

102. Leone M, D'Amico D, Moschiano F, Fraschini F, Bussone G. Melatonin versus placebo in the prophylaxis of cluster headache: a double-blind pilot study with parallel groups. Cephalalgia. 1996;16:494–6.

103. Pringsheim T, Magnoux E, Dobson CF, Hamel E, Aube M. Melatonin as adjunctive therapy in the prophylaxis of cluster headache: a pilot study. Headache. 2002;42:787–92.

104. Kowacs PA, et al. Warfarin as a therapeutic option in the control of chronic cluster headache: a report of three cases. J Headache Pain. 2005;6:417–9.

105. Hakim SM. Warfarin for refractory chronic cluster headache: a randomized pilot study. Headache. 2011;51:713–25.

106. Jürgens TP, et al. Long-term effectiveness of sphenopalatine ganglion stimulation for cluster headache. Cephalalgia. 2017;37:423–34. Together with Ref. 78, these studies show the effectiveness of modulating the parasympathetic SPG in patients with cluster headache, which has spurred interest in this structure as part of the pathophysiology of cluster headache.

107. Silberstein SD, et al. Non-invasive vagus nerve stimulation for the acute treatment of cluster headache: findings from the randomized, double-blind, sham-controlled ACT1 study. Headache. 2016;56:1317–32.

108. Torkamani M, et al. The neuropsychology of cluster headache: cognition, mood, disability, and quality of life of patients with chronic and episodic cluster headache. Headache. 2015;55:287–300.

109. D'Amico D, et al. Health-related quality of life in patients with cluster headache during active periods. Cephalalgia. 2002;22:818–21.

110. Saunders K, Merikangas K, Low NCP, Von Korff M, Kessler RC. Impact of comorbidity on headache-related disability. Neurology. 2008;70:538–47.

111. Jürgens TP, et al. Impairment in episodic and chronic cluster headache. Cephalalgia. 2011;31:671–82.

112. Donnet A, et al. Chronic cluster headache: a French clinical descriptive study. J Neurol Neurosurg Psychiatry. 2007;78:1354–8.

113. Romero-Reyes M, Pardi V, Akerman S. A potent and selective calcitonin gene-related peptide (CGRP) receptor antagonist, MK-8825, inhibits responses to nociceptive trigeminal activation: role of CGRP in orofacial pain. Exp Neurol. 2015;271:95–103.
114. Crowley BM, et al. Novel oxazolidinone calcitonin gene-related peptide (CGRP) receptor antagonists for the acute treatment of migraine. Bioorg Med Chem Lett. 2015;25:4777–81.
115. Bigal ME, et al. Safety, tolerability, and efficacy of TEV-48125 for preventive treatment of high-frequency episodic migraine: a multicentre, randomised, double-blind, placebo-controlled, phase 2b study. Lancet Neurol. 2015;14:1081–90.
116. Sun H, et al. Safety and efficacy of AMG 334 for prevention of episodic migraine: a randomised, double-blind, placebo-controlled, phase 2 trial. Lancet Neurol. 2016;15:382–90.
117. Zidverc-Trajkovic J, Markovic K, Radojicic A, Podgorac A, Sternic N. Cluster headache: is age of onset important for clinical presentation? Cephalalgia. 2014;34:664–70.
118. Russell MB. Epidemiology and genetics of cluster headache. Lancet Neurol. 2004;3(5):279–83. https://doi.org/10.1016/S1474-4422(04)00735-5.
119. Rozen TD. Cluster headache clinical phenotypes: tobacco nonexposed (never smoker and no parental secondary smoke exposure as a child) versus tobacco-exposed: results from the United States Cluster headache survey. Headache. 2018;58(5):688–99.
120. Barloese M, Jennum P, Lund N, et al. Reduced CSF hypocretin-1 levels are associated with cluster headache. Cephalalgia. 2015;35(10):869–76.
121. May A, Bahra A, Buchel C, et al. Hypothalamic activation in cluster headache attacks. Lancet. 1998;352(9124):275–8. https://doi.org/10.1016/S0140-6736(98)02470-2.
122. May A, Ashburner J, Buchel C, et al. Correlation between structural and functional changes in brain in an idiopathic headache syndrome. Nat Med. 1999;5:836–8.
123. Morelli N, Pesaresi I, Cafforio G, et al. Functional magnetic resonance imaging in episodic cluster headache. J Headache Pain. 2009;10:11–4.
124. Schurks M, Kurth T, de Jesus J, et al. Cluster headache: clinical presentation, lifestyle features, and medical treatment. Headache. 2006;46:1246–54.
125. Irimia P, Cittadini E, Paemeleire K, et al. Unilateral photophobia or phonophobia in migraine compared with trigeminal autonomic cephalalgias. Cephalalgia. 2008;28:626–30.
126. Nesbitt AD, Goadsby PJ. Cluster headache. BMJ. 2012;344:e2407.
127. Wilbrink LA, Ferrari MD, Kruit MC, et al. Neuroimaging in trigeminal autonomic cephalgias: when, how, and of what? Curr Opin Neurol. 2009;22:247–53.
128. Ljubisavljevic S, Prazic A, Lazarevic M, et al. The rare painful phenomena—chronic paroxysmal hemicrania-tic syndrome as a clinically isolated syndrome of the central nervous system. Pain Physician. 2017;20(2):315–22.
129. Voiticovschi-Iosob C, et al. Diagnostic and therapeutic errors in cluster headache: a hospital-based study. J Headache Pain. 2014;15:56.
130. Robbins MS. The psychiatric comorbidities of cluster headache. Curr Pain Headache Rep. 2013;17:313.
131. Chervin RD, Zellek N, Lin X, et al. Sleep disordered breathing in patients with cluster headache. Neurology. 2000;54:2302–6.
132. Barloese M, Jennum P, Knudsen S, et al. Cluster headache and sleep, is there a connection? A review. Cephalalgia. 2012;32(6):481–91.
133. Matharu M, et al. Cluster headache. Clin Evid. 2010;02:1212.
134. Cittadini E, May A, Straube A, et al. Effectiveness of intranasal zolmitriptan in acute cluster headache. A randomized, placebo-controlled, double-blind crossover study. Arch Neurol. 2006;63:1537–42.
135. Loomba V, Upadhyay A, Kaveeshvar H. Radiofrequency ablation of the sphenopalatine ganglion using cone beam computed tomography for intractable cluster headache. Pain Physician. 2016;19(7):E1093–6.
136. Naegel S, Holle D, Desmarattes N, et al. Cortical plasticity in episodic and chronic cluster headache. Neuroimage Clin. 2014;6:415–23. https://doi.org/10.1016/j.nicl.2014.10.003.

137. Seifert CL, Magon S, Staehle K, et al. A case-control study on cortical thickness in episodic cluster headache. Headache. 2012;52(9):1362–8. https://doi.org/10.1111/j.1526-4610.2012.02217.x.

138. Teepker M, Menzler K, Belke M, et al. Diffusion tensor imaging in episodic cluster headache. Headache. 2012;52(2):274–82. https://doi.org/10.1111/j.1526-4610.2011.02000.x.

139. Sprenger T, Ruether KV, Boecker H, et al. Altered metabolism in frontal brain circuits in cluster headache. Cephalalgia. 2007;27(9):1033–42. https://doi.org/10.1111/j.1468-2982.2007.01386.x.

140. Tekeli H, Altundag A, Salihoglu M, et al. The applicability of the "Sniffin' Sticks" olfactory test in a Turkish population. Med Sci Monit. 2013;19:1221–6. https://doi.org/10.12659/MSM.889838.

141. Boger HD, Bode-Boger SM. The clinical pharmacology of l-arginine. Annu Rev Pharmacol Toxicol. 2001;41:79–99.

142. Danielson TJ, Boulton AA, Robertson HS. m-Octopamine, p-octopamine and phenylethylamine in mammalian brain: a sensitive specific assay and effects of drugs. J Neurochem. 1977;29:1131–11.

143. May A, Bahra A, Buchel C, Frackowiak RS, Goadsby PJ. PET and MRA findings in in cluster headache and MRA in experimental pain. Neurology. 2000;55:1328–35.

144. Piacentino M, D'Andrea G, Perini F, Volpin L. Drug-resistant cluster headache: long-term evaluation of pain control by posterior hypothalamic deep-brain stimulation. World Neurosurg. 2014;81(2):442.

145. D'Andrea G, Bussone G, Di Fiore P, Perini F, Gucciardi A, et al. Pathogenesis of chronic cluster headache and bouts: role of tryptamine, arginine metabolism and α1 agonists. Neurol Sci. 2018;38(Suppl 1):S37–43.

146. Reddy DS, Estes WA. Clinical potential of neurosteroids for CNS disorders. Trends Pharmacol Sci. 2016;37:543–61.

147. Hosie AM, Wilkins ME, Smart TG. Neurosteroid binding sites on GABAA receptors. Pharmacol Ther. 2007;116:7–19.

148. Friess E, Schiffelholz T, Steckler T, Steiger A. Dehydroepiandrosterone-a neurosteroid. Eur J Clin Investig. 2000;30(Suppl):46–50.

149. Aguila ME, Rebbeck T, Leaver AM, Lagopoulos J, Brennan PC, Hübscher M, et al. The association between clinical characteristics of migraine and brain GABA levels: an exploratory study. J Pain. 2016;17:1058–67.

150. Lionetto L, De Andrés F, Capi M, Curto M, Sabato D, Simmaco M, et al. LC-MS/MS simultaneous analysis of allopregnanolone, epiallopregnanolone, pregnanolone, dehydroepiandrosterone and dehydroepiandrosterone 3-sulfate in human plasma. Bioanalysis. 2017;9:527–39.

151. Negro A, Martelletti P. Chronic migraine plus medication overuse headache: two entities or not? J Headache Pain. 2011;12:593–601.

152. Naylor JC, Kilts JD, Strauss JL, Szabo ST, Dunn CE, Wagner HR, et al. An exploratory pilot investigation of neurosteroids and self-reported pain in female Iraq/Afghanistan-era veterans. J Rehabil Res Dev. 2016;53:499–510.

153. Wang MD, Bäckström T, Landgren S. The inhibitory effects of allopregnanolone and pregnanolone on the population spike, evoked in the rat hippocampal CA1 stratum pyramidale in vitro, can be blocked selectively by epiallopregnanolone. Acta Physiol Scand. 2000;169:333–41.

154. Rocca MA, Valsasina P, Absinta M, Colombo B, Barcella V, Falini A, Comi G, Filippi M. Central nervous system dysregulation extends beyond the pain-matrix network in cluster headache. Cephalalgia. 2010;30(11):1383–91.

155. Thompson MD, Xhaard H, Sakurai T, Rainero I, Kukkonen JP. OX(1) and OX(2) orexin/hypocretin receptor pharmacogenetics. Front Neurosci. 2014;8:57. https://doi.org/10.3389/fnins.2014.00057.

156. Rainero I, et al. Association between the G1246A polymorphism of the hypocretin receptor 2 gene and cluster headache: a meta-analysis. J Headache Pain. 2007;8(3):152–6.

157. Ashkenazi A, Schwedt T. Cluster headache—acute and prophylactic therapy. Headache. 2011;51:272–86. https://doi.org/10.1111/j.1526-4610.2010.01830.x.
158. Fischera M, Marziniak M, Gralow I, Evers S. The incidence and prevalence of cluster headache: a meta-analysis of population-based studies. Cephalalgia. 2008;28(6):614–8. https://doi.org/10.1111/j.1468-2982.2008.01592.x.
159. Goadsby PJ. Pathophysiology of cluster headache: a trigeminal autonomic cephalgia. Lancet Neurol. 2002;1(4):251–7. https://doi.org/10.1016/S1474-4422(02)00104-7.
160. May A. Cluster headache: pathogenesis, diagnosis, and management. Lancet. 2005;366:843–55. https://doi.org/10.1016/S0140-6736(05)67217-0.
161. Leone M, Proietti Cecchini A. Advances in the understanding of cluster headache. Expert Rev Neurother. 2017;17:165–72. https://doi.org/10.1080/14737175.2016.1216796.
162. Goadsby PJ, Edvinsson L. Human in vivo evidence for trigeminovascular activation in cluster headache. Neuropeptide changes and effects of acute attacks therapies. Brain. 1994;117:427–34.
163. Rainero I, De Martino P, Pinessi L. Hypocretins and primary headaches: neurobiology and clinical implications. Expert Rev Neurother. 2008b;8:409–16. https://doi.org/10.1586/14737175.8.3.409.
164. Thompson MD, Sakurai T, Rainero I, Maj MCKJ. Orexin receptor multimerization versus functional interactions: neuropharmacological implications for opioid and cannabinoid signalling and pharmacogenetics. Pharmaceuticals. 2017;10:79. https://doi.org/10.3390/ph10040079.
165. Rainero I, Gallone S, Valfre W, et al. A polymorphism of the hypocretin receptor 2 gene is associated with cluster headache. Neurology. 2004;63:1286–8. https://doi.org/10.1212/01.WNL.0000142424.65251.DB.
166. Baumber L, et al. A genome-wide scan and *HCRTR2* candidate gene analysis in a European cluster headache cohort. Neurology. 2006;66(12):1888–93.
167. Schurks M, et al. Cluster headache is associated with the G1246A polymorphism in the hypocretin receptor 2 gene. Neurology. 2006;66(12):1917–9.
168. Weller CM, et al. Cluster headache and the hypocretin receptor 2 reconsidered: a genetic association study and meta-analysis. Cephalalgia. 2015;35(9):741–7.
169. Fourier C, Ran C, Steinberg A, Sjöstrand C, Waldenlind E, Belin AC. Analysis of HCRTR2 gene variants and cluster headache in Sweden. Headache. 2019;59:410–7. https://doi.org/10.1111/head.13462.
170. Klenke S, Kussmann M, Siffert W. The GNB3 C825T polymorphism as a pharmacogenetic marker in the treatment of hypertension, obesity, and depression. Pharmacogenet Genomics. 2011;21(9):594–606. https://doi.org/10.1097/FPC.0b013e3283491153.
171. Banaś A, Płońska E, Larysz B, et al. Influence of 825 C>T polymorphism of G protein β3 subunit gene (GNB3) on hemodynamic response during dobutamine stress echocardiography. Pharmacol Rep. 2012;64:123–8. https://doi.org/10.1016/S1734-1140(12)70738-7.
172. Edenberg HJ. The genetics of alcohol metabolism: role of alcohol dehydrogenase and aldehyde dehydrogenase variants. Alcohol Res Health. 2007;30:5–13.
173. Cederbaum AI. Alcohol metabolism. Clin Liver Dis. 2012;16:667–85. https://doi.org/10.1016/j.cld.2012.08.002.
174. Rainero I, et al. Cluster headache is associated with the alcohol dehydrogenase 4 (ADH4) gene. Headache. 2010;50(1):92–8.
175. Luo X, Kranzler HR, Zuo L, Lappalainen J, Yang BZ, Gelernter J. ADH4 gene variation is associated with alcohol dependence and drug dependence in European Americans: results from HWD tests and case–control association studies. Neuropsychopharmacology. 2006;31:1085–95. https://doi.org/10.1038/sj.npp.1300925.
176. Katsarou M-S, Karakonstantis K, Demertzis N, Vourakis E, Skarpathioti A, Nosyrev AE, Tsatsakis A, Kalogridis T, Drakoulis N. Effect of single-nucleotide polymorphisms in ADH1B, ADH4, ADH1C, OPRM1, DRD2, BDNF, and ALDH2 genes on alcohol depen-

dence in a Caucasian population. Pharmacol Res Perspect. 2017;5(4):e00326. https://doi.org/10.1002/prp2.326.

177. Zarrilli F, et al. Molecular analysis of cluster headache. Clin J Pain. 2015;31(1):52–7.

178. Fourier C, Ran C, Steinberg A, Sjöstrand C, Waldenlind E, Carmine Belin A. Screening of two ADH4 variations in a Swedish cluster headache case-control material. Headache. 2016;56:835–40. https://doi.org/10.1111/head.12807.

179. Fan Z, Hou L, Wan D, Ao R, Zhao D, Yu S. Genetic association of HCRTR2, ADH4 and CLOCK genes with cluster headache: a Chinese population-based case-control study. J Headache Pain. 2018;19:1. https://doi.org/10.1186/s10194-017-0831-1.

180. Katsarou M-S, Papasavva M, Latsi R, Toliza I, Gkaros AP, Papakonstantinou S, Gatzonis S, Mitsikostas DD, Kovatsi L, Izotov BN, Tsatsakis AM, Drakoulis N. Population-based analysis of cluster headache-associated genetic polymorphisms. J Mol Neurosci. 2018;65:367–76. https://doi.org/10.1007/s12031-018-1103-5.

181. Rodriguez S, Gaunt TR, Day INM. Hardy-Weinberg equilibrium testing of biological ascertainment for Mendelian randomization studies. Am J Epidemiol. 2009;169:505–14. https://doi.org/10.1093/aje/kwn359.

182. Rainero I, Rivoiro C, Gallone S, Valfre W, Ferrero M, Angilella G, Rubino E, De Martino P, Savi L, Lo Giudice R, Pinessi L. Lack of association between the 3092 T-->C clock gene polymorphism and cluster headache. Cephalalgia. 2005;25:1078–81.

183. Cevoli S, et al. Investigation of the T3111C CLOCK gene polymorphism in cluster headache. J Neurol. 2008;255(2):299–300.

184. Fourier C, Ran C, Zinnegger M, Johansson AS, Sjöstrand C, Waldenlind E, Steinberg A, Belin AC. A genetic CLOCK variant associated with cluster headache causing increased mRNA levels. Cephalalgia. 2017; https://doi.org/10.1177/0333102417698709.

185. Buture A, Gooriah R, Nimeri R, Ahmed F. Current understanding on pain mechanism in migraine and cluster headache. Anesthesiol Pain Med. 2016;6:e35190. https://doi.org/10.5812/aapm.35190.

186. Eyles DW, Smith S, Kinobe R, et al. Distribution of the Vitamin D receptor and 1α-hydroxylase in human brain. J Chem Neuroanat. 2005;29:21–30. https://doi.org/10.1016/j.jchemneu.2004.08.006.

187. Jirikowski GF, Kauntzer UW, Dief AEE, Caldwell JD. Distribution of vitamin D binding protein expressing neurons in the rat hypothalamus. Histochem Cell Biol. 2009;131:365–70. https://doi.org/10.1007/s00418-008-0540-6.

188. Liampas I, Siokas V, Brotis A, Dardiotis E. Vitamin D serum levels in patients with migraine: a meta-analysis. Rev Neurol (Paris). 2020;176:560–70. https://doi.org/10.1016/j.neurol.2019.12.008.

189. Motaghi M, Haghjooy Javanmard S, Haghdoost F, et al. Relationship between vitamin D receptor gene polymorphisms and migraine without aura in an Iranian population. Biomed Res Int. 2013;2013:351942. https://doi.org/10.1155/2013/351942.

190. Berridge MJ. Vitamin D, reactive oxygen species and calcium signalling in ageing and disease. Philos Trans R Soc B Biol Sci. 2016;371:20150434. https://doi.org/10.1098/rstb.2015.0434.

191. Robbins MS, Starling AJ, Pringsheim TM, et al. Treatment of cluster headache: the American Headache Society evidence-based guidelines. Headache. 2016;56(7):1093–106.

192. Mulder EJ, Van Baal C, Gaist D, et al. Genetic and environmental influences on migraine: a twin study across six countries. Twin Res. 2003;6:422–31.

193. The International Headache Society (IHS). The international classification of headache disorders: 2nd edition. Cephalalgia. 2004;24(Suppl 1):9–160.

194. Ran C, Graae L, Magnusson PKE, Pedersen NL, Olson L, Belin AC. A replication study of GWAS findings in migraine identifies association in a Swedish case-control sample. BMC Med Genet. 2014;15:38.

195. Anttila V, Stefansson H, Kallela M, et al. Genome-wide association study of migraine implicates a common susceptibility variant on 8q22.1. Nat Genet. 2010;42:869–73.

196. van Oosterhout WPJ, Schoonman GG, van Zwet EW, et al. Female sex hormones in men with migraine. Neurology. 2018;91:e374–81.

197. Frederiksen HH, Lund NL, Barloese MC, Petersen AS, Jensen RH. Diagnostic delay of cluster headache: a cohort study from the Danish Cluster Headache Survey. Cephalalgia. 2020;40(1):49–56. https://doi.org/10.1177/0333102419863030.

198. Launer LJ, Terwindt GM, Ferrari MD. The prevalence and characteristics of migraine in a population-based cohort: the GEM study. Neurology. 1999;53:537–42.

199. Wilbrink LA, Weller CM, Cheung C, et al. Stepwise web-based questionnaires for diagnosing cluster headache: LUCA and QATCH. Cephalalgia. 2013;33:924–31.

200. Chou K-H, Yang F-C, Fuh J-L, Kuo C-Y, Wang Y-H, Lirng J-F, Lin Y-Y, Wang S-J, Lin C-P. Bout-associated intrinsic functional network changes in cluster headache: a longitudinal resting-state functional MRI study. Cephalalgia. 2017;37(12):1152–63.

201. Pringsheim T. Cluster headache: evidence for a disorder of circadian rhythm and hypothalamic function. Can J Neurol Sci. 2002;29(1):33–40.

202. Leone M, Bussone G. A review of hormonal findings in cluster headache. Evidence for hypothalamic involvement. Cephalalgia. 1993;13:309–17. https://doi.org/10.1046/j.1468-2982.1993.1305309.x.

203. Schulte LH, May A. The migraine generator revisited: continuous scanning of the migraine cycle over 30 days and three spontaneous attacks. Brain. 2016;139(7):1987–93.

204. Lund N, Barloese M, Petersen A, Haddock B, Jensen R. Chronobiology differs between men and women with cluster headache, clinical phenotype does not. Neurology. 2017;88(11):1069–76. https://doi.org/10.1212/WNL.0000000000003715.

205. Qiu E, Wang Y, Ma L, Tian L, Liu R, Dong Z, Xu X, Zou Z, Yu S. Abnormal brain functional connectivity of the hypothalamus in cluster headaches. PLoS One. 2013;8(2):e57896.

206. Yang F-C, Chou K-H, Fuh J-L, Lee P-L, Lirng J-F, Lin Y-Y, Lin C-P, Wang S-J. Altered hypothalamic functional connectivity in cluster headache: a longitudinal resting-state functional MRI study. J Neurol Neurosurg Psychiatry. 2015;86(4):437–45.

207. Apkarian AV, Bushnell MC, Treede R-D, Zubieta J-K. Human brain mechanisms of pain perception and regulation in health and disease. Eur J Pain. 2005;9(4):463–84.

208. Shin KJ, Lee HJ, Park KM. Alterations of individual thalamic nuclei volumes in patients with migraine. J Headache Pain. 2019;20(1):112. https://doi.org/10.1186/s10194-019-1063-3.

209. Ha SY, Park KM. Alterations of structural connectivity in episodic cluster headache: a graph theoretical analysis. J Clin Neurosci. 2019;62:60–5. https://doi.org/10.1016/j.jocn.2019.01.007.

210. Arkink EB, Schmitz N, Schoonman GG, van Vliet JA, Haan J, van Buchem MA, Ferrari MD, Kruit MC. The anterior hypothalamus in cluster headache. Cephalalgia. 2017;37(11):1039–50. https://doi.org/10.1177/0333102416660550.

211. Jenkinson M, Smith S. A global optimisation method for robust affine registration of brain images. Med Image Anal. 2001;5(2):143–56.

212. Pruim RH, Mennes M, van Rooij D, Llera A, Buitelaar JK, Beckmann CF. ICA-AROMA: a robust ICA-based strategy for removing motion artifacts from fMRI data. NeuroImage. 2015;112:267–77.

213. Cittadini E, Matharu MS, Goadsby PJ. Paroxysmal hemicrania: a prospective clinical study of 31 cases. Brain. 2008;131:1142–55. https://doi.org/10.1093/brain/awn010.

214. Leone M, Bussone G. Pathophysiology of trigeminal autonomic cephalalgias. Lancet Neurol. 2009;8:755–64. https://doi.org/10.1016/S1474-4422(09)70133-4.

215. Svensson D, Ekbom K, Pedersen N, Träff H, Waldenlind E. A note on cluster headache in a population-based twin register. Cephalalgia. 2003;23:376–80. https://doi.org/10.1046/j.1468-2982.2003.00521.x.

216. Sjöstrand C, Modin H, Masterman T, Ekbom K, Waldenlind E, Hillert J. Analysis of nitric oxide synthase genes in cluster headache. Cephalalgia. 2002;22:758–64.

217. Sjöstrand C, Giedratis V, Ekbom K, Waldenlind E, Hillert J. CACNA1A gene polymorphisms in cluster headache. Cephalalgia. 2001;21:953–8. https://doi.org/10.1046/j.1468-2982.2001.00281.x.

218. Schürks M, Kurth T, Geissler I, Tessmann G, Diener HC, Rosskopf D. The G1246A polymorphism in the hypocretin receptor 2 gene is not associated with treatment response in cluster headache. Cephalalgia. 2007;27:363–7. https://doi.org/10.1111/j.1468-2982.2007.01287.x.

219. Leone M, Franzini A, Bussone G. Stereotactic stimulation of posterior hypothalamic gray matter in a patient with intractable cluster headache. N Engl J Med. 2001;345:1428–9. https://doi.org/10.1056/NEJM200111083451915.

220. Leone M, Franzini A, Proietti Cecchini A, Bussone G. Success, failure, and putative mechanisms in hypothalamic stimulation for drug-resistant chronic cluster headache. Pain. 2013;154:89–94. https://doi.org/10.1016/j.pain.2012.09.011.

221. Nager W, Münte TF, Marco-Pallares J, Heldmann M, Dengler R, Holger Capelle H, Lütjens G, Krauss JK, Nager ÁF, Münte WT, Marco-Pallares ÁJ, Dengler WRNÁ, Münte TF, Marco-Pallares J, Heldmann M, Capelle ÁG, Lütjens ÁJK, Krauss HH. Beta-oscillations in the posterior hypothalamus are associated with spontaneous cluster headache attack. J Neurol. 2010;257:1743–4. https://doi.org/10.1007/s00415-010-5586-4.

222. Bartsch T, Pinsker MO, Rasche D, Kinfe T, Hertel F, Diener HC, Tronnier V, Mehdorn HM, Volkmann J, Deuschl G, Krauss JK. Hypothalamic deep brain stimulation for cluster headache: experience from a new multicase series. Cephalalgia. 2008;28:285–95. https://doi.org/10.1111/j.1468-2982.2007.01531.x.

223. Leone M, Franzini A, Broggi G, Mea E, Cecchini AP, Bussone G. Acute hypothalamic stimulation and ongoing cluster headache attacks. Neurology. 2006;67:1844–5. https://doi.org/10.1212/01.wnl.0000247273.93084.49.

224. Matharu MS, Cohen AS, Frackowiak RSJ, Goadsby PJ. Posterior hypothalamic activation in paroxysmal hemicrania. Ann Neurol. 2006;59:535–45. https://doi.org/10.1002/ana.20763.

225. May A, Bahra A, Büchel C, Turner R, Goadsby PJ. Functional magnetic resonance imaging in spontaneous attacks of SUNCT: short-lasting neuralgiform headache with conjunctival injection and tearing. Ann Neurol. 1999;46:791–4. https://doi.org/10.1002/1531-8249(199911)46:5<791::aid-ana18>3.0.co;2-8.

226. Matharu MS, Cohen AS, McGonigle DJ, Ward N, Frackowiak RS, Goadsby PJ. Posterior hypothalamic and brainstem activation in hemicrania continua. Headache. 2004;44:747–61. https://doi.org/10.1111/j.1526-4610.2004.04141.x.

227. Bartsch T, Levy MJ, Knight YE, Goadsby PJ. Differential modulation of nociceptive dural input to [hypocretin] orexin A and B receptor activation in the posterior hypothalamic area. Pain. 2004;109:367–78. https://doi.org/10.1016/j.pain.2004.02.005.

228. Matharu MS, Goadsby PJ. Persistence of attacks of cluster headache after trigeminal nerve root section. Brain. 2002;125:976–84. https://doi.org/10.1093/brain/awf118.

229. Guo S, et al. Cranial parasympathetic activation induces autonomic symptoms but no cluster headache attacks. Cephalalgia. 2017; https://doi.org/10.1177/0333102417738250.

230. Möller M, Haji AA, Hoffmann J, May A. Peripheral provocation of cranial autonomic symptoms is not sufficient to trigger cluster headache attacks. Cephalalgia. 2017; https://doi.org/10.1177/0333102417738248.

231. Narouze SN. Role of sphenopalatine ganglion neuroablation in the management of cluster headache. Curr Pain Headache Rep. 2010;14:160–3. https://doi.org/10.1007/s11916-010-0100-3.

232. Edvinsson L, Tajti J, Szalárdy L, Vécsei L. PACAP and its role in primary headaches. J Headache Pain. 2018;19:21. https://doi.org/10.1186/s10194-018-0852-4.

233. Nielsen T, May A, Jürgens TP. Some observations about the origin of the pain in cluster headache. In: Leone M, May A, editors. Cluster headache and other trigeminal autonomic cephalgias. Cham: Springer; 2020. p. 91–101.

234. Jarrar RG, Black DF, Dodick DW, Davis DH. Outcome of trigeminal nerve section in the treatment of chronic cluster headache. Neurology. 2003;60:1360–2. https://doi.org/10.1212/01.WNL.0000055902.23139.16.
235. Lin H, Dodick DW. Tearing without pain after trigeminal root section for cluster headache. Neurology. 2005;65:1650–1. https://doi.org/10.1212/01.wnl.0000184522.12998.11.
236. Schuster NM, Rapoport AM. New strategies for the treatment and prevention of primary headache disorders. Nat Rev Neurol. 2016;12:635–50.
237. Russell MB, Hilden J, Sorensen SA, et al. Familial occurrence of migraine without aura and migraine with aura. Neurology. 1993;43:1369–73.
238. Sutherland HG, Griffiths LR. Genetics of migraine: insights into the molecular basis of migraine disorders. Headache. 2017;57:537–69.
239. Afridi SK, Matharu MS, Lee L, et al. A PET study exploring the laterality of brainstem activation in migraine using glyceryl trinitrate. Brain. 2005;128:932–9.
240. Mainero C, Boshyan J, Hadjikhani N. Altered functional magnetic resonance imaging resting-state connectivity in periaqueductal gray networks in migraine. Ann Neurol. 2011;70:838–45.
241. Schwedt TJ, Schlaggar BL, Mar S, et al. Atypical resting-state functional connectivity of affective pain regions in chronic migraine. Headache. 2013;53:737–51.
242. Boran HE, Bolay H. Pathophysiology of migraine. Noro Psikiyatr Ars. 2013;50:S1–7.
243. Coppola G, Di Lorenzo C, Schoenen J, et al. Habituation and sensitization in primary headaches. J Headache Pain. 2013;14:65.
244. Kiraly A, Szabo N, Pardutz A, et al. Macro- and microstructural alterations of the subcortical structures in episodic cluster headache. Cephalalgia. 2018;38:662–73.
245. Farago P, Szabo N, Toth E, et al. Ipsilateral alteration of resting state activity suggests that cortical dysfunction contributes to the pathogenesis of cluster headache. Brain Topogr. 2017;30:281–9.
246. Chen W-T, Wang S-J, Fuh J-L, et al. Persistent ictal-like visual cortical excitability in chronic migraine. Pain. 2011;152:254–8.
247. Chong CD, Dumkrieger GM, Schwedt TJ. Structural co-variance patterns in migraine: a cross-sectional study exploring the role of the Hippocampus. Headache. 2017;57:1522–31.
248. Yang F-C, Chou K-H, Kuo C-Y, et al. The pathophysiology of episodic cluster headache: insights from recent neuroimaging research. Cephalalgia. 2017;38:970–83.
249. Xue T, Yuan K, Zhao L, et al. Intrinsic brain network abnormalities in migraines without aura revealed in resting-state fMRI. PLoS One. 2012;7:e52927.
250. Xue T, Yuan K, Cheng P, et al. Alterations of regional spontaneous neuronal activity and corresponding brain circuit changes during resting state in migraine without aura. NMR Biomed. 2013;26:1051–8.
251. Lassen LH, Thomsen LL, Olesen J. Histamine induces migraine via the H1-receptor. Support for the NO hypothesis of migraine. Neuroreport. 1995;6:1475–9.
252. Krabbe AA, Olesen J. Headache provocation by continuous intravenous infusion of histamine. Clinical results and receptor mechanisms. Pain. 1980;8:253–9.
253. Horton BT. Histaminic cephalgia: differential diagnosis and treatment. Proc Staff Meet Mayo Clin. 1956;31:325–33.
254. Vollesen LH, Snoer A, Beske RP, Guo S, Hoffmann J, Jensen RHAM. Infusion of calcitonin gene-related peptide provokes cluster headache attacks. JAMA Neurol. 2018;75(10):1187–97.
255. Singhal AB, Maas MB, Goldstein JN, et al. High-flow oxygen therapy for treatment of acute migraine: a randomized crossover trial. Cephalalgia. 2017;37:730–6.
256. Jürgens TP, Schulte LH, May A. Oxygen treatment is effective in migraine with autonomic symptoms. Cephalalgia. 2013;33:65–7.
257. Leone M, Giustiniani A, Cecchini AP. Cluster headache: present and future therapy. Neurol Sci. 2017;38:45–50.

258. Tassorelli C, Grazzi L, de Tommaso M, et al. Noninvasive vagus nerve stimulation as acute therapy for migraine. Neurology. 2018; https://doi.org/10.1212/WNL.0000000000005857.
259. Lipton RB, Dodick DW, Silberstein SD, et al. Single-pulse transcranial magnetic stimulation for acute treatment of migraine with aura: a randomised, double-blind, parallel-group, sham-controlled trial. Lancet Neurol. 2010;9:373–80.
260. Cosentino G, Brighina F, Brancato S, et al. Transcranial magnetic stimulation reveals cortical hyperexcitability in episodic cluster headache. J Pain. 2015;16:53–9.
261. Edvinsson L. The Trigeminovascular pathway: role of CGRP and CGRP receptors in migraine. Headache. 2017;57:47–55.
262. Khan S, Olesen A, Ashina M. CGRP, a target for preventive therapy in migraine and cluster headache: systematic review of clinical data. Cephalalgia. 2019;39:374–89.
263. Schytz HW. Investigation of carbachol and PACAP38 in a human model of migraine. Dan Med Bull. 2010;57:B4223.
264. Patrick M. Behind Amgen's plans to penetrate the migraine segment. 2016. http://marketrealist.com/2016/05/amgen-plans-penetrate-migraine-segment-multiple-investigational-drugs/. Accessed 27 Feb 2017.
265. Bussone G. Strictly unilateral headaches: considerations of a clinician. Neurol Sci. 2014;35(1):71–5. https://doi.org/10.1186/1750-1172-3-20.
266. Bahra A, Goadsby PJ. Diagnostic delays and mis-management in cluster headache. Acta Neurol Scand. 2004;109(3):175–9. https://doi.org/10.1046/j.1600-0404.2003.00237.x.
267. Van Alboom E, et al. Diagnostic and therapeutic trajectory of cluster headache patients in Flanders. Acta Neurol Belg. 2009;109(1):10–7.
268. Van Vliet JA, et al. Features involved in the diagnostic delay of cluster headache. J Neurol Neurosurg Psychiatry. 2003;74(8):1123–5.
269. Bangash TH. Trigeminal neuralgia: frequency of occurrence in different nerve branches. Anesth Pain Med. 2011;1(2):70–2. https://doi.org/10.5812/kowsar.22287523.2164.
270. Ji Lee M, Cho SJ, Wook Park J, et al. Increased suicidality in patients with cluster headache. Cephalalgia. 2019;2019:333102419845660.
271. Olesen J. The International Classification of Headache Disorders, 2nd edition: application to practice. Funct Neurol. 2005;20:61–8.
272. Fischera M, Marziniak M, Gralow I. The incidence and prevalence of cluster headache: a meta-analysis of population-based studies. Cephalalgia. 2008;28:614–8.
273. Baharav A, Shinar Z, Akselrod S, Mosek A, Davrath LR. Cluster headache patients have normal circadian and sleep time autonomic nervous system function. IEEE. 2005;2005:263–6.
274. Barloese M, Lund N, Petersen A, Rasmussen M, Jennum P, Jensen R. Sleep and chronobiology in cluster headache. Cephalalgia. 2015;35(11):969–78.
275. Holland PR, Goadsby PJ. Cluster headache, hypothalamus, and orexin. Curr Pain Headache Rep. 2009;13(2):147–54.
276. Barloese M, Jennum P, Knudsen S, Jensen R. Cluster headache and sleep, is there a connection? A review. Thousand Oaks: SAGE Publications; 2012.
277. Dexter JD, Weitzman ED. The relationship of nocturnal headaches to sleep stage patterns. Neurology. 1970;20(5):513–8.
278. Kudrow L, McGinty D, Phillips ER, Stevenson M. Sleep apnea in cluster headache. Cephalalgia. 1984;4:33–8. https://doi.org/10.1046/j.1468-2982.1984.0401033.x.
279. Zaremba S, Holle D, Wessendorf TE, Diener HC, Katsarava Z, Obermann M. Cluster headache shows no association with rapid eye movement sleep. Cephalalgia. 2012;32(4):289–96.
280. de Tommaso M, Delussi M. Circadian rhythms of migraine attacks in episodic and chronic patients: a cross sectional study in a headache center population. BMC Neurol. 2018;18:94–103.
281. Lund NLT, Snoer AH, Jensen RH. The influence of lifestyle and gender on cluster headache. Curr Opin Neurol. 2019;32(3):443–8.

282. Rozen T, Fischman R. Female cluster headache in the United States of America? What are the gender differences? Results from the United States Cluster Headache Survey. J Neurol Sci. 2012;317:17–28.

283. Taga A, Manzoni GC, Russo M, Paglia MV, Torelli P. Childhood-onset cluster headache: observations from a personal case-series and review of the literature. Headache. 2018;58(3):443–54.

284. Lund N, Barloese M, Petersen A, Haddock B, Jensen R. Chronobiology differs between men and women with cluster headache, clinical phenotype does not. Neurology. 2016;88(11):1069–76.

285. Martins IP, Gouveia RG, Parreira E. Cluster headache without autonomic symptoms: why is it different? Headache. 2005;45:190–5. https://doi.org/10.1111/j.1526-4610.2005.05043.x.

286. Kroenke K, Spitzer R. The PHQ-9: a new depression diagnostic and severity measure. Psychiatr Ann. 2002;32:509–21. https://doi.org/10.3928/0048-5713-20020901-06.

287. Spitzer RL, Kroenke K, Williams JB, Löwe B. A brief measure for assessing generalized anxiety disorder: the GAD-7. Arch Intern Med. 2006;166:1092–7. https://doi.org/10.1001/archinte.166.10.1092.

288. Gil-Martínez A, Navarro-Fernández G, Mangas-Guijarro MÁ, Díaz-de-Terán J. Hyperalgesia and central sensitization signs in patients with cluster headache: a cross-sectional study. Pain Med. 2019;20(12):2562–70.

289. Ashkenazi A. Allodynia in cluster headache. Curr Pain Headache Rep. 2010;14(2):140–4.

290. Holroyd KA, Drew JB, Cottrell CK, Romanek KM, Heh V. Impaired functioning and quality of life in severe migraine: the role of catastrophizing and associated symptoms. Cephalalgia. 2007;27(10):1156–65.

291. Pedler A. The pain catastrophising scale. J Physiother. 2010;56(3):137.

292. Szende A, Janssen B, Cabasés J, editors. Self-reported population health: an international perspective based on EQ-5D. Berlin: Springer; 2014.

293. Kim BS, Park JW, Sohn JH, Lee MJ, Kim BK, Chu MK, et al. Associated factors and clinical implication of cutaneous allodynia in patients with cluster headache: a prospective multicentre study. Sci Rep. 2019;9(1):1–8.

294. Sullivan MJL, Thorn B, Haythornthwaite JA, Keefe F, Martin M, Bradley LA, Lefebvre JC. Theoretical perspectives on the relation between catastrophizing and pain. Clin J Pain. 2001;17(1):52–64.

295. Snoer A, Lund N, Beske R, Hagedorn A, Jensen RH, Barloese M. Cluster headache beyond the pain phase: a prospective study of 500 attacks. Neurology. 2018;91(9):e822–31. https://doi.org/10.1212/01.wnl.0000542491.92981.03.

296. Snoer A, Lund N, Beske R, Jensen R, Barloese M, et al. Cephalalgia. 2017; https://doi.org/10.1177/0333102417726498. This study describes frequent symptoms that may precede attacks. Identification and recognition of pre-attack symptoms will help delineate cluster headache pathophysiology and may enable earlier abortive treatment

297. Bjorner JB, Kosinski M, Ware JE Jr. Using item response theory to calibrate the Headache Impact Test (HIT) to the metric of traditional headache scales. Qual Life Res. 2003;12:981–1002.

298. Bjorner JB, Kosinski M, Ware JE Jr. Calibration of an item pool for assessing the burden of headaches: an application of item response theory to the headache impact test (HIT). Qual Life Res. 2003;12:913–33.

299. Sohn JH, et al. Clinical features of probable cluster headache: a prospective, cross-sectional multicenter study. Front Neurol. 2018;9:908. https://doi.org/10.3389/fneur.2018.00908.

300. Robbins MS, Bronheim R, Lipton RB, et al. Depression and anxiety in episodic and chronic cluster headache: a pilot study. Headache. 2012;52:600–11.

301. Horton BTMA, Craig WM. A new syndrome of vascular headache: results of treatment with histamine: preliminary report. Mayo Clin Proc. 1939;14:257.

302. Nock MK, Borges G, Bromet EJ, Cha CB, Kessler RC, Lee S. Suicide and suicidal behavior. Epidemiol Rev. 2008;30:133–54.
303. Ashkenazi A, Young WB. Dynamic mechanical (brush) allodynia in cluster headache. Headache. 2004;44:1010–2. https://doi.org/10.1111/j.1526-4610.2004.04195.x.
304. Young WB, Richardson ES, Shukla P. Brush allodynia in hospitalized headache patients. Headache. 2005;45:999–1003. https://doi.org/10.1111/j.1526-4610.2005.05180.x.
305. Ladda J, Straube A, Förderreuther S, Krause P, Eggert T. Quantitative sensory testing in cluster headache: increased sensory thresholds. Cephalalgia. 2006;26:1043–50.
306. Huber G, Lampl C. Oxygen therapy influences episodic cluster headache and related cutaneous brush and cold allodynia. Headache. 2009;49:134–6. https://doi.org/10.1111/j.1526-461 0.2008.01187.x.
307. Marmura MJ, Abbas M, Ashkenazi A. Dynamic mechanical (brush) allodynia in cluster headache: a prevalence study in a tertiary headache clinic. J Headache Pain. 2009;10:255–8. https://doi.org/10.1007/s10194-009-0124-4.
308. Riederer F, Selekler HM, Sandor PS, Wober C. Cutaneous allodynia during cluster headache attacks. Cephalalgia. 2009;29:796–8. https://doi.org/10.1111/j.1468-2982.2008.01794.x.
309. Wilbrink LA, Louter MA, Teernstra OPM, Van Zwet EW, Huygen FJPM, Haan J, et al. Allodynia in cluster headache. Pain. 2017;158(6):1113–7.
310. Bigal ME, et al. Prevalence and characteristics of allodynia in headache sufferers: a population study. Neurology. 2008;70:1525–33. https://doi.org/10.1212/01.wnl.0000310645.31020.b1.
311. Nicholson RA, Gramling SE, Ong JC, Buenevar L. Differences in anger expression between individuals with and without headache after controlling for depression and anxiety. Headache. 2003;43:651–63.
312. Materazzo F, Cathcart S, Pritchard D. Anger, depression, and coping interactions in headache activity and adjustment: a controlled study. J Psychosom Res. 2000;49:69–75.
313. Venable VL, Carlson CR, Wilson J. The role of anger and depression in recurrent headache. Headache. 2001;41:21–30.
314. Slavin-Spenny O, Lumley MA, Thakur ER, Nevedal DC, Hijazi AM. Effects of anger awareness and expression training versus relaxation training on headaches: a randomized trial. Ann Behav Med. 2012;46:181–92.
315. Fernandez E, Milburn TW. Sensory and affective predictors of overall pain and emotions associated with affective pain. Clin J Pain. 1994;10:3–9.
316. Nicholson RA, Gramling SE, Ong JC. The role of anger in predicting headache-related disability. Chicago: American Headache Society; 2003.
317. Bruehl COY, Burns JW. Anger expression and pain: an overview of findings and possible mechanisms. J Behav Med. 2006;29:593–606.
318. Luerding R, Henkel K, Gaul C, et al. Aggressiveness in different presentations of cluster headache: results from a controlled multicentric study. Cephalalgia. 2012;32:528–36.
319. Schenk LAM, Andrasik F. Behavioral and psychological aspects of cluster headache: an overview. Neurol Sci. 2019;40:3–7.
320. Montagna P, Pierangeli G, Cortelli P. The primary headaches as a reflection of genetic Darwinian adaptive behavioral responses. Headache. 2010;50:273–89.
321. Burns JW, Gerhart JI, Bruehl S, Peterson KM, Smith DA, Porter LS, Schuster E, Kinner E, Buvanendran A, Fras AM, Keefe FJ. Anger arousal and behavioral anger regulation in everyday life among patients with chronic low back pain: relationships to patient pain and function. Health Psychol. 2015;34:547–55.
322. Santos-Lasaosa S, Bellosta-Diago E, López-Bravo A, Viloria-Alebesque A, Garrido-Fernández A, Pilar Navarro-Pérez M. Cognitive performance in episodic cluster headache. Pain Med. 2018; https://doi.org/10.1093/pm/pny238.
323. Govare A, Leroux E. Licit and illicit drug use in cluster headache. Curr Pain Headache Rep. 2014;18:413. https://doi.org/10.1007/x11916-014-0413-8.

324. Choong CK, Ford JH, Nyhuis AW, Joshi SG, Robinson RL, Aurora SK, et al. Clinical characteristics and treatment patterns among patients diagnosed with cluster headache in U.S. healthcare claims data. Headache. 2017;57(9):1359–74.

325. Trejo-Gabriel-Galan JM, Aicua-Rapún I, Cubo-Delgado E, Velasco-Bernal C. Suicide in primary headaches in 48 countries: a physician-survey based study. Cephalalgia. 2018;38(4):798–803. https://doi.org/10.1177/0333102417714477.

326. Schenck LA-M, Raggi A, D'Amico D, Checchini AP, Andrasik F. Behavioral and psychological aspects, quality of life, and disability and impact of cluster headache. In: Leone M, May A, editors. Cluster headache and other trigeminal autonomic cephalalgias. Cham: Springer International Publishing AG; 2019.

327. Andrasik F. Behavioral treatment approaches to chronic headache. Neurol Sci. 2003;24:S80–5.

328. Blanchard EB, Andrasik F, Jurish SE, Teders SJ. The treatment of cluster headache with relaxation and thermal biofeedback. Biofeedback Self Regul. 1982;7:185–91.

329. Lifting The Burden in collaboration with the European Headache Federation. Aids to management of common headache disorders in primary care. J Headache Pain. 2007;8(Suppl 1):1–47.

330. Lifting The Burden. The Global Campaign against Headache. www.l-t-b.org.

331. Goadsby PJ. Trigeminal autonomic cephalalgias. Continuum (Minneap Minn). 2012;18(4):883–95.

332. Schor L. Cluster headache: investigating severity of pain, suicidality, personal burden, access to effective treatment, and demographics among a large international survey sample. Cephalalgia. 2017;37(1S):172–208.

333. May A, Leone M, Afra J, Linde M, Sándor PS, Evers S, Goadsby PJ, EFNS Task Force. EFNS guidelines on the treatment of cluster headache and other trigeminal-autonomic cephalalgias. Eur J Neurol. 2006;13(10):1066–77. https://doi.org/10.1111/j.1468-1331.2006.01566.x.

334. Cohen AS, Burns B, Goadsby PJ. High flow oxygen for treatment of cluster headache. A randomized trial. JAMA. 2009;302:2451–7.

335. Fogan L. Treatment of cluster headache. A double-blind comparison of oxygen v air inhalation. Arch Neurol. 1985;42(4):362–3.

336. Schindler EAD, Wright DA, Weil MJ, Gottschalk CH, Pittman BP, Sico JJ. Survey analysis of the use, effectiveness, and patient-reported tolerability of inhaled oxygen compared with injectable sumatriptan for the acute treatment of cluster headache. Headache. 2018;58(10):1568–78.

337. Geerlings RP, Haane DY, Koehler PJ. Rebound following oxygen therapy in cluster headache. Cephalalgia. 2011;31(10):1145–9.

338. Igarashi H, Sakai F, Kanda T, Tazaki Y, Saitoh Y. The mechanism by which oxygen interrupts cluster headache. Cephalalgia. 1991;11:238–9.

339. Petersen AS, Barloese MC, Lund NL, Jensen RH. Oxygen therapy for cluster headache. A mask comparison trial. A single-blinded, placebo-controlled, crossover study. Cephalalgia. 2017;37(3):214–24. https://doi.org/10.1177/0333102416637817.

340. The Sumatriptan Cluster Headache Study Group. Treatment of acute cluster headache with sumatriptan. N Engl J Med. 1991;325(5):322–6.

341. Ekbom K, Monstad I, Prusinski A, Cole JA, Pilgrim AJ, Noronha D. Subcutaneous sumatriptan in the acute treatment of cluster headache: a dose comparison study. The Sumatriptan Cluster Headache Study Group. Acta Neurol Scand. 1993;88(1):63–9.

342. Ekbom K, Krabbe A, Micieli G, Prusinski A, Cole JA, Pilgrim AJ, et al. [corrected to Micieli G] Cluster headache attacks treated for up to three months with subcutaneous sumatriptan (6 mg). Sumatriptan Cluster Headache Long-term Study Group. Cephalalgia. 1995;15(3):230–6.

343. National Clinical Guideline Centre. Headaches in over 12s: diagnosis and management. National Institute for Health and Clinical Excellence; 2012. http://www.nice.org.uk/guidance/cg150. Accessed 16 Apr 2020

344. Akerman S, Williamson DJ, Goadsby PJ. Voltage-dependent calcium channels are involved in neurogenic dural vasodilatation via a presynaptic transmitter release mechanism. Br J Pharmacol. 2003;140(3):558–66.

345. Bussone G, Leone M, Peccarisi C, Micieli G, Granella F, Magri M, et al. Double blind comparison of lithium and verapamil in cluster headache prophylaxis. Headache. 1990;30:411–7. https://doi.org/10.1111/j.1526-4610.1990.hed3007411.x.

346. Steiner TJ, Hering R, Couturier EG, Davies PT, Whitmarsh TE. Double-blind placebo-controlled trial of lithium in episodic cluster headache. Cephalalgia. 1997;17(6):673–5.

347. Ambrosini A, Vandenheede M, Rossi P, Aloj F, Sauli E, Pierelli F, et al. Suboccipital injection with a mixture of rapid- and long-acting steroids in cluster headache: a double-blind placebo-controlled study. Pain. 2005;118(1–2):92–6. https://doi.org/10.1016/j.pain.2005.07.015.

348. Leroux E, Valade D, Taifas I, Vicaut E, Chagnon M, Roos C, et al. Suboccipital steroid injections for transitional treatment of patients with more than two cluster headache attacks per day: a randomised, double-blind, placebo-controlled trial. Lancet Neurol. 2011;10:891–7. https://doi.org/10.1016/S1474-4422(11)70186-7. A randomised, double-blind, and placebo-controlled trial concluded that suboccipital steroid injections can relieve CH rapidly in patients having frequent daily attacks, irrespective of type (chronic or episodic).

349. Gelfand AA, Goadsby PJ. The role of melatonin in the treatment of primary headache disorders. Headache. 2016;56(8):1257–66.

350. Schuh-Hofer S, Israel H, Neeb L, Reuter U, Arnold G. The use of gabapentin in chronic cluster headache patients refractory to first-line therapy. Eur J Neurol. 2007;14:694–6. https://doi.org/10.1046/j.1526-4610.2002.02181.x.

351. Vollesen ALH, Snoer A, Beske RP, Guo S, Hoffmann J, Jensen RH, Ashina M. Effect of infusion of calcitonin gene-related peptide on cluster headache attacks: a randomized clinical trial. JAMA Neurol. 2018;75:1187–97. https://doi.org/10.1001/jamaneurol.2018.1675.

352. National Clinical Guideline Centre. gammaCore. National Institute for Health and Clinical Excellence; 2019. http://www.nice.org.uk/guidance/mtg46. Accessed 16 Apr 2020

353. Goadsby PJ, Sahai-Srivastava S, Kezirian EJ, Calhoun AH, Matthews DC, McAllister PJ, et al. Safety and efficacy of sphenopalatine ganglion stimulation for chronic cluster headache: a double-blind, randomised controlled trial. Lancet Neurol. 2019;18(12):1081–90.

354. Kandel SA, Mandiga P. Cluster headache. [Updated 2020 Jun 30]. In: StatPearls [Internet]. Treasure Island (FL): StatPearls Publishing; 2021 Jan. https://www.ncbi.nlm.nih.gov/books/NBK544241/. Great overview of CH.

355. Hoffmann J, May A. Diagnosis, pathophysiology, and management of cluster headache. Lancet Neurol. 2018;17(1):75–83. https://doi.org/10.1016/S1474-4422(17)30405-2.

356. Carmine Belin A, Ran C, Edvinsson L. Calcitonin gene-related peptide (CGRP) and cluster headache. Brain Sci. 2020;10(1):30. https://doi.org/10.3390/brainsci10010030. Great paper on CGRP and its role in CH.

357. Grangeon L, O'Connor E, Danno D, Ngoc TMP, Cheema S, Tronvik E, et al. Is pituitary MRI screening necessary in cluster headache? Cephalalgia. 2021;41:779–88. https://doi.org/10.1177/0333102420983303. New findings regarding work up for CH.

358. Matharu MS, Levy MJ, Meeran K, Goadsby PJ. Subcutaneous octreotide in cluster headache: randomized placebo-controlled double-blind crossover study. Ann Neurol. 2004;56(4):488–94. https://doi.org/10.1002/ana.20210. Erratum in: Ann Neurol. 2004 Nov;56(5):751.

359. Paemeleire K, Evers S, Goadsby PJ. Medication-overuse headache in patients with cluster headache. Curr Pain Headache Rep. 2008;12(2):122–7. https://doi.org/10.1007/s11916-008-0023-4.

360. Headache Classification Subcommittee of the International Headache Society. The International Classification of Headache Disorders: 2nd edition. Cephalalgia. 2004;24(Suppl 1):9–160.

361. Sjaastad O. Cluster headache syndrome. London: Saunders Companu Ltd.; 1992.

362. Van Vliet JA, Bahra A, Martin V, et al. Intranasal sumatriptan in cluster headache—randomized placebo-controlled double-blind study. Neurology. 2003;60:630–3.
363. Horton BT, Ryan R, Reynolds JL. Clinical observations on the use of E.C. 110, a new agent for the treatment of headache. Proc Staff Meet Mayo Clin. 1948;23:105–8.
364. Andersson PG, Jespersen LT. Dihydroergotamine nasal spray in the treatment of attacks of cluster headache. A double-blind trial versus placebo. Cephalalgia. 1986;6:51–4. https://doi.org/10.1046/j.1468-2982.1986.0601051.x.
365. Curran DA. Methysergide. Res Clin Stud Headache. 1967;1:74–122.
366. Krabbe A. Limited efficacy of methysergide in cluster headache: a clinical experience. Cephalalgia. 1989;9(Suppl 10):S404–5.
367. Leone M, Dodick D, Rigamonti A, D'Amico D, Grazzi L, Mea E, et al. Topiramate in cluster headache prophylaxis: an open trial. Cephalalgia. 2003;23:1001–2. https://doi.org/10.1046/j.1468-2982.2003.00665.x.
368. Pascual J, Láinez MJA, Dodick D, Hering-Hanit R. Antiepileptic drugs for the treatment of chronic and episodic cluster headache: a review. Headache. 2007;47:81–9. https://doi.org/10.1111/j.1526-4610.2007.00653.x.
369. Tay BA, Ngan Kee WD, Chung DC. Gabapentin for the treatment and prophylaxis of cluster headache. Reg Anesth Pain Med. 2001;26:373–5. https://doi.org/10.1053/rapm.2001.24404.
370. Nesbitt AD, Marin JC, Tompkins E, Ruttledge MH, Goadsby PJ. Initial use of a novel noninvasive vagus nerve stimulator for cluster headache treatment. Neurology. 2015;84(12):1249–53.
371. Magis D, Schoenen J. Advances and challenges in neurostimulation for headaches. Lancet Neurol. 2012;11:708–19. https://doi.org/10.1016/S1474-4422(12)70139-4.
372. Leone M, Proietti Cecchini A, Messina G, Franzini A. Long-term occipital nerve stimulation for drug-resistant chronic cluster headache. Cephalalgia. 2016; https://doi.org/10.1177/0333102416652623.
373. Jurgens TP, Barloese M, May A, et al. Long-term effectiveness of sphenopalatine ganglion stimulation for cluster headache. Cephalalgia. 2017;37(5):423–34. https://doi.org/10.1177/0333102416649092.
374. Leone M, Proietti Cecchini A. Deep brain stimulation in headache. Cephalalgia. 2016;36:1143–8. https://doi.org/10.1177/0333102415607176.
375. Lasaosa SS, Diago EB, Calzada JN, Benito AV. Cardiovascular risk factors in cluster headache. Pain Med. 2017;18(6):1161–7.
376. Couch JR, Ziegler DK. Prednisone therapy for cluster headache. Headache. 1978;18:219–21.
377. Gabai IJ, Spierings EL. Prophylactic treatment of cluster headache with verapamil. Headache. 1989;29(3):167–8.
378. Leandri M, Luzzani M, Cruccu G, Gottlieb A. Drug-resistant cluster headache responding to gabapentin: a pilot study. Cephalalgia. 2001;21:744–6.
379. Granata L, Niebergall H, Langner R, Agosti R, Sakellaris L. Ketamine i. v. for the treatment of cluster headaches: an observational study. Schmerz. 2016;30(3):286–8.
380. Moisset X, Giraud P, Meunier E, Conde S, Perie M, Picard P, et al. Ketamine-magnesium for refractory chronic cluster headache: a case series. Headache. 2020;60(10):2537–43.
381. Lampl C, Rudolph M, Brautigam E. OnabotulinumtoxinA in the treatment of refractory chronic cluster headache. J Headache Pain. 2018;19(1):45.
382. Sjöstrand C, Alexanderson K, Josefsson P, Steinberg A. Sickness absence and disability pension days in patients with cluster headache and matched references. Neurology. 2020;94(21):e2213–21.
383. Goadsby PJ, May A. PET demonstration of hypothalamic activation in cluster headache. Neurology. 1999;52(7):1522.
384. May A, Goadsby PJ. Hypothalamic involvement and activation in cluster headache. Curr Pain Headache Rep. 2001;5(1):60–6. https://doi.org/10.1007/s11916-001-0011-4.
385. Sprenger T, Boecker H, Tolle TR, Bussone G, May A, Leone M. Specific hypothalamic activation during a spontaneous cluster headache attack. Neurology. 2004;62(3):516–7.

386. Edvardsson B. Symptomatic cluster headache: a review of 63 cases. Springerplus. 2014;3(1):64.
387. Leone M, D'Amico D, Frediani F, Moschiano F, Grazzi L, Attanasio A, et al. Verapamil in the prophylaxis of episodic cluster headache: a double-blind study versus placebo. Neurology. 2000;54(6):1382–5. https://doi.org/10.1212/wnl.54.6.1382.
388. Hering R, Kuritzky A. Sodium valproate in the treatment of cluster headache: an open clinical trial. Cephalalgia. 1989;9:195–8. https://doi.org/10.1046/j.1468-2982.1989.0903195.x.
389. Anthony M. Arrest of attacks of cluster headache by local steroid injection of the occipital nerve. In: Clifford Rose F, editor. Clinical and research advances 5th International Symposium, London, September 1984. Basel: Karger; 1985. p. 169–73.
390. O'Connor TP, van der Kooy D. Enrichment of a vasoactive neuropeptide (calcitonin gene related peptide) in the trigeminal sensory projection to the intracranial arteries. J Neurosci. 1988;8:2468–76.
391. Li J, Vause CV, Durham PL. Calcitonin gene-related peptide stimulation of nitric oxide synthesis and release from trigeminal ganglion glial cells. Brain Res. 2008; https://doi.org/10.1016/j.brainres.2007.12.028.
392. Csati A, Tajti J, Tuka B, Edvinsson L, Warfvinge K. Calcitonin gene-related peptide and its receptor components in the human sphenopalatine ganglion - interaction with the sensory system. Brain Res. 2012;1435:29–39. https://doi.org/10.1016/j.brainres.2011.11.058.
393. Walker CS, Eftekhari S, Bower RL, Wilderman A, Insel PA, Edvinsson L, Waldvogel HJ, Jamaluddin MA, Russo AF, Hay DL. A second trigeminal CGRP receptor: function and expression of the AMY1 receptor. Ann Clin Transl Neurol. 2015;2:595–608. https://doi.org/10.1002/acn3.197.
394. Fanciullacci M, Alessandri M, Figini M, Geppetti P, Michelacci S. Increase in plasma calcitonin gene-related peptide from the extracerebral circulation during nitroglycerin-induced cluster headache attack. Pain. 1995;60(2):119–23.
395. Fanciullacci M, Alessandri M, Sicuteri R, Marabini S. Responsiveness of the trigeminovascular system to nitroglycerine in cluster headache patients. Brain. 1997;120(Pt 2):283–8.
396. Messlinger K. The big CGRP flood - sources, sinks and signalling sites in the trigeminovascular system. J Headache Pain. 2018;19(22):22. https://doi.org/10.1186/s10194-018-0848-0.
397. Feindel W, Penfield W, McNaughton F. The tentorial nerves and localization of intracranial pain in man. Neurology. 1960;10:555–63.
398. Johnston MM, Jordan SE, Charles AC. Pain referral patterns of the C1 to C3 nerves: implications for headache disorders. Ann Neurol. 2013;74:145–8.
399. Horton BT. Histaminic cephalgia. J Lancet. 1952;72:92–8.
400. Neeb L, Anders L, Euskirchen P, Hoffmann J, Israel H, Reuter U. Corticosteroids alter CGRP and melatonin release in cluster headache episodes. Cephalalgia. 2015;35(4):317–26. https://doi.org/10.1177/0333102414539057.
401. Jónsdóttir M, Meyer JS, Rogers RL. Efficacy, side effects and tolerance compared during headache treatment with three different calcium blockers. Headache. 1987;27:364–9.
402. Lipton RB, et al. Efficacy and safety of fremanezumab for the prevention of episodic cluster headache: results of a randomized, double-blind, placebo-controlled, phase 3 study. Cephalalgia. 2019;39:358–9.
403. Silberstein SD, Mechtler LL, Kudrow DB, Calhoun AH, McClure C, Saper JR, et al. Non-invasive vagus nerve stimulation for the acute treatment of cluster headache: findings from the randomized, double-blind, sham-controlled ACT1 study. Headache. 2016;56(8):1317–32.
404. Goadsby PJ, de Coo IF, Silver N, Tyagi A, Ahmed F, Gaul C, et al. Non-invasive vagus nerve stimulation for the acute treatment of episodic and chronic cluster headache: a randomized, double-blind, sham-controlled ACT2 study. Cephalalgia. 2018; https://doi.org/10.1177/0333102417744362.
405. de Coo IF, Marin JC, Silberstein SD, Friedman DI, Gaul C, McClure CK, et al. Differential efficacy of non-invasive vagus nerve stimulation for the acute treatment of

episodic and chronic cluster headache: a meta-analysis. Cephalalgia. 2019; https://doi.org/10.1177/0333102419856607.

406. Schytz HW, et al. Experimental activation of the sphenopalatine ganglion provokes cluster-like attacks in humans. Cephalalgia. 2013;33:831–41.

407. Franzini A, Ferroli P, Leone M, Broggi G. Stimulation of the posterior hypothalamus for treatment of chronic intractable cluster headaches: first reported series. Neurosurgery. 2003;52:1095–1099, discussion 1099–1101.

408. Burns B, Watkins L, Goadsby PJ. Treatment of medically intractable cluster headache by occipital nerve stimulation: long-term follow-up of eight patients. Lancet. 2007;369:1099–106.

409. Fontaine D, et al. Treatment of refractory chronic cluster headache by chronic occipital nerve stimulation. Cephalalgia. 2011;31:1101–5.

410. Magis D, Gerard P, Schoenen J. Invasive occipital nerve stimulation for refractory chronic cluster headache: what evolution at long-term? Strengths and weaknesses of the method. J Headache Pain. 2016;17:8.

411. Fontaine D, Blond S, Lucas C, Regis J, Donnet A, Derrey S, et al. Occipital nerve stimulation improves the quality of life in medically-intractable chronic cluster headache: results of an observational prospective study. Cephalalgia. 2017;37(12):1173–9.

412. Wei DY, Goadsby PJ. Comprehensive clinical phenotyping of nitroglycerin infusion induced cluster headache attacks. Cephalalgia. 2021; https://doi.org/10.1177/0333102421989617.

413. Kudrow L. Response of cluster headache attacks to oxygen inhalation. Headache. 1981;21(1):1–4.

414. Goadsby PJ, Bartsch T. On the functional neuroanatomy of neck pain. Cephalalgia. 2008;28(Suppl 1):1–7. https://doi.org/10.1111/j.1468-2982.2008.01606.x.

415. Chua NH, Vissers KC, Wilder-Smith OH. Quantitative sensory testing may predict response to sphenopalatine ganglion pulsed radiofrequency treatment in cluster headaches: a case series. Pain Pract. 2011;11(5):439–45.

416. Van Bets B, Raets I, Gypen E, Mestrum R, Heylen R, Van Zundert J. Pulsed radiofrequency treatment of the pterygopalatine (sphenopalatine) ganglion in cluster headache: a 10 year retrospective analysis. Eur J Anaesthesiol. 2014;31:233. https://doi.org/10.1097/00003643-201406001-00672.

417. Bendersky DC, Hem SM, Yampolsky CG. Unsuccessful pulsed radiofrequency of the sphenopalatine ganglion in patients with chronic cluster headache and subsequent successful thermocoagulation. Pain Pract. 2015;15(5):E40–5. https://doi.org/10.1111/papr.12288.

418. Fang L, Jingjing L, Ying S, Lan M, Tao W, Nan J. Computerized tomography-guided sphenopalatine ganglion pulsed radiofrequency treatment in 16 patients with refractory cluster headaches: twelve- to 30-month follow-up evaluations. Cephalalgia. 2016;36(2):106–12. https://doi.org/10.1177/0333102415580113.

419. Mathew NT, Hurt W. Percutaneous radiofrequency trigeminal gangliorhizolysis in intractable cluster headache. Headache. 1988;28(5):328–31.

420. Bordini EC, Bordini CA, Woldeamanuel YW, Rapoport AM. Indomethacin responsive headaches: exhaustive systematic review with pooled analysis and critical appraisal of 81 published clinical studies. Headache. 2016;56:422–35. https://doi.org/10.1111/head.12771.

421. Prakash S, Shah ND, Chavda BV. Cluster headache responsive to indomethacin: case reports and a critical review of the literature. Cephalalgia. 2010;30:975–82. https://doi.org/10.1177/0333102409357642.

422. Buzzi M, Formisano R. A patient with cluster headache responsive to indomethacin: any relationship with chronic paroxysmal hemicrania? Cephalalgia. 2003;23:401–4. https://doi.org/10.1046/j.1468-2982.2003.00558.x.

423. Geaney DP. Indomethacin-responsive episodic cluster headache. J Neurol Neurosurg Psychiatry. 1983;46:860–1. https://doi.org/10.1136/jnnp.46.9.860.

424. Klimek A. Indomethacin-responsive episodic cluster headache. J Neurol Neurosurg Psychiatry. 1984;47:1058–9. https://doi.org/10.1136/jnnp.47.9.1058-a.

425. Prakash S, Dholakia S, Shah K. A patient with chronic cluster headache responsive to high-dose indomethacin: is there an overlap with chronic paroxysmal hemicrania? Cephalalgia. 2008;28:778–81. https://doi.org/10.1111/j.1468-2982.2008.01581.x.

426. Lisotto C, Mainardi F, Maggioni F, Zanchin G. O004. Refractory chronic cluster headache responding absolutely to indomethacin. J Headache Pain. 2015;16(Suppl 1):A96.

427. May A, Schwedt TJ, Magis D, Pozo-Rosich P, Evers S, Wang S-J. Cluster headache. Nat Rev Dis Primers. 2018;4(1):1–17.

428. D'Amico D, Centonze V, Grazzi L, Leone M, Ricchetti G, Bussone G. Coexistence of migraine and cluster headache: report of 10 cases and possible pathogenetic implications. Headache. 1997;37(1):21–5.

429. Dodick DW, Goadsby PJ, Lucas C, Jensen R, Bardos JN, Martinez JM, Zhou C, Aurora SK, Yang JY, Conley RR, Oakes T. Phase 3 randomized, placebo-controlled study of galcanezumab in patients with chronic cluster headache: results from 3-month double-blind treatment. Cephalalgia. 2020;40(9):935–48. https://doi.org/10.1177/0333102420905321.

430. Lipton RB. How useful is the HIT-6 for measuring headache-related disability? Nat Clin Pract Neurol. 2006;2:70–1. https://doi.org/10.1038/ncpneuro0122.

431. Sohn JH, Park JW, Lee MJ, Chung PW, Chu MK, Chung JM, Ahn JY, Kim BS, Kim SK, Choi YJ, Kim D, Song TJ, Oh K, Moon HS, Park KY, Kim BK, Bae DW, Chung CS, Cho SJ. Clinical factors influencing the impact of cluster headache from a prospective multicenter study. Sci Rep. 2020;10:2428.

432. Silvestro M, Tessitore A, Scotto di Clemente F, Tedeschi G, Russo A. Erenumab efficacy on comorbid cluster headache in patients with migraine: a real-world case series. Headache. 2020;60:1187–95.

433. Ruscheweyh R, Broessner G, Gossrau G, Heinze-Kuhn K, Jurgens TP, Kaltseis K, Kamm K, Peikert A, Raffaelli B, Rimmele F, Evers S. Effect of calcitonin gene-related peptide (-receptor) antibodies in chronic cluster headache: results from a retrospective case series support individual treatment attempts. Cephalalgia. 2020;40:1574–84.

434. Goadsby PJ, Edvinsson L, Ekman R. Release of vasoactive peptides in the extracerebral circulation of humans and the cat during activation of the trigeminovascular system. Ann Neurol. 1988;23:193–6. https://doi.org/10.1002/ana.410230214.

435. Goadsby PJ, Edvinsson L, Ekman R. Vasoactive peptide release in the extracerebral circulation of humans during migraine headache. Ann Neurol. 1990;28:183–7.

436. Edvinsson L, et al. Perivascular peptides relax cerebral arteries concomitant with stimulation of cyclic adenosine monophosphate accumulation or release of an endothelium-derived relaxing factor in the cat. Neurosci Lett. 1985;58(2):213–7.

437. Edvinsson L, Haanes KA, Warfvinge K, Krause DN. CGRP as the target of new migraine therapies—successful translation from bench to clinic. Nat Rev Neurol. 2018;14:338–50.

438. Oakes TMM, et al. Safety of galcanezumab in patients with episodic migraine: a randomized placebo-controlled dose-ranging phase 2b study. Cephalalgia. 2018;38(6):1015–25.

439. Stauffer VL, et al. Evaluation of Galcanezumab for the prevention of episodic migraine: the EVOLVE-1 randomized clinical trial. JAMA Neurol. 2018;75(9):1080–8.

440. Skljarevski V, et al. Efficacy and safety of galcanezumab for the prevention of episodic migraine: results of the EVOLVE-2 phase 3 randomized controlled clinical trial. Cephalalgia. 2018;38(8):1442–54.

441. Detke HC, et al. Galcanezumab in chronic migraine: the randomized, double-blind, placebo-controlled REGAIN study. Neurology. 2018;91(24):e2211–21.

442. Goadsby PJ, Dodick DW, Leone M, Bardos JN, Oakes TM, Millen BA, Zhou C, Dowsett SA, Aurora SK, Ahn AH, Yang J-YY, Conley RR, Martinez JM. Trial of galcanezumab in prevention of episodic cluster headache. N Engl J Med. 2019;381:132–41. https://doi.org/10.1056/NEJMoa1813440.

443. Dodick DW, et al. Safety and efficacy of LY2951742, a monoclonal antibody to calcitonin gene-related peptide, for the prevention of migraine: a phase 2, randomised, double-blind, placebo-controlled study. Lancet Neurol. 2014;13(9):885–92.

444. Camporeale A, et al. A phase 3, long-term, open-label safety study of Galcanezumab in patients with migraine. BMC Neurol. 2018;18(1):188.
445. Zhu Y, et al. The efficacy and safety of calcitonin gene-related peptide monoclonal antibody for episodic migraine: a meta-analysis. Neurol Sci. 2018;39(12):2097–106.
446. Xu D, et al. Safety and tolerability of calcitonin-gene-related peptide binding monoclonal antibodies for the prevention of episodic migraine - a meta-analysis of randomized controlled trials. Cephalalgia. 2019;39(9):1164–79.
447. Peres MF, Stiles MA, Siow HC, Rozen TD, Young WB, Silberstein SD. Greater occipital nerve blockade for cluster headache. Cephalalgia. 2002;22(7):520–2.
448. Gaul C, Diener H-C, Silver N, Magis D, Reuter U, Andersson A, et al. Non-invasive vagus nerve stimulation for PREVention and Acute treatment of chronic cluster headache (PREVA): a randomised controlled study. Cephalalgia. 2016;36:534–46. https://doi.org/10.1177/0333102415607070. A prospective, multicenter, open-label, and randomized study concluded that adjunctive prophylactic nVNS is a well-tolerated novel treatment for chronic CH, offering clinical benefits beyond standard of care.
449. Trescot AM, Abipp F. Peripheral nerve entrapments: clinical diagnosis and management. Berlin: Springer; 2016.
450. Manchikanti L, Falco FJE, Singh V, et al. An Update of comprehensive evidence-based guidelines for interventional techniques in chronic spinal pain. Part I: Introduction and general considerations. Pain Physician. 2013;16:S1–48.
451. Manchikanti L, Abdi S, Atluri S, et al. An update of comprehensive evidence-based guidelines for interventional techniques in chronic spinal pain. Part II: Guidance and recommendations. Pain Physician. 2013;16:S49–283.
452. Manchikanti L. Evidence-based medicine, systematic reviews, and guidelines in interventional pain management, Part I: Introduction and general considerations. Pain Physician. 2008;11:161–86.
453. Manchikanti L, Hirsch JA, Smith HS. Evidence-based medicine, systematic reviews, and guidelines in interventional pain management: Part 2: Randomized controlled trials. Pain Physician. 2008;11:717–73.
454. Manchikanti L, Benyamin RM, Helm S, et al. Evidence-based medicine, systematic reviews, and guidelines in interventional pain management: Part 3: Systematic reviews and meta-analyses of randomized trials. Pain Physician. 2009;12:35–72.
455. Manchikanti L, Singh V, Smith HS, et al. Evidence-based medicine, systematic reviews, and guidelines in interventional pain management: Part 4: Observational studies. Pain Physician. 2009;12:73–108.
456. Manchikanti L, Derby R, Wolfer LR, et al. Evidence-based medicine, systematic reviews, and guidelines in interventional pain management: Part 5. Diagnostic accuracy studies. Pain Physician. 2009;12:517–40.
457. Manchikanti L, Datta S, Smith HS, et al. Evidence-based medicine, systematic reviews, and guidelines in interventional pain management: Part 6. Systematic reviews and meta-analyses of observational studies. Pain Physician. 2009;12:819–50.
458. Manchikanti L, Derby R, Wolfer L, et al. Evidence-based medicine, systematic reviews, and guidelines in interventional pain management: Part 7: Systematic reviews and meta-analyses of diagnostic accuracy studies. Pain Physician. 2009;12:929–63.
459. Liberati A, Altman DG, Tetzlaff J, et al. The PRISMA statement for reporting systematic reviews and meta-analyses of studies that evaluate health care interventions: explanation and elaboration. Ann Intern Med. 2009;151:W1–30.
460. van Tulder M, Furlan A, Bombardier C, et al. Updated method guidelines for systematic reviews in the Cochrane collaboration back review group. Spine. 2003;28:1290–9.
461. Furlan AD, Pennick V, Bombardier C, et al. Updated method guidelines for systematic reviews in the Cochrane Back Review Group. Spine (Phila Pa 1976). 2009;34:1929–41.

462. Manchikanti L, Singh V, Helm S, et al. An introduction to an evidence-based approach to interventional techniques in the management of chronic spinal pain. Pain Physician. 2009;12:E1–33.

463. Guyatt GH, Oxman AD, Vist GE, et al. GRADE: an emerging consensus on rating quality of evidence and strength of recommendations. BMJ. 2008;336:924–6.

464. Morton S, Berg A, Levit L, et al. Finding what works in health care: standards for systematic reviews: committee on standards for systematic reviews of comparative effectiveness research. Institute of Medicine, National Academies Press; 2011.

465. Agency for Healthcare Research and Quality. Methods guide for effectiveness and comparative effectiveness reviews. Rockville: Agency for Healthcare Research and Quality; 2017.

466. García-Bermejo P, De-la-Cruz-Torres B, Romero-Morales C. Ultrasound-guided percutaneous neuromodulation in patients with unilateral anterior knee pain: a randomized clinical trial. Appl Sci. 2020;10:4647.

467. Gokyildiz S, Beji NK, Yalcin O, et al. Effects of percutaneous tibial nerve stimulation therapy on chronic pelvic pain. Gynecol Obstet Investig. 2012;73:99–105.

468. Kabay S, Kabay SC, Yucel M, et al. Efficiency of posterior tibial nerve stimulation in category IIIB chronic prostatitis/chronic pelvic pain: a Sham-Controlled Comparative Study. Urol Int. 2009;83:33–8.

469. Oswald J, Shahi V, Chakravarthy KV. Prospective case series on the use of peripheral nerve stimulation for focal mononeuropathy treatment. Pain Manag. 2019;9:551–8.

470. Campbell JN, Long DM. Peripheral nerve stimulation in the treatment of intractable pain. J Neurosurg. 1976;45:692–9.

471. Strege DW, Cooney WP, Wood MB, et al. Chronic peripheral nerve pain treated with direct electrical nerve stimulation. J Hand Surg. 1994;19:931–9.

472. Mobbs RJ, Nair S, Blum P. Peripheral nerve stimulation for the treatment of chronic pain. J Clin Neurosci. 2007;14:216–21.

473. Picaza JA, Hunter SE, Cannon BW. Pain suppression by peripheral nerve stimulation. Appl Neurophysiol. 1977;40:223–34.

474. Law JD, Swett J, Kirsch WM. Retrospective analysis of 22 patients with chronic pain treated by peripheral nerve stimulation. J Neurosurg. 1980;52:482–5.

475. Van Balken MR, Vandoninck V, Messelink BJ, et al. Percutaneous tibial nerve stimulation as neuromodulative treatment of chronic pelvic pain. Eur Urol. 2003;43:158–63.

476. Warner NS, Schaefer KK, Eldrige JS, et al. Peripheral nerve stimulation and clinical outcomes: a retrospective case series. Pain Pract. 2021;21:411–8.

477. Wilson R, Gunzler D, Bennett M, et al. Peripheral nerve stimulation compared with usual care for pain relief of hemiplegic shoulder pain: a randomized controlled trial (Erratum vol 95, pg E29, 2016). Am J Phys Med Rehabil. 2014;93:17–28.

478. Eisenberg E, Waisbrod H, Gerbershagen HU. Long-term peripheral nerve stimulation for painful nerve injuries. Clin J Pain. 2004;20:143–5.

479. Chmiela MA, Hendrickson M, Hale J, et al. Direct peripheral nerve stimulation for the treatment of complex regional pain syndrome: a 30–year review. Neuromodulation. 2020; https://doi.org/10.1111/ner.13295.

480. Finch P, Price L, Drummond P. High-frequency (10 kHz) electrical stimulation of peripheral nerves for treating chronic pain: a double-blind trial of presence vs absence of stimulation. Neuromodulation. 2019;22:529–36.

481. Eldabe S, Buchser E, Duarte RV. Complications of spinal cord stimulation and peripheral nerve stimulation techniques: a review of the literature. Pain Med. 2016;17:325–36.

482. Wall PD, Sweet WH. Temporary abolition of pain in man. Science. 1967;155:108–9.

483. Harris RP, Helfand M, Woolf SH, et al. Current methods of the US preventive services task force: a review of the process. Am J Prev Med. 2001;20:21–35.

484. Reverberi C, Dario A, Barolat G, et al. Using peripheral nerve stimulation (PNS) to treat neuropathic pain: a clinical series. Neuromodulation. 2014;17:777–83.

485. Ertsey C, et al. Health-related and condition-specific quality of life in episodic cluster headache. Cephalalgia. 2004;24(3):188–96.
486. Kosinski M, et al. A six-item short-form survey for measuring headache impact: the HIT-6™. Qual Life Res. 2003;12(8):963–74.
487. Liang MH. Longitudinal construct validity: establishment of clinical meaning in patient evaluative instruments. Med Care. 2000;38(9 Suppl):II84–90.
488. Cohen J. Statistical power analysis for the behavioral sciences. Academic press; 2013.
489. Lambru G, Abu Bakar N, Stahlhut L, McCulloch S, Miller S, Shanahan P, et al. Greater occipital nerve blocks in chronic cluster headache: a prospective open-label study. Eur J Neurol. 2014;21:338–43. https://doi.org/10.1111/ene.12321.
490. Morelli N, et al. Brainstem activation in cluster headache: an adaptive behavioural response? Cephalalgia. 2013;33(6):416–20.
491. Qiu E, et al. Abnormal brain functional connectivity of the hypothalamus in cluster headaches. PLoS One. 2013;8(2):e57896.
492. Magis D, et al. Central modulation in cluster headache patients treated with occipital nerve stimulation: an FDG-PET study. BMC Neurol. 2011;11(1):25.
493. Ziv M, et al. Individual sensitivity to pain expectancy is related to differential activation of the hippocampus and amygdala. Hum Brain Mapp. 2010;31(2):326–38.
494. Qiu E, et al. Abnormal coactivation of the hypothalamus and salience network in patients with cluster headache. Neurology. 2015;84(14):1402.
495. Matharu MS, Goadsby PJ. Trigeminal autonomic Cephalalgias: diagnosis and management. In: Silberstein SD, Lipton R, Dodick D, editors. Wolff's headache other head pain. 8th ed. New York: Oxford University Press; 2008.
496. Lanteri-Minet M, Silhol F, Piano V, Donnet A. Cardiac safety in cluster headache patients using the very high dose of verapamil (>/=720 mg/day). J Headache Pain. 2011;12(2):173–6.
497. Schoenen J, Jensen RH, Lanteri-Minet M, Lainez MJ, Gaul C, Goodman AM, et al. Stimulation of the sphenopalatine ganglion (SPG) for cluster headache treatment. Pathway CH-1: a randomized, sham-controlled study. Cephalalgia. 2013;33(10):816–30.
498. Barloese MC, Jürgens TP, May A, Lainez JM, Schoenen J, Gaul C, Goodman AM, Caparso A, Jensen RH. Cluster headache attack remission with sphenopalatine ganglion stimulation: experiences in chronic cluster headache patients through 24 months. J Headache Pain. 2016;17(1):67. https://doi.org/10.1186/s10194-016-0658-1.
499. Eller M, Goadsby P. Trigeminal autonomic cephalalgias. Oral Dis. 2016;22(1):1–8.
500. Franzini A, Moosa S, D'Ammando A, Bono B, Scheitler-Ring K, Ferroli P, Messina G, Prada F, Franzini A. The neurosurgical treatment of craniofacial pain syndromes: current surgical indications and techniques. Neurol Sci. 2019;40:159–68. https://doi.org/10.1007/s10072-019-03789-4.
501. Donnet A, Carron R, Regis J. Predilection to deafferentation pain syndrome after radiosurgery in cluster headache. Cephalalgia. 2012;32:635–40. https://doi.org/10.1177/0333102412445219.
502. Donnet A, Tamura M, Valade D, Regis J. Trigeminal nerve radiosurgical treatment in intractable chronic cluster headache: unexpected high toxicity. Neurosurgery. 2006;59:1252–1257; discussion 1257. https://doi.org/10.1227/01.NEU.0000245612.86484.7.
503. Goadsby PJ, Lipton RB. A review of paroxysmal hemicranias, SUNCT syndrome and other short-lasting headaches with autonomic feature, including new cases. Brain J Neurol. 1997;120(1):193–209.
504. Cohen AS. Short-lasting unilateral neuralgiform headache attacks with conjunctival injection and tearing. Cephalalgia. 2007;27(7):824–32. https://doi.org/10.1111/j.1468-2982.2007.01352.x.
505. Williams MH, Broadley SA. SUNCT and SUNA: clinical features and medical treatment. J Clin Neurosci. 2008;15(5):526–34. https://doi.org/10.1016/j.jocn.2006.09.006.
506. D'Andrea G, Granella F, Ghiotto N, Nappi G. Lamotrigine in the treatment of SUNCT syndrome. Neurology. 2001;57(9):1723–5.

507. Cação G, Correia FD, Pereira-Monteiro J. SUNCT syndrome: a cohort of 15 Portuguese patients. Cephalalgia. 2016;36(10):1002–6.
508. Etemadifar M, Maghzi A, Ghasemi M, Chitsaz A, Esfahani MK. Efficacy of gabapentin in the treatment of SUNCT syndrome. Cephalalgia. 2008;28(12):1339–42.
509. Weng H-Y, Cohen AS, Schankin C, Goadsby PJ. Phenotypic and treatment outcome data on SUNCT and SUNA, including a randomised placebo-controlled trial. Cephalalgia. 2017;38(9):1554–63. https://doi.org/10.1177/0333102417739304. A clinical description of 102 SUNCT and SUNA patients with both phenotypical descriptions and summary of attempted treatments.
510. Benoliel R, Sharav Y. Paroxysmal hemicrania: case studies and review of the literature. Oral Surg Oral Med Oral Pathol Oral Radiol Endod. 1998;85(3):285–92.
511. Blankenburg M, Hechler T, Dubbel G, Wamsler C, Zernikow B. Paroxysmal hemicrania in children—symptoms, diagnostic criteria, therapy and outcome. Cephalalgia. 2009;29(8):873–82.
512. Antonaci F, Pareja JA, Caminero AB, Sjaastad O. Chronic paroxysmal hemicrania and hemicrania continua: lack of efficacy of sumatriptan. Headache. 1998;38(3):197–200.
513. Zidverc-Trajkovic J, Pavlovic A, Mijajlovic M, Jovanovic Z, Sternic N, Kostic V. Cluster headache and paroxysmal hemicrania: differential diagnosis. Cephalalgia. 2005;25(4):244–8.
514. Prakash S, Belani P, Susvirkar A, Trivedi A, Ahuja S, Patel A. Paroxysmal hemicrania: a retrospective study of a consecutive series of 22 patients and a critical analysis of the diagnostic criteria. J Headache Pain. 2013;14(1):26.
515. Pareja JA, Caminero AB, Franco E, Casado JL, Pascual J, Sanchez D, del Rio M. Efficacy and tolerability of long-term indomethacin treatment of chronic paroxysmal hemicrania and hemicrania continua. Cephalalgia. 2001;21(9):906–10. https://doi.org/10.1046/j.1468-2982.2001.00287.x.
516. Boes CJ, Dodick DW. Refining the clinical spectrum of chronic paroxysmal hemicrania: a review of 74 patients. Headache. 2002;42(8):699–708. https://doi.org/10.1046/j.1526-4610.2002.02171.x.
517. Evers S, Husstedt IW. Alternatives in drug treatment of chronic paroxysmal hemicrania. Headache. 1996;36(7):429–32. https://doi.org/10.1046/j.1526-4610.1996.3607429.x.
518. Tso AR, Marin J, Goadsby PJ. Noninvasive vagus nerve stimulation for treatment of indomethacin-sensitive headaches. JAMA Neurol. 2017;74(10):1266–7. https://doi.org/10.1001/jamaneurol.2017.2122. The first larger study describing treatment of PH and CH with non-invasive vagus nerve stimulation.
519. Kamourieh S, Lagrata S, Matharu MS. Non-invasive vagus nerve stimulation is beneficial in chronic paroxysmal hemicrania. J Neurol Neurosurg Psychiatry. 2019;90(9):1072–4. https://doi.org/10.1136/jnnp-2018-319538. A recent larger study describing treatment of PH with non-invasive vagus nerve stimulation.
520. Antonaci F, Pareja JA, Caminero AB, Sjaastad O. Chronic paroxysmal hemicrania and hemicrania continua. Parenteral indomethacin: the 'indotest'. Headache. 1998;38(2):122–8. https://doi.org/10.1046/j.1526-4610.1998.3802122.x.
521. Antonaci F, Pareja JA, Caminero AB, Sjaastad O. Chronic paroxysmal hemicrania and hemicrania continua: anaesthetic blockades of pericranial nerves. Funct Neurol. 1997;12(1):11–5.
522. Hryvenko I, Cervantes-Chavarría AR, Law AS, Nixdorf DR. Hemicrania continua: case series presenting in an orofacial pain clinic. Cephalalgia. 2018;38(13):1950–9.
523. Spears RC. Is gabapentin an effective treatment choice for hemicrania continua? J Headache Pain. 2009;10(4):271–5.
524. Cittadini E, Goadsby PJ. Hemicrania continua: a clinical study of 39 patients with diagnostic implications. Brain. 2010;133:1973–86. https://doi.org/10.1093/brain/awq137.
525. Pareja JA, Sjaastad O. Chronic paroxysmal hemicrania and hemicrania continua. Interval between indomethacin administration and response. Headache. 1996;36(1):20–3.
526. Guerrero AL, Herrero-Velázquez S, Penas ML, Mulero P, Pedraza MI, Cortijo E, et al. Peripheral nerve blocks: a therapeutic alternative for hemicrania continua. Cephalalgia. 2012;32(6):505–8.

527. Peres MF, Silberstein SD. Hemicrania continua responds to cyclooxygenase-2 inhibitors. Headache. 2002;42(6):530–1. https://doi.org/10.1046/j.1526-4610.2002.02131.x.
528. Akerman S, Holland PR, Summ O, Lasalandra MP, Goadsby PJ. A translational in vivo model of trigeminal autonomic cephalalgias: therapeutic characterization. Brain. 2012;135(12):3664–75.
529. Hoskin KL, Zagami AS, Goadsby PJ. Stimulation of the middle meningeal artery leads to Fos expression in the trigeminocervical nucleus: a comparative study of monkey and cat. J Anat. 1999;194(4):579–88.
530. Summ O, Andreou AP, Akerman S, Goadsby PJ. A potential nitrergic mechanism of action for indomethacin, but not of other COX inhibitors: relevance to indomethacin-sensitive headaches. J Headache Pain. 2010;11(6):477–83. https://doi.org/10.1007/s10194-010-0263-7.
531. Goadsby PJ, Uddman R, Edvinsson L. Cerebral vasodilatation in the cat involves nitric oxide from parasympathetic nerves. Brain Res. 1996;707(1):110–8.
532. Miller S, Watkins L, Matharu M. Long-term follow up of intractable chronic short lasting unilateral neuralgiform headache disorders treated with occipital nerve stimulation. Cephalalgia. 2017;38(5):933–42. https://doi.org/10.1177/0333102417721716. A study of 31 SUNHA patients treated with ONS.
533. Fuad F, Jones NS. Paroxysmal hemicrania and cluster headache: two discrete entities or is there an overlap? Clin Otolaryngol Allied Sci. 2002;27(6):472–9. https://doi.org/10.1046/j.1365-2273.2002.00615.x.
534. Miller S, Lagrata S, Matharu M. Multiple cranial nerve blocks for the transitional treatment of chronic headaches. Cephalalgia. 2019;39(12):1488–99.
535. Porta-Etessam J, Cuadrado M, Rodríguez-Gómez O, García-Ptacek S, Valencia C. Are cox-2 drugs the second line option in indomethacin responsive headaches? J Headache Pain. 2010;11(5):405–7.
536. Prakash S, Rana K. Topiramate as an indomethacin-sparing agent in hemicrania continua: a report of 2 cases. Headache. 2019;59(3):444–5. https://doi.org/10.1111/head.13490.
537. Paul Weyker M, Christopher Webb M, Leena MM. Radiofrequency ablation of the supra-orbital nerve in the treatment algorithm of hemicrania continua. Pain Physician. 2012;15:E719–E24.
538. Olesen J. Headache Classification Committee of the International Headache Society (IHS). The International Classification of Headache Disorders, Abtracts. Cephalalgia. 2018;38:1–211.
539. Cittadini E, Goadsby PJ. Update on hemicrania continua. Curr Pain Headache Rep. 2011;15:51–6.
540. Headache Classification Subcommittee of the International Headache Society. The International Classification of Headache Disorders, 2nd ed. Cephalalgia. 2004;24:1–154.
541. Costa A, Antonaci F, Ramusino M, Nappi G. The neuropharmacology of cluster headache and other trigeminal autonomic cephalalgias. Curr Neuropharmacol. 2015;13:304–23. https://doi.org/10.2174/1570159X13666150309233556.
542. Viana M, Tassorelli C, Allena M, Nappi G, Sjaastad O, Antonaci F. Diagnostic and therapeutic errors in trigeminal autonomic cephalalgias and hemicrania continua: a systematic review. J Headache Pain. 2013;14:14.
543. Lipscomb GR, Wallis N, Armstrong G, Rees WDW. Gastrointestinal tolerability of meloxicam and piroxicam: a double-blind placebo-controlled study. Br J Clin Pharmacol. 1998;46:133–7.
544. Prakash S, Shah ND, Soni RK. Secondary hemicrania continua: case reports and a literature review. J Neurol Sci. 2009;280(1–2):29–34. https://doi.org/10.1016/j.jns.2009.01.011. Excellent article explaining Secondary HC, its causes and management.
545. Jurgen TP, Schulte LH, May A. Indomethacin-induced de novo headache in hemicrania continua-fighting fire with fire? Cephalalgia. 2013;33:1203–5.
546. Rozen TD. How effective is melatonin as a preventive treatment for hemicrania continua? A clinic-based study. Headache. 2015;55:430–6.

547. Peres MFP. Hemicrania continua: recent treatment strategies and diagnostic evaluation. Curr Neurol Neurosci Rep. 2002;2:108–13.
548. Silberstein SD, Peres MF. Hemicrania continua. Arch Neurol. 2002;59:1029–30.
549. Prakash S, Patel P. Hemicrania continua: clinical review, diagnosis and management. J Pain Res. 2017;10:1493–509. https://doi.org/10.2147/jpr.s128472. An excellent review of HC providing the reader with an in-depth understanding of the clinical, diagnostic and management of HC.
550. Prakash S, Adroja B. Hemicrania Continua. Ann Indian Acad Neurol. 2018;21(Suppl 1):S23–30.
551. Vikelis M, Xifaras M, Magoufis G, Gekas G, Mitsikostas DD. Headache attributed to unruptured saccular aneurysm, mimicking hemicrania continua. J Headache Pain. 2005;6:156–8.
552. Tepper SJ. CGRP and headache: a brief review. Neurol Sci. 2019;40(Suppl 1):99–105.
553. Giani L, Proietti C, Leone M. Anti-CGRP in cluster headache therapy. Neurol Sci. 2019;40(Suppl 1):129–35.
554. Pozo-Rosich P, Coppola G, Pascual J, Schwedt TJ. How does the brain change in chronic migraine? Developing disease biomarkers. Cephalalgia. 2021;41:613–30.
555. Benoliel R, Sharav Y, Haviv Y, Almoznino G. Tic, triggering, and tearing: from CTN to SUNHA. Headache. 2017;57(6):997–1009. https://doi.org/10.1111/head.13040.
556. Meyers SL. Cluster headache and trigeminal autonomic cephalalgias. Dis Mon. 2015;61(6):236–9. https://doi.org/10.1016/j.disamonth.2015.03.007.
557. Wober C. Tics in TACs: a step into an avalanche? Systematic literature review and conclusions. Headache. 2017;57(10):1635–47. https://doi.org/10.1111/head.13099.
558. Lambru G, Matharu MS. SUNCT, SUNA and trigeminal neuralgia: different disorders or variants of the same disorder? Curr Opin Neurol. 2014;27(3):325–31. https://doi.org/10.1097/wco.0000000000000090.
559. Miller S, Akram H, Lagrata S, Hariz M, Zrinzo L, Matharu M. Ventral tegmental area deep brain stimulation in refractory short-lasting unilateral neuralgiform headache attacks. Brain. 2016;139(Pt 10):2631–40. https://doi.org/10.1093/brain/aww204.
560. Matharu MS, Zrinzo L. Deep brain stimulation in cluster headache: hypothalamus or midbrain Tegmentum? Curr Pain Headache Rep. 2010;14(2):151–9.
561. Martins IP, Viana P, Lobo PP. Familial SUNCT in mother and son. Cephalalgia. 2016;36:993–7. https://doi.org/10.1177/0333102415616879.
562. Zhang Y, Zhang H, Lain YJ, Ma YQ, Xie NC, Chen X, Zhang L. Botulinum toxin a for the treatment of a child with SUNCT syndrome. Pain Res Manag. 2016; https://doi.org/10.1155/2016/8016065.
563. Zabalza RJ. Sustained response to botulinum toxin in SUNCT syndrome. Cephalalgia. 2012;32:869–72.
564. Baraldi C, Pellesi L, Guerzoni S, Cainazzo MM, Pini LA. Therapeutical approaches to paroxysmal hemicrania, hemicrania continua and short lasting unilateral neuralgiform headache attacks: a critical appraisal. J Headache Pain. 2017;18(1):71. https://doi.org/10.1186/s10194-017-0777-3. Recent comprehensive review of the treatment of TACs.
565. Favoni V, Grimaldi D, Pierangeli G, Cortelli P, Cevoli S. SUNCT/SUNA and neurovascular compression: new cases and critical literature review. Cephalalgia. 2013;33(16):1337–48. https://doi.org/10.1177/0333102413494273.
566. Kitahara I, Fukuda A, Imamura Y, Ikawa M, Yokochi T. Pathogenesis, surgical treatment, and cure for SUNCT syndrome. World Neurosurg. 2015;84(4):1080–3. https://doi.org/10.1016/j.wneu.2015.05.024.
567. Kang JK, Ryu JW, Choi JH, Merrill RL, Kim ST. Application of ICHD-II criteria for headaches in a TMJ and orofacial pain clinic. Cephalalgia. 2010;30:37–41.
568. Hryvenko I, Cervantes-Chavarria AR, Law AS, Nixdorf DR. Hemicrania continua: case series presenting in an orofacial pain clinic. Cephalalgia. 2018;38:1950–9.

569. Headache Classification Committee of the International Headache Society (IHS). The International Classification of Headache Disorders, 3rd edition (beta version). Cephalalgia. 2013;33(9):629–808.
570. Afridi SK, Shields KG, Bhola R, Goadsby PJ. Greater occipital nerve injection in primary headache syndromes – prolonged effects from a single injection. Pain. 2006;122(1–2):126–9. https://doi.org/10.1016/j.pain.2006.01.016.
571. Martelletti P, Giamberardino MA, Mitsikostas DD. Greater occipital nerve as target for refractory chronic headaches: from corticosteroid block to invasive neurostimulation and back. Expert Rev Neurother. 2016;16(8):865–6.
572. Inan LE, Inan N, Karadas O, Gul HL, Erdemoglu AK, Turkel Y, et al. Greater occipital nerve blockade for the treatment of chronic migraine: a randomized, multicenter, double-blind, and placebo-controlled study. Acta Neurol Scand. 2015;132(4):270–7.
573. Gelfand AA, Reider AC, Goadsby PJ. Outcomes of greater occipital nerve injections in pediatric patients with chronic primary headache disorders. Pediatr Neurol. 2014;50(2):135–9.
574. Goadsby PJ, et al. Pathophysiology of migraine: a disorder of sensory processing. Physiol Rev. 2017;97:553–622.
575. Schulman E. Refractory migraine - a review. Headache. 2013;53(4):599–613.
576. Macedo A, Banos JE, Farre M. Placebo response in the prophylaxis of migraine: a meta-analysis. Eur J Pain. 2008;12(1):68–75.

# Chapter 3
# Other Non-migraine Primary Headache Disorders

## 3.1 Introduction

This chapter has the important function to describe the other primary headache disorders like thunderclap headache, exercise headache and sexual headache and other primary forms, but above all as forms that must alert the clinician because they can also be signs of secondary forms. The educational target is clinicians that, observing very violent and unusual forms of headache, can immediately orient themselves in the definition of primary or secondary forms, since errors in this diagnostic process could be life-threatening.

## 3.2 Machine-Generated Summaries

Machine generated keywords: airplane, travel, headache attribute, exercise, airplane headache, attribute, intracranial, airplane travel, ichd, benign, ascent, case report, adult, secondary, trigger.

### *Other Primary Headaches. Cough Headache, Nummular Headache and Primary Exercise Headache: A Secondary Point of View*

DOI: https://doi.org/10.1007/s10072-020-04689-8

**Cough Headache**
According to this statement, for a definite diagnosis, a neuroimaging study is suggested, considering that the proportion of patients affected by cough headache who

© The Author(s), under exclusive license to Springer Nature Switzerland AG 2023
P. Martelletti (ed.), *Non-Migraine Primary Headaches in Medicine*,
https://doi.org/10.1007/978-3-031-20894-2_3

have a structural brain lesion (secondary cough headache) varied between 11 and 59% in recent series.

The lifetime prevalence of primary cough headache is about 1% and most often affect people older than 40 years.

The most frequent causes of secondary cough headaches are Chiari type I malformation (caudal displacement of one cerebellar tonsil by >5 mm or both tonsils by 3–5 mm below the foramen magnum), posterior fossa lesions (i.e. arachnoid cysts or meningiomas) and acquired tonsillar descent due to low intracranial pressure (i.e. after lumboperitoneal shunt).

## Nummular Headache

The term nummular headache is referred to a rare headache characterized by a well-circumscribed oppressive pain in a small, elliptical or oval-shaped area on the head.

To stress this possibility, we describe the case of a 29-year-old female patient, with no prior history of headache, referred to our headache centre for a 2 months history of focal pain located in a circular area with the diameter of about 4 cm on the right parietal region.

This clinical history supports the peripheral origin of secondary nummular headache (pain stemming from terminal branches of sensory nerves in periosteum, the pain-sensitive structure of the diploe), considering that headache ceased soon after the symptomatic area was removed.

Trophic changes in the site of nummular headache, distinct boundaries of pain area and increased mechanical pain sensitivity restricted in the symptomatic area may all support this theory [1].

## Primary Exercise Headache

Primary exercise headache is brought on by and occurs during or immediately after strenuous physical exercise.

The episodes last from 5 min to 48 h and usually occur at the peak of the exercise.

Primary exercise headache was associated to pheochromocytoma, reversible cerebral vasoconstriction syndrome, idiopathic intracranial hypertension, cerebral venous sinus thrombosis and cervical artery dissection [2].

And particularly for a first episode, a careful neurological examination and evaluation by MRI is strongly suggested to exclude secondary pathologies.

## [Section 4]

According to the 2018 classification of International Headache Society (IHS), a group of clinically heterogeneous headache phenotypes are defined as "other primary headaches".

They are classified in a specific syndromic way, grouped and coded as primary headaches in Section 4 of the IHS classification.

Primary cough headache (4.1), primary exercise headache (4.2), primary headache associated with sexual activity (4.3), primary thunderclap headache (4.4), cold stimulus headache (4.5), external pressure headache (4.6), primary stabbing headache (4.7), nummular headache (4.8), hypnic headache (4.9) and new daily persistent headache (4.10) are recognized and classified with specific diagnostic criteria as peculiar entities.

When in daily practice a diagnosis of a new headache is challenging on clinical basis, a neuroimaging approach is warmly suggested [3].

**Acknowledgement**
*A machine generated summary based on the work of Colombo, Bruno; Filippi, Massimo. 2020 in Neurological Sciences.*

## *Exercise Headache: A Review*

DOI: https://doi.org/10.1007/s11910-018-0840-8

**Abstract-Summary**
Although secondary causes must be excluded, most cases of exercise headache are benign, idiopathic, and self-limited.

This article reviews the revised diagnostic criteria for primary exercise headache (PEH) and discusses recent research into the clinical presentation, epidemiology, pathophysiology, suggested workup, and treatment of this condition.

A secondary cause is thought to be present infrequently, but should be explored in all patients with a first or atypical presentation of exercise headache.

Red flags for potential secondary causes may include older age at onset and more prolonged headache duration.

No recent trials have been conducted, but experts suggest that avoidance of triggers coupled with short-term NSAID and/or beta-blocker treatment may be effective for patients diagnosed with PEH.

Larger studies are needed to provide high-quality evidence regarding the pathophysiology and treatment of PEH.

**Introduction**
In the most recent revision of the International Classification of Headache Disorders (ICHD) criteria, ICHD-3, this entity has been moved from the Appendix to Section 4: Other Primary Headache Disorders, indicating a shift both in the acceptance of this entity as a primary headache disorder and in the recognition that in most cases, exercise headache is not due to a sinister secondary pathology [4].

Distinguishing between exercise-induced headache and migraine may be straightforward in a patient whose headaches are exclusively triggered by exercise, which should not be the case for migraines, but it may require more careful history-taking to distinguish a migraine from an exercise headache in a patient with a history of migraines.

Exercise headaches may have migrainous features such as a pulsating quality, as will be discussed in greater detail below, but if an exercise-induced headache otherwise meets diagnostic criteria for migraine, it should be considered as a migraine.

## Clinical Presentation and Epidemiology

Methods of ascertaining prevalence of exercise headache have varied widely, with some studies using ICHD-II criteria, few utilizing the updated ICHD-III criteria, and still others having much more broad inclusion criteria such as including patients with headache induced by straining or Valsalva, which under the ICHD-3 is classified under primary cough headache (PCH) as mentioned above.

Patients who develop exercise headache when embarking upon a new exercise routine or activity often self-identify triggering activities and avoid these; thus, lifetime prevalence and point prevalence may be quite different, although many studies do not clearly draw this distinction.

An Iranian study from 2015, using ICHD-II criteria (with the subsequent inclusion of both pulsating and compressive-type headaches after the publication of the ICHD-III during the study period) in a face-to-face, questionnaire-based survey of 2076 randomly identified community-dwelling adults, found a 1-year prevalence of exercise headache of 7.3% (152 patients) [5].

## Pathophysiology

A small radiological study did not find an increased preponderance of transverse sinus and/or internal jugular vein stenosis in patients with PEH [6].

This study included 36 patients and used magnetic resonance (MR) venography in patients with ICHD-II criteria PEH (10 patients), PCH (7 patients), or primary headache associated with sexual activity (PHASA) (19 patients), with 16 controls from patients undergoing MR venography for non-headache reasons.

They found a significant increase in transverse sinus and/or internal jugular vein stenosis in the PCH (5/7 patients) and PHASA groups (12/19 patients), but not in the group with PEH (2/10 patients) or in controls (0/16 patients).

Given our recent shift in classifying many other primary headache disorders as non-vascular in origin, whether a vascular origin for PEH will be borne out by future studies remains to be seen.

## Investigations

As with any new, exertional headache, patients presenting with a first episode of exercise-induced headache should undergo a directed workup to exclude secondary causes.

Older patients (typically those over 50), patients with vascular risk factors, and those with unusual associated symptoms such as chest pain or sweating should undergo cardiac workup, including ECG, echocardiography, and consideration of referral to cardiology for more invasive testing.

The European Headache Federation guidelines from 2015 recommend that patients with a new presentation consistent with PEH (i.e., a headache precipitated by physical activity) undergo investigations including brain magnetic resonance imaging (MRI) and magnetic resonance angiography (MRA), carotid and vertebral MRA, and lumbar puncture and cardiological evaluation in specific conditions [7].

Magnetic resonance venography is recommended in the evaluation of PHASA but not included in the PEH workup suggestions; this may be included at the physician's discretion, especially in patients with overlap syndromes and headache provoked by both sexual activity and exercise.

### Treatment

PEH also seems more frequent in hot weather and at high altitude, so avoiding these potentially aggravating factors may also be prudent when feasible [5, 8, 9].

From a pharmacological perspective, small studies have suggested a role for indomethacin 25 mg tid, while other experts recommend indomethacin 25–50 mg, or other NSAIDs such as naproxen, taken as needed 30–60 min prior to exercise [10, 11].

Other medication classes of potential use in PEH include beta-blockers such as nadolol or propranolol at 1–2 mg/kg/day [12].

Pharmacological prevention of PEH with ergotamine tartrate or flunarizine has also been proposed, but further studies are needed on the topic of both acute and prophylactic treatment of PEH [13].

### Conclusions

Previous studies on PEH are limited by their methodology, including many with questionnaire-based retrospective data, the potential for recall bias, small sample sizes, and varying definitions of PEH.

PEH appears to have overlap or at the very least is comorbid with other primary headache disorders, and thus, studying it in isolation presents a major problem.

Identifying patients with PEH is fraught with difficulty as many of these patients may not present to medical attention, or the typically self-limited course of the condition may influence patient recall and reporting.

### Acknowledgement

*A machine generated summary based on the work of Sandoe, Claire H.; Kingston, William. 2018 in Current Neurology and Neuroscience Reports.*

## *Primary Exercise Headache*

DOI: https://doi.org/10.1007/s11910-020-01028-4

### Abstract-Summary

Its presentation can remain vague, often confused with other primary and secondary headache disorders and thus undertreated.

This review aims to discuss primary exercise headache in the context of epidemiology, presentation, pathophysiology, differential diagnosis, and treatment.

While large-scale epidemiological studies have aided in further characterization and determining varying prevalence, a lack of randomized clinical trials in the treatment of primary exercise headache remains.

## Introduction

One of the first studies examining this type of headache was in 1968 [14].

The prevalence of PEH varies greatly from one study to another; however, among all headaches, it is relatively rare.

In another prospective study of over 6000 patients seen over 10 years for headaches, only 1.5% were considered provoked and 11% of those were considered exertional [12].

In a 2015 epidemiology study of 2076 patients in Iran, the 1-year prevalence of PEH was seen at 7.3%, with a significant preponderance for females (10% vs 5.4% men) and a mean age of 32 years (±12 years) [5].

A 2015 Japanese study evaluated 2546 patients with headache and identified 30 patients with PEH using the current guideline classifications [15].

PEH was comorbid with migraine without aura in most patients (20 out of 30), headache with sexual activity (7 patients), or cough headaches (5 patients) [15].

## Symptomatology/Presentation and Diagnosis

Clinical descriptions of patients with PEH in the literature is minimal and largely from small case series.

These episodes can last anywhere from 5 min to 48 h and always precipitated by strenuous exercise [14–17].

The International Classification of Headache Disorders, 3rd edition defines PEH as patients having at least two headache episodes that last less than 48 h and precipitated by or during strenuous exercise and must also not be better accounted for by another ICHD-3 diagnosis [4].

## Differential Diagnosis

Wei published a case series describing cardiac cephalgia, emphasizing the importance of ruling out cardiac disease in patients with exertional headaches and risk factors [18].

Curter and others described a patient with new-onset headache, without associated chest pain or EKG changes, who underwent myocardial perfusion imaging (MPI) as part of a cardiac evaluation due to exertional nature of pain.

This patient underwent cardiac stenting after discovering cardiac ischemia; post-procedure, the patient no longer experienced an exertional type of headache [19].

Exertional headache with associated fever, shortness of breath, chest pain, or focal neurologic deficits should point to cardiac, pulmonary, neurologic, or systemic involvement.

## Pathophysiology and Etiology

Tinel describes how incompetent internal jugular valves in the context of Valsalva maneuvers can increase intrathoracic pressure and decrease cerebral venous drainage, thus playing a role in the cause of PEH [20].

Retrograde flow from incompetent venous vasculature may lead to a transient increase in blood flow, causing an increase in intracranial pressure leading to head pain [21].

Seventy percent of exertional headache patients demonstrated venous retrograde flow and thus valvular incompetence [21].

Transient spikes in blood pressure via exertion in a system without adequate autoregulation could lead to similar increases in intracranial pressure and thus pain [22].

## Management

In one early study of 15 patients with PEH, successful control of headache with continuous use of indomethacin was noted [10].

Overlap between other headache disorders can lend alternate therapeutic considerations as in the case of headache with sexual activity.

In one case series of 45 patients, 9 patients experienced both PEH and headache with sexual activity within 72 h of each other.

In terms of management, this study found benefit in a cohort of patients with sexual headache with either propranolol at 40–80 mg daily or atenolol 50 mg.

## Cases

In this patient, given his history of MVA and significant family history of heart disease, an MRA of his head and neck was obtained and primary evaluation of his cardiac function was done.

The decision made with his primary physician to start low-dose propranolol helped reduce the length and severity of his headaches.

This patient presents with headache after prolonged strenuous exercise and once even with sexual activity.

If headaches were not improved, up-titration of propranolol or the use of indomethacin as needed prior to strenuous activity could be reasonable treatment strategies.

She reports that now after every weightlifting session, she suffers a crushing bilateral headache lasting 2 h. Her primary physician started her on low-dose atenolol daily and indomethacin prior to weightlifting.

This case demonstrates the importance of the evaluation of secondary etiologies of headache and re-evaluation in the treatment of refractory cases of suspected primary exercise headaches.

## Conclusion

Primary exercise headache presents during or after strenuous activity with pain lasting upwards of 48 h. Investigations of secondary pathologies that may also worsen with exertion or manifest in a temporal manner, including cerebrovascular and cardiac etiologies, should be evaluated before diagnosis.

Patients that fail to respond with beta-blockade or indomethacin should warrant reassessment for secondary causes.

## Acknowledgement

*A machine generated summary based on the work of Upadhyaya, Parth; Nandyala, Arathi; Ailani, Jessica. 2020 in Current Neurology and Neuroscience Reports.*

# *Other Primary Headaches: Thunderclap-, Cough-, Exertional-, and Sexual Headache*

DOI: https://doi.org/10.1007/s00415-020-09728-0

## Abstract-Summary

This article reviews the disorders of thunderclap, cough, exertional and sexual headache.

Thunderclap headache is the most frequently reported headache syndrome associated with a secondary pathology.

Discussed are the complexities of whether all patients with thunderclap headache should have further investigation if timely computerised tomography is normal and, the relevance of abnormal imaging in these disorders, differentiating what is deemed to be secondary and managing the pain.

## Introduction

A primary headache is synonymous with a headache disorder having no clear correlating aetiology on examination of the patient nor on structural imaging.

The International Classification of Headache Disorders (ICHD) has been successful in refining phenotypes which, based upon history alone, provides well-defined clinical syndromes [23] likely to respond to specific treatments.

Knowledge of the primary headaches comes largely from the work in the most prevalent disorders, namely tension-type headache, migraine, and cluster headache.

In patients presenting with tension-type headache, or migraine with and without typical aura and a normal neurological examination, the prevalence of an underlying brain lesion is the same as that in an asymptomatic population [24, 25].

Part I of the ICHD orders the primary headaches into four sections: migraine, tension-type headache, the trigeminal autonomic cephalalgias and a fourth groups of miscellaneous, largely paroxysmal headache disorders.

Each disorder can occur in primary and secondary forms.

## Thunderclap Headache

Thunderclap headache (TCH) describes a sudden severe explosive onset headache.

Isolated thunderclap onset headache is the most consistently reported presentation of a secondary headache, with the time frame of the pathology and onset of the headache supporting an association [26].

One hundred and sixty cases of sudden and severe headache were reported in association with infection, 44% affecting the CNS and the remainder systemic with likely CNS involvement or, encompassed within the terminology of a 'viral illness' without further elaboration.

This will capture up to 75% of primary and secondary thunderclap headache, while altering this definition to escalation within 5 min will capture 95% of cases [27].

TCH is the most common headache syndrome associated with a secondary precipitating pathology.

Primary and secondary thunderclap headache, however, cannot be reliably differentiated clinically thus, all patients should be investigated.

## Cough Headache

Mathew first reported the response to Indomethacin in a double-blind placebo controlled manner in two patients with cough headache resistant to other tried preventatives [28].

In the case report of Buzzi, a 54 year-old patient presented with a 10 year history of cough headache as an isolated presentation.

This is particularly pertinent in the cases of patients presenting with valsalva headache, normal neurological examination and a Chiari I. It is clear that not all patients with a Chiari I develop cough headache [29].

In Symond's original cohort of cough headache patients, one patient developed symptoms after successful treatment for an acoustic neuroma.

There is a single case report of cough headache, without precipitating thunderclap headache, associated with bilateral acute parietal infarcts and reversible vasoconstriction [30].

Not only can secondary cough headache respond to medical treatment, but the disorder can also go into spontaneous remission, occur coincidentally and be precipitated by surgical intervention.

## Exertional Headache

The exertional precipitant is usually a sustained strenuous effort which precipitates the headache during or after exertion.

Silbert reports that in his cohort of 45 patients with benign sexual headache 27 (60%) also reported experiencing exertional headache [31].

Bougea reported on three patients with comorbid exertional-, cough-, and sexual headache [32].

Diamond reported on the complete resolution of symptoms with Indomethacin in 13 of his 15 patients within 1–4 weeks; medication was withdrawn after 3–12 months with all but one patient remaining asymptomatic, suggesting natural remission [10].

Five of nine patients in a later cohort, responded to prophylactic nadolol or propranolol over a period ranging from 2 to 6 months [33]. The main forms of exertional headache associated with a secondary pathology are those where exertion precipitates a TCH.

## Cardiac Cephalgia

Cardiac cephalgia is a rare exertional headache secondary to cardiac ischaemia and responds to treatment of the cardiac ischaemia.

Half of the cases were precipitated by exertion, sexual activity and emotional fluctuation.

This is a particularly useful indicator, given that in headaches of a similar phenotype, namely migraine and tension-type headache, nitroglycerine precipitates the headache [34].

Most cases had an abnormal baseline ECG and elevated cardiac enzymes.

Of those who had indicators for cardiac ischemia, three had a normal baseline ECG, one a normal exercise stress test and two normal angiography.

## Sexual Headache

Pornography precipitated headache has been reported in a 40 year old man who experienced pre-orgasmic headache within 10 min of watching pornography, only on the internet.

In Frese's cohort of 51 patients, the sexual headache most commonly occurred with sexual activity with the usual partner (94%), but also during masturbation (35%), with a new partner (14%), and only during an extramarital affair in one patient.

Twenty patients (40%) could terminate the headache by stopping sexual activity.

Thirteen patients had recurrent bouts of sexual headache interspersed by remissions lasting up to 10 years [35].

Frese reported benefit with triptans for the headache precipitated by sexual activity if attacks usually lasted longer than 2 h. The paper also reported on the preventative benefit of rizatriptan, almotriptan and sumatriptan, 30 min before sexual intercourse [36].

Lundberg reported on 4–12% of patients, confirmed to have subarachnoid haemorrhage, presenting with sexual thunderclap headache [37].

## Summary

Thunderclap, cough, exertional and sexual headache can occur as both primary and secondary headache disorders, the primary headaches predominating.

A regular pattern of bouts and remissions, as seen in cluster headache, is not characteristic.

Patients tend to be more likely to have other comorbid headache disorders than would be expected based on population prevalence.

The infrequency with which each disorder is seen, based upon prevalence but also remission periods, makes it more difficult to address the issue of what proportion with the isolated headache syndrome have a primary headache or are secondarily precipitated.

The issue is more difficult with cough, exertional and sexual headache because of the risk of identifying an incidental lesion.

The report of two families with sexual headache, suggests that, as with the other primary headache disorders, these disorders may also occur in those genetically predisposed.

## Acknowledgement

*A machine generated summary based on the work of Bahra, Anish. 2020 in Journal of Neurology.*

# *Narrative Review: Headaches After Reversible Cerebral Vasoconstriction Syndrome*

DOI: https://doi.org/10.1007/s11916-020-00908-1

## Abstract-Summary

Patients may report headaches after the resolution of RCVS while relative studies were scarce.

Patients with prior migraine history and patients whose thunderclap headaches are elicited by sexual activity or exertion are at higher risk for RCVS recurrence.

Several retrospective studies and case reports reported that chronic headaches are common in RCVS patients after the resolution of acute bouts.

The chronic headaches after RCVS are sometimes disabling in certain patients.

Medical attention and examinations are warranted in patient with RCVS who reported recurrence of thunderclap headaches or chronic headaches after RCVS.

## Introduction

RCVS is a syndrome characterized by recurrent thunderclap headaches that clustering within 2–3 weeks, accompanying with vasospasm of intracranial arteries revealed by neuroimaging techniques, including computed tomography (CT) or magnetic resonance (MR) angiography, or transcranial Doppler scan.

In most patients, certain triggers, including defecation, exertion, bathing, coughing, and sexual activity, may elicit their thunderclap headaches during the acute phase of RCVS.

Despite the heterogeneity of the etiologies, some phenomena are rather similar in patients with RCVS with different ethnicities: female predominant, middle aged (40–50 years old), and acute, severe headaches (even if not thunderclap at onset).

Several studies investigated the functional outcomes of patients with RCVS.

Despite its potentially fatal complications, RCVS leads to favorable functional outcome in most patients [38–40].

## Recurrence of RCVS

One of the sixteen patients with benign angiopathy of the central nervous system (CNS) that Hajj-Ali and others [41] reported in 2002 had a recurrence of RCVS 14 months after the first bout.

Patients, nine (5.4%) were confirmed to have recurrent RCVS during the follow-up period.

Thunderclap headaches triggered by sexual activity or exercise during the initial RCVS presentation were reported to be significant in predicting RCVS recurrence, with hazard ratio of 5.68 [42] and 8.4 [43], respectively.

Having any complications during the initial RCVS presentation did not predict RCVS recurrence in both studies.

Biotet and others [43] reported five women with postpartum RCVS who had new pregnancies, and none of these patients had recurrent post-partum RCVS.

The recurrence rate in patients who were re-exposed to the vasoactive agents, especially illicit drugs, that triggered their initial RCVS remained an unsolved but potentially significant issue.

## Chronic Headache After RCVS

Fifty-three percent (24/45) of patients continued to have chronic headaches after RCVS resolution.

Although studies were still limited, chronic headache after RCVS has drawn more attention.

Prospective studies that investigate the prevalence of chronic headaches after RCVS resolution are still lacking.

Patients with RCVS do develop chronic headaches after the recovery of intracranial vasospasm; part of them would need long-term medical attention due to chronic headaches that follow the acute bouts of RCVS.

Consistent with the unusual phenotype reported by Rozen and his colleagues [44, 45], we did recognize few patients who developed daily persistent headaches after RCVS onset.

The pathophysiology of chronic headaches after RCVS is unknown.

These findings suggested that some patients may remain subclinically abnormal even after the resolution of RCVS, providing the physiological basis of persistent headaches after RCVS.

## Conclusion

Headaches after RCVS, including RCVS recurrence and chronic persistent headache that developed after RCVS resolution, are not uncommon but usually overseen.

Research regarding the pathophysiology of headaches after RCVS is lacking.

Studies that elucidate the underlying mechanism of recurrent RCVS or chronic headaches after RCVS may help us demystify the pathophysiology of RCVS itself.

## Acknowledgement

*A machine generated summary based on the work of Ling, Yu-Hsiang; Chen, Shih-Pin. 2020 in Current Pain and Headache Reports.*


# *Thunderclap Headache in Children and Adolescents*

DOI: https://doi.org/10.1007/s11916-022-01020-2

## Abstract-Summary

This work aimed to review the epidemiology, clinical criteria, and primary and secondary diagnoses of pediatric thunderclap headache and to compare to adult thunderclap headache.

Thunderclap headache among children aged 6–18 years are rare; this headache presented in 0.08% of the patients admitted to a pediatric emergency department in a tertiary pediatric center.

Contrary to adults, in children, most thunderclap headaches are due to either a primary thunderclap headache or another type of primary headache.

Three-year data from a pediatric emergency department of one center did not find these reasons to be causes of secondary thunderclap headache.

Four of the 19 patients with thunderclap headache reported in that single study had secondary thunderclap; the causes were infection in three and malignant hypertension in one.

More research is needed to investigate pediatric thunderclap headache.
Extended:

More research is needed to examine if neurovascular and neurological non-vascular causes are related to thunderclap headache in pediatric patients presenting to primary, secondary, and tertiary emergency departments.

**Introduction**

The purpose of this paper was to review the epidemiology, clinical criteria, and primary and secondary diagnoses of pediatric thunderclap headache, and to compare to adult thunderclap headache.

Four patients (9.5%) for whom a secondary cause was adequately excluded were diagnosed with primary headache: 1 with primary thunderclap, 2 with headache associated with sexual activity, and 1 with primary cough headache [46].

A number of studies have reported that for about half of adult patients who experience thunderclap headache, imaging and laboratory investigation do not clearly reveal the causes of the pain [46–50].

In a systematic review that included 214 patients with adult reversible cerebral vasoconstriction syndrome, 94% presented with thunderclap headache, which was often recurrent in the first week of presentation [51, 52].

According to the systematic review [48], 7% of adult thunderclap headache are due to infectious causes.

**Thunderclap Headache in the Pediatric and Adolescent Population**

This would bias thunderclap headache to a lower prevalence [53].

This can bias to a lower prevalence of thunderclap headache in the pediatric population.

According to the cohort study described above, 52% of the patients in a tertiary pediatric emergency department with thunderclap headache were females [53].

The mean duration of headache attack was 9.1 ± 8.7 h, the median was 6 h. In comparison, among adults, the mean age of patients in an emergency department with thunderclap headache was 43.1 ± 17.1 years.

**Criteria of Thunderclap Headache in Pediatric Patients According to the ICHD-3**

The visual analogue scale (VAS), which measures pain according to number and color intensity increment, is useful for children aged 7 years or older.

For younger children or children with developmental delay, or children who do not understand the explanation of VAS, the pain scale used in the pediatric emergency department, the Faces Pain Scale—Revised, can be used.

Abrupt Onset, Reaching a Maximum of <1 min: according to our experience, children and their parents usually do not report that the pain reaches its maximum intensity in less than 1 min, but report a sudden or abrupt severe headache.

Children usually do not describe the time of pain in minutes but use the terms "abrupt" and "sudden."

This criterion is legitimate since even for young children who may not have a reliable estimation of time, parents can report the duration of the pain.

**Pediatric Primary Thunderclap Headache and Thunderclap Headache Due to Primary Headache**

As in adults, 50% of pediatric thunderclap are classified as primary headaches or as primary thunderclap headache [48].

Nineteen children were diagnosed with thunderclap headache in a pediatric emergency department during 3 years [53].

Fifteen (79%) were diagnosed as having primary thunderclap or another type of primary headache, of whom six were with migraine and eight were classified as having primary thunderclap headache.

**Secondary Pediatric Thunderclap Headache**

In the largest systematic review of thunderclap headache in 2345 adult patients [48], 517 (22%) had neurovascular and neurological non-vascular diagnoses and 234 (10%) vasoconstriction causes [48].

In the single cohort study in a pediatric emergency department [53], thunderclap headache was not found to be due to cerebral reversible vasoconstriction syndrome in any of the patients.

Only a few reports described other severe causes of pediatric and adolescent thunderclap headache.

None of the patients [53] during a 3-year period presented with thunderclap headache due to hemorrhagic stroke and intracranial aneurysms.

Among our 2290 pediatric patients with headache, only two had intracranial bleeding, neither had thunderclap [53].

Of the 19 patients diagnosed with thunderclap in the cohort study conducted in a pediatric emergency department [53], only 4 (21%) [53] were with secondary thunderclap headache.

In the systematic review of adult thunderclap headache [48], 50% had secondary headache, only 7% had causes related to infectious disease.

**Conclusions**

Thunderclap headache was rare among pediatric patients aged 6–18 years presenting at a pediatric emergency department in a tertiary center.

Validated pain scales suitable for the pediatric and adolescent age groups are mandatory to diagnose severe pain.

Most pediatric patients with thunderclap have primary thunderclap due to primary headache or primary thunderclap headache.

More research is needed to examine if neurovascular and neurological non-vascular causes are related to thunderclap headache in pediatric patients presenting to primary, secondary, and tertiary emergency departments.

**Acknowledgement**

*A machine generated summary based on the work of Levinsky, Yoel; Eidlitz-Markus, Tal. 2022 in Current Pain and Headache Reports.*

## *Headache Attributed to Airplane Travel: A Review of Literature*

DOI: https://doi.org/10.1007/s11916-018-0701-9

**Abstract-Summary**
Headaches due to airplane travel are rare but documented in the literature.

Airplane headache is classified as unilateral, stabbing, orbito-frontal pain, lasting under 30 min, and occurs during ascent or descent of a plane.

There are no randomized controlled trials regarding treatment, but case reports suggest headache prevention with pre-treatment with naproxen, decongestants, and triptans prior to air travel.

Some non-pharmacological therapies reported include Valsalva maneuvers, chewing, relaxation techniques, and pressure at the pain area.

As more cases of headache attributed to airplane travel are reported, epidemiological data can be obtained to further understand the incidence and prevalence of this condition, which can lead to improved treatment options for patients.

Extended:
Diagnostic workup included magnetic resonance imaging of brain and computerized tomography of the maxillofacial sinuses did not reveal any pathology that could explain symptoms.

**Introduction**
While to date there is no clear epidemiologic data on the incidence of headache attributed to airplane travel, a significant amount of case reports has been presented in the literature.

A recent systematic review from cumulative prior case reports found 275 patients [54] for which extensive description of the condition was presented.

Initial case reports were mostly in males [54, 55] but as more cases where identified, the condition was found to be present in females with similar incidence [54].

Episode initially began while traveling during plane ascent.

After initial episode, during subsequent travel, episodes recurred causing significant anxiety and fear of flying.

**Clinical Presentation**
Diagnosis is mostly clinical and mostly made by history and associated symptoms described by patients [56].

There are usually no associated symptoms but there have been reports of some associated congestion [55] and tearing [57].

Some other associated symptoms that infrequently have been reported include ipsilateral tearing, conjunctival injection, ptosis, nasal congestion, and nasal discharge [57].

There is no literature about epidemiology of this disorder, but a systematic review published in 2017 by Bui and others provides good analysis about patient demographics for this condition as more cases emerge [58].

Most patients do not have any associated primary headache disorder, but some reported prior history of migraine headache, retinal migraine, exercise induced headache, and tension type headache [55, 58].

Few cases have reported an association with sinus infection and chronic rhinosinusitis [58].

## Diagnosis

Formal diagnostic criteria were first proposed by Mainardi and others in 2007 [59] after presenting the first Italian case.

At the time, there were only 7 cases reported but all sharing similar clinical features which prompted the authors to propose formal diagnostic criteria into the ICHD [59].

There is also an ICHD comment suggesting the nasal congestion, stuffy feeling of the face, or tearing can occur ipsilaterally (in 5% of cased) [60], despite these symptoms not being included in formal diagnostic criteria.

## Diagnostic Workup

Diagnostic workup has included magnetic resonance imaging of the brain, magnetic resonance angiography of the crania vessels, and computerized tomography of sinuses.

There is a case report by Kim and others [61] where cranial computerized tomography showed ethmoidal sinus mucosal thickening.

The author recommends obtaining magnetic resonance imaging of the brain to evaluate for secondary causes of headache at initial presentation.

There appears to be no reason to order magnetic resonance angiography of the head after reviewing the literature, but it would be reasonable to order if suspicious finding on magnetic resonance imaging.

## Pathophysiology

The exact mechanism of airplane headaches still remains unclear; however, there has been several different proposed hypotheses [58, 62–64].

The most common suspected mechanism of airplane headache in current literature includes the changes in cabin pressure which is seen during take-off and landing periods [58, 62–64] and its effects.

Imbalances of pressure between the atmosphere and sinuses can cause direct nasal tissue damage, also known as paranasal barotrauma which is similar to this proposed mechanism [58].

In a person who suffers from airplane headache, it is proposed there is possible structural variations causing reduced patency of the nasal pathways, making it difficult to equalize pressure [58, 62].

One study found that $PGE_2$ infusions can induce vasodilation of the cerebral arteries and directly cause headaches in healthy subjects [58, 64].

Studies have shown a direct correlation between higher amounts of cortisol and patients who experience various types of headaches [64].

**Treatment**

Some patients have pre-treated with simple analgesics (paracetamol), non-steroidal anti-inflammatory drugs (ibuprofen and naproxen), and triptans [56, 58].

Based on reported patient experience with pre-treatment, Mainardi and others [56] suggest application of decongestant nasal spray along with a non-steroidal anti-inflammatory drug 30–60 min before the expected onset of pain, but their data did not allow them to draw definitive therapeutic conclusions.

Ipekdal and others [65] reported 5 cases where pre-treatment with a triptan 30–45 min before travel resulted in pain freedom.

While these case reports do not provide sufficient evidence for a formal recommendation of triptans as prevention of headache attributed to airplane, they do assist in selecting triptans for patients that have failed other analgesics and provide way to consider further randomized trials for triptans as prevention of this disorder.

Use of non-pharmacological treatments have been reported with minimal efficacy [56].

**Conclusion**

While this is an unusual type of headache, there have been an increase in number of cases being reported in part from patients suffering from the condition that have reached to authors.

Airplane travel is very common these times and patients that suffer this condition can suffer significant discomfort that in some instances can limit travel.

The ability of properly diagnosing is helpful in performing further studies that would help better understand this condition in order to provide optimal treatment and minimize pain passengers with this condition suffer during airplane travel.

**Acknowledgement**

*A machine generated summary based on the work of Nierenburg, Hida; Jackfert, Katelin. 2018 in Current Pain and Headache Reports.*

# *Headache Attributed to Airplane Travel: Diagnosis, Pathophysiology, and Treatment—A Systematic Review*

DOI: https://doi.org/10.1186/s10194-017-0788-0

**Abstract-Summary**

Headache attributed to airplane travel, also named "airplane headache" (AH) is a headache that occurs during take-off and landing.

There are still uncertainties about the pathophysiology and treatment of AH.

This systematic review was performed to facilitate identification of the existing literature on AH in order to discuss the current evidence and areas that remain to be investigated in AH.

Main findings revealed that AH attacks are clinically stereotyped and appear mostly during landing phases.

Nonsteroidal anti-inflammatory drugs and triptans have been taken by passengers with AH, to relieve the headache.

Systematic review, further studies seem required to investigate underlying mechanisms in AH and also to investigate the biological effects of nonsteroidal anti-inflammatory drugs and triptans for alleviating of AH.

These studies would advance our understanding of AH pathogenesis and potential use of treatments that are not yet established.

Extended:

Headache attributed to airplane travel, also named "airplane headache" (AH) occurs in a population of passengers during airplane travels.

Systematic review, it is now evident that further studies are required to investigate AH systematically.

## Introduction

Despite its occurrence rate and high impact, only limited is known about AH, and this type of headache has only been defined and included in the headache classification since 2013 by International Headache Society (IHS), which provides headache classifications and maintains related updates [66].

Previous reports, before inclusion of AH in classification, could be based on diversity in diagnosis, which makes it difficult to determine whether reported patients suffered from AH or other conditions [62, 66].

Current knowledge about pathophysiology and treatment of AH is limited that calls for further investigation on both epidemiological aspects of AH, pathophysiology and treatment options.

Considering challenges and limitation of AH studies under real-time conditions, it might be an option to study this headache under controlled experimental conditions.

This model [67] can also serve for testing treatment options for AH.

To provide a better overview of existing literature on diagnosis, pathophysiology, and treatment of AH, this systematic review was performed.

## Methods

Both authors (SBDB and PG) contributed in performing the systematic literature search in PubMed, Scopus, and Embase by using the terms "airplane headache" and "aeroplane headache" (airplane OR aeroplane AND headache).

Due to limited information available about AH, all types of studies and levels of evidence about AH were considered eligible for inclusion, including, i.e. case series, case reports, conference abstracts, and all types of publications providing knowledge on diagnosis, pathophysiology, or treatment of AH.

Papers were excluded if they were not available in English.

All data from the included papers were reviewed and tabulated according to authors of study, year, study type, demographic data on the patients, and main outcomes.

**Results**

Based on available evidences, landing appears to be the phase of the flight during which most of patients experience AH-attack with a duration within 30 min.

In few cases, patients have had experienced a second mild phase headache after the AH-attack that resolved within 4–24 h (n = 2/275).

The frequencies of the AH-attacks were reported by some patients: 42 patients experienced AH in every flight travel, while AH occurred in more than 50% of the flight travels in 39 patients.

The stress hormone cortisol has also been shown to be significantly elevated in AH-patients during a simulated flight when compared to healthy subjects indicating a physiological response during an AH-attack [67].

A small group of AH-patients (n = 35) has used self-administered maneuvers such as pressure on the headache pain site (n = 19/35), Valsalva maneuver (n = 11/35), relaxation methods (n = 3/35), chewing (n = 1/35), and extension of the ear lobes (n = 1/35) [62].

**Discussion**

Based on the findings, AH was found to occur in 138 patients (n = 138/275) [59, 68–73] since their first flight experience.

One of the substances investigated in that study was $PGE_2$, where $PGE_2$ levels were significantly higher in a group of AH-patients compared with healthy subjects during a simulated flight in a pressure chamber [67].

For future studies, it would be valuable to use imaging techniques during a real or simulated flight travel to investigate whether vasoconstriction or vasodilation occurs in the cerebral arteries during an AH-attack.

It has been shown that cortisol levels were significantly higher before and during a simulated flight in a small group of AH-patients compared with a healthy matched group tested in a pressure chamber [67].

Some AH-patients reported that they felt stressed and had anxiety during the simulated flight [67].

**Conclusions**

Systematic review, it is now evident that further studies are required to investigate AH systematically.

Future experimental studies are also essential to further investigate proposed mechanisms underlying AH; barotrauma and vasodilation in the cerebral arteries, and also to investigate the biological effects of most used medications, ibuprofen, naproxen and triptans for alleviating of AH-attacks.

These studies would advance our understanding of AH pathogenesis and value of treatment options that are not yet established.

**Acknowledgement**

*A machine generated summary based on the work of Bui, Sebastian Bao Dinh; Gazerani, Parisa. 2017 in The Journal of Headache and Pain.*

## *Diving Headache*

DOI: https://doi.org/10.1007/s11916-019-0787-8

### Abstract-Summary

This review will focus on the most recent information regarding the ICHD-3 definition of diving headache as well as other important causes of diving headache that are not listed in the ICHD-3 classification system.

Other causes of diving headache range from decompression sickness to external compression headache to primary headache disorders, such as migraine.

Correctly determining the underlying cause of the diving headache is critical to management and relies on history taking and physical exam.

Further investigation may yield more information regarding management as well as possible insight into other headache disorders.

### Introduction

We review the ICHD-3 diagnosis of diving headache, the etiology of which is thought to be due to hypercapnia.

It is also important to consider secondary causes of and contributors to diving headache.

We will discuss diving ascent headache, a more recently described phenomenon not yet listed in ICHD-3 which may have different pathophysiological mechanisms.

### Epidemiology of Headache in Diving

There are few epidemiological studies to determine the prevalence of headache in SCUBA divers.

The best data available come from a 2011 study examining 201 professional male divers and the prevalence of common primary headache disorders (as defined by ICHD-2 criteria), migraine with and without aura and tension-type headache.

A primary headache diagnosis was present in 16% of divers vs 22% of matched controls.

Divers can be prone to other headache types (to be discussed further below), but likewise, there was no assessment for them in this study.

### ICHD-3 Diving Headache

It is thought that each of these syndromes likely has a similar pathophysiologic mechanism, headache attributed to hypoxia and/or hypercapnia.

Diving headache is defined as occurring during or after a dive to a depth greater than 10 m, often with symptoms of carbon dioxide ($CO_2$) intoxication, and in the absence of another ICHD-3 diagnosis or cause of the headache.

Physiologically, $CO_2$ causes relaxation of cerebrovascular smooth muscle; thus, hypercapnia can lead to cerebral vasodilatation with resultant increased intracranial pressure (ICP) and headache pain.

High-altitude headache may share pathophysiology with diving headache in the form of increased ICP from hypercapnia-induced cerebral vasodilation.

Whether this increase leads directly to ICP elevation and pain remains under debate based on recent studies [74].

Headache attributed to travel in space is surprisingly prevalent (12 of 17 astronauts surveyed) and may also be due to increased ICP from fluid and pressure shifts in microgravity.

Microgravity alone can induce hypoxia and subsequently increased ICP.

## Other Diving-Related Headaches

Decompression sickness (DCS), where dissolved nitrogen returns to gaseous form within the tissues, is a dreaded complication of overly rapid ascent and can be affected by dehydration also, with headache as presenting symptom in 24% of divers [75].

Primary headache disorders, including migraine and tension-type headache, should also be considered, particularly in divers who carry those pre-existing diagnoses.

Tension-type headache attacks can also occur during a dive, and those who experience primary exertional headache may be at increased risk of experiencing pain with vigorous underwater swimming [76].

A case series of 200 patients affected by headache attributed to airplane travel found that of the 46 patients who had diving experience, 21 (45.6%) reported experiencing a nearly identical headache during or shortly after ascent from free diving, snorkeling, or SCUBA diving [77].

## Diagnosis and Management

Determining the cause may be as straightforward as noticing that equipment is ill-fitting; however, the physical exam is important in evaluating the head for trauma and to check for reproducible pain, such as by palpation of the supraorbital notch in a patient with goggle-related headache.

Barotrauma is the most common diving-related injury and can occur in the lungs, ears, sinuses, and dental fillings, with headache often a significant symptom in the latter three scenarios.

Divers who breathe continuously with slow, deep breaths and avoid prolonged vigorous exertion underwater are significantly less likely to experience diving headache.

No specific treatment is well-described, but those who have had a history of headache with airplane travel, or who have previously noted headache with rapid descents from high altitude, should be aware that they may experience a similar phenomenon with diving ascent [77].

## Conclusion

Headache while diving is a commonly experienced phenomenon with multiple etiologies.

Research continues into further elucidating the pathophysiology of diving-related headache syndromes.

Diving ascent headache appears to share commonalities with airplane headache, the pathophysiology of which remains under investigation, having been theorized to be due to differences in pressure inside the sinuses compared with the airplane cabin pressure.

Prevention is a key part of diving headache; good diver education/training, as an appropriate screening of divers for PFO and proper equipment management, can often prevent poor outcomes.

## Acknowledgement

*A machine generated summary based on the work of Burkett, John Glenn; Nahas-Geiger, Stephanie J. 2019 in Current Pain and Headache Reports.*

# *Sherpas, Coca Leaves, and Planes: High Altitude and Airplane Headache Review with a Case of Post-LASIK Myopic Shift*

DOI: https://doi.org/10.1007/s11910-019-1013-0

## Abstract-Summary

High altitude headache is a common neurological symptom that is associated with ascent to high altitude.

We review recent clinical and insights into the pathophysiological mechanisms of high altitude and airplane headache.

Headache attributed to airplane travel is a severe typically unilateral orbital headache that usually improves after landing.

Recent studies have helped identify this as a distinct headache disorder.

Physiologic, hematological, and biochemical biomarkers have been identified in recent high altitude studies.

There have been recent advance in identification of molecular mechanisms underlying neurophysiologic changes secondary to hypoxia.

Recent epidemiological studies indicate that the prevalence of airplane headache may be more common than we think in the adult as well at the pediatric population.

Although research is limited, there have been advances in both clinical and pathophysiological mechanisms associated with high altitude and airplane headache.

Extended:

High altitude headache (HAH) is coded in the International Classification of Headache Disorders, 3rd edition (ICHD-3) among headaches attributed to headache disorders of homeostasis [4].

## Personal Case of Post-LASIK Myopic Shift at High Altitude from Author LM

When the opportunity came to climb Mt. Kilimanjaro in Tanzania, Africa, for a fundraiser with my patients and colleagues, I did not want to climb with glasses or contact lenses, so I began considering laser-assisted in situ keratomileusis (LASIK) surgery.

I was 48 years old at the time and did not have any visual issues up until approximately 500 feet. from the summit.

At 19,000 feet, I started noticing blurry vision.

That day, we started climbing at midnight and, essentially, we were summiting during sunrise.

The guide told me that I should return to base but I whispered to him to hold my arm and take me to the summit, which was another 340 feet.

When I reached the camp at 5000 feet, my vision was 80–90% returned.

For the first time in my life, essentially, I am without corrective lenses.

## Introduction

Diagnostic criteria (HAH): A. Headache fulfilling criterion C B. Ascent to altitude above 2500 m has occurred C. Evidence of causation demonstrated by at least two of the following:

Headache has at least two of the following three characteristics a) Bilateral location b) Mild or moderate intensity c) Aggravated by exertion, movement, straining, coughing, and/or bending D. Not better accounted for by another ICHD-3 diagnosis Headache attributed to airplane travel (AH) is typically unilateral, orbital, severe, and caused by airplane travel and improves after landing [4].

HAH occurred in 39% of hikers and AMS in 26% of hikers even though the median elevation for the residence for the subjects was 1697 m. History of migraine resulted in any headaches at altitude (OR 2.49, 95% CI 1.62–3.65), whereas there was a stronger association with migraine (OR 14.05, 95% CI 5.49–35.93).

## Pathophysiology of High Altitude Headaches

Between 1500 and 3500 m (high altitude), one may experience AMS, high altitude cerebral edema (HACE), slowing to complex reactions, and psychomotor slowing.

Between 3500 and 5500 m (very high) learning and spatial memory impairment, >5500 m (extreme altitude) recall impairment, MRI white matter changes above 7000 m and hallucinations above 7500 m. As a reference, the peak of Mt. Kilimanjaro is 5895 m and Mt. Everest 8848 m. HACE is typically treated with rapid decent and dexamethasone.

There is increased blood brain barrier permeability at higher altitude.

Underlying mechanism of HACE may be due to a combination of cytotoxic (intracellular) and/or vasogenic (extracellular) edema.

PET studies suggest that indigenous persons living at higher altitude have lower glucose metabolism in the frontal cortex, suggesting a protective mechanism from chronic low oxygen states [78].

A prospective study of 77 volunteers simulated high altitude (4500 m) by regulated normobaric hypoxia ($F_IO_2 = 12.6\%$) to evaluate AMS.

## Treatment

There is no data currently to suggest that newer migraine CGRP monoclonal antibodies can have a protective benefit for HAH.

A systemic review and meta-analysis suggest that ibuprofen with doses of up to 600 mg three times daily may be a preventive alternative to acetazolamide or dexamethasone [79].

Acetazolamide is a carbonic anhydrase inhibitor and may result in metabolic acidosis.

Typical doses for acetazolamide are 125–250 mg twice per day.

A recent study looking at administration of acetazolamide the day of ascent showed a slightly higher rate of AMS [80].

Acetazolamide has been found to increase cerebral oxygenation in OSA patients [81].

Other diuretics such as furosemide are more useful for acute treatment of cerebral edema versus prevention.

While acetazolamide is used to prevent AMS, dexamethasone can also be used to treat cerebral edema.

**Personal Anecdote from Author SJ**

I embarked on a classical 4-day trek through the Andes, on the famous Inca Trail to Machu Picchu, Peru.

This consisted basically of a few coca leaves in hot water.

During the trek, we also periodically chewed on the leaves.

Coca leaf products, in the form of raw leaves chewed or as tea, were used by 62.8% vs. 16.6% of travelers who took acetazolamide to prevent AMS.

Use of coca leaves was associated with increased frequency [82].

Indigenous persons living at higher altitudes for centuries have used coca leaves.

A small study looked at biochemical and physiologic changes of chewing coca leaves.

They found that coca leaves blocked glycolytic pathways resulting in increase in glucose and pyruvate.

Chewing coca leaves during exercise was thought to provide sustained benefits [83].

**Airplane Headache**

A recent multiheadache center Italian population–based study identified the prevalence of AH to be 4.0% (30/733).

AH is not uncommon in the pediatric populations.

In a multicenter study, out of 320 children with a history of a primary headache disorder, 4.7% had AH.

There appeared to be no relationship between migraine and AH in this study [84].

**Pathophysiology of Airplane Headaches**

AH patients (14) matched with health controls (7) entered a pressure chamber that simulated an airplane flight.

Prostaglandin $E_2$ ($PGE_2$), cortisol, and saturation pulse oxygenation (SPO) alterations were observed in the AH group vs. controls, suggesting a potential role as biomarkers.

There was a higher increase in $PGE_2$, in the AH group post-stimulation.

Cortisol levels were elevated for the AH group during simulation, possibly related to greater anxiety in the group.

The oxygen saturation dropped lower for the AH group in the chamber.

It was unclear if there is a relationship between low saturation and headache or if the AH group is more sensitive to atmospheric pressure changes.

RCVS is under diagnosed in the general population, and it may be possible that "low-grade" RCVS is an underlying mechanism for AH with atypical longer duration symptoms.

**Treatment of Airplane Headache**
Non-pharmacological approach, including applying pressure to painful area to chewing and extension of the earlobe, has been tried to alleviate the pain associated with AH with limited success [62].

Pharmacological agents such as naproxen, ibuprofen, and triptans have been used with some efficacy; however, rigorous clinical trials are needed [62, 65, 84, 85].

Mechanisms may be related to their anti-inflammatory effects on $PGE_2$ and cyclooxygenase.

**Conclusion**
Recent identifications of physiologic and biochemical biomarkers in HAH may allow for better preparedness and development of specific treatments.

Potential underlying pathophysiological mechanisms such as low-grade RCVS need to be further studied.

There is no current data on the use of CGRP antibodies for the treatment or prevention of AH or HAH.

Larger multicenter studies are needed in order to better characterize both airplane and high altitude headaches.

**Acknowledgement**
*A machine generated summary based on the work of Joshi, Shivang G.; Mechtler, Laszlo L. 2019 in Current Neurology and Neuroscience Reports.*

## *Simulated Airplane Headache: A Proxy Towards Identification of Underlying Mechanisms*

DOI: https://doi.org/10.1186/s10194-017-0724-3

**Abstract-Summary**
Simulation of AH was achieved by entering a pressure chamber with similar characteristics of an airplane flight.

Selected potential biomarkers including salivary prostaglandin $E_2$ ($PGE_2$), cortisol, facial thermo-images, blood pressure, pulse, and saturation pulse oxygen (SPO) were defined and values were collected before, during and after flight simulation in the pressure chamber.

All participants in the AH-group experienced a headache attack similar to AH experience during flight.

The non-AH-group did not experience any headaches.

Our data showed that the values for $PGE_2$, cortisol and SPO were significantly different in the AH-group in comparison with the non-AH-group during the flight simulation in the pressure chamber.

The pressure chamber proved useful not only to provoke AH-like attack but also to study potential biomarkers for AH in this study.

$PGE_2$, and cortisol levels together with SPO presented dysregulation during the simulated AH-attack in affected individuals compared with healthy controls.

We propose to use pressure chamber as a model to induce AH, and thus assess new potential biomarkers for AH in future studies.

Extended:

All participants in the AH-group experienced a headache under simulated condition suggesting that the model works.

All participants in this study were healthy volunteers, who experienced HAH, while situated in an elevated position.

The pressure chamber has been expanded to accommodate 7 participants instead of 6; hence, the number of recruited participants for each group was limited to 7.

The pressure chamber succeeded in inducing an AH-like attack in the AH-group, which gives rise to the possibility of using the pressure chamber as a model to simulate AH on the ground and thereby facilitating assessment of other potential biomarkers or further AH investigations in general.

These findings were then collected and compared with the international guidelines for AH in order to ensure matching the criteria set by IHS.

## Background

Airplane Headache (AH) occurs in a subset of general population during flights.

If AH and HAH share a common mechanism, changes in cabin pressure might alter saturation pulse oxygen (SPO) and contribute in development of AH.

Cortisol, released at higher concentrations during stressful conditions, has been proposed to play a role in development of headaches including AH [62].

To test whether pressure changes would lead to alteration in serum oxygen and circulating $PGE_2$ concentration, and if cortisol levels might be a factor in development of AH, this study was designed to simulate AH as a proxy towards identification of underlying mechanisms.

It was proposed that pressure chamber would cause a headache with similar characteristics to AH and that it would be correlated with some alterations in some biomarkers such as alterations in blood perfusion, SPO, $PGE_2$ and cortisol concentrations.

## Methods

The applied criteria were maintained to ensure a high safety level for the participants and a controlled simulation of AH headache if occurred in the pressure chamber.

No participant was allowed in stepping the pressure chamber if a headache occurred in the trial day due to any reason.

Participants seated in the pressure chamber for approximately one hour to experience a simulated airplane flight by altering the pressure and air composition similar to what occurs during a real flight [86].

Assessments were conducted in the middle of the simulated flight, when the participants had been present in the chamber for 30 min, where the maximal altitude and pressure had been achieved.

All participants were asked to report the possible occurrence of headache and its characteristics before, during, and after their stay in the pressure chamber.

**Statistical Analysis**

Data handling was conducted in Excel 2010 (Microsoft Corp., Seattle, WA, USA).

All statistical tests were conducted in SPSS version 22.0 (IBM Corp., Armonk, NY, USA).

Data normality was assessed by Shapiro-Wilk's Test of Normality.

**Results**

Between group comparison showed that cortisol level was not statistically different in the non-AH-group (1.94 ± 3.15 ng/ml) compared to the AH-group (4.62 ± 2.29 ng/ml) at pre-simulated flight (p = 0.062).

Between group comparison showed that $PGE_2$ was not statistically different in the non-AH-group (41.43 ± 6.03 pg/mL) compared to the AH-group (38.93 ± 25.55 pg/mL) at pre-simulated flight (p = 0.82).

Between group comparison showed that SPO was not statistically different in the non-AH-group (97.43 ± 1.51%) compared to the AH-group (98.00 ± 1.00%) at pre-simulated flight (p = 0.49).

Between group comparison showed that the pulse did not show any significant difference in the non-AH-group (70.43 ± 17.85 bpm) compared to the AH-group (74.14 ± 10.51 bpm) at pre-simulated flight (p = 0.62).

**Discussion**

The concentration of cortisol was elevated during the simulated flight for the AH-group, whereas it dropped for all members of the non-AH-group during the stay in the pressure chamber.

The average SPO for the healthy participants was found decreased in both groups during the simulated flight in the pressure chamber.

Our data indicate a gradual increase in pulse for both groups of non-AH-group and AH-group during the simulation trial in the pressure chamber, even though the increase did not reach to a significant change statistically.

A non-significant increased pulse was observed in our AH-group during the simulated flight, but this gradual increasing has potentially been insufficient to evoke an attack or might be just indicating that elevated pulse might not be a trigger for AH.

**Conclusion**

These biomarkers can attribute to a better understanding of the underlying mechanisms in AH.

The pressure chamber succeeded in inducing an AH-like attack in the AH-group, which gives rise to the possibility of using the pressure chamber as a model to simulate AH on the ground and thereby facilitating assessment of other potential biomarkers or further AH investigations in general.

### Acknowledgement

*A machine generated summary based on the work of Bui, Sebastian Bao Dinh; Petersen, Torben; Poulsen, Jeppe Nørgaard; Gazerani, Parisa. 2017 in The Journal of Headache and Pain.*

## *Headache and Barometric Pressure: A Narrative Review*

DOI: https://doi.org/10.1007/s11916-019-0826-5

### Abstract-Summary

The purpose of this review article is to investigate the association of barometric pressure with headache, classifying into two broad categories primary headache disorders (barometric pressure triggering migraine or tension-type headache) and secondary headache disorders (barometric pressure triggering high-altitude headache and headache attributed to airplane travel), discussing the pathophysiology and possible treatments.

Multiple studies have been performed with inconsistent results regarding the directionality of the association between atmospheric pressure changes and triggering of primary headache disorders, chiefly headaches.

Atmospheric pressure is also a trigger of two secondary headache disorders, i.e., high-altitude headache and headache attributed to airplane travel.

Greater understanding of pathophysiology may enable both acute and preventive treatments for headaches triggered by changes in barometric pressure.

### Introduction

Box 1 ICHD-3 diagnostic criteria of high-altitude headache (HAH) [87]. Box 2 ICHD-3 diagnostic criteria of high-altitude headache (HAH) [87]. Barometric pressure is a possible trigger of primary headache disorders, chiefly migraine.

In another study, analysis of 2–24 months of daily headache diaries collected from 77 people with migraine as per the ICHD-1 criteria seen in an American headache clinic reported a positive association of weather variables as collected from the United States National Weather Service with headache and that more patients noted weather as a contributory factor to their headaches (mean = 4.33, SE = 0.130) when compared with the control group (mean = 3.86, SE = 0.125) (p = 0.014).

The researchers in this study determined that only 12.9% of participants had headache sensitivity to barometric pressure, while 33.7% of the participants were sensitive to absolute temperature and humidity and 14.3% were sensitive to changing weather patterns [88].

**Studies' Finding That Decrease in Barometric Pressure Increases Headache**
A large study of 7054 patients seen over 7 years in the emergency department demonstrated that lower barometric pressure in the preceding 48–72 h was linked to an increased risk of presentation for acute headache (OR 0.939 per 5 mmHg; 95% CI 0.902–0.978; p = 0.002) [89].

A study of 34 patients performed in 2015 in the Isehara region of Japan revealed that migraine occurred most frequently when the barometric pressure decreased by 6–10 hPA relative to the standard pressure (range 1003–1007 hPa).

The study reported increased frequency of migraine in the weather-sensitive group (18/28 patients) when the difference in atmospheric pressure was lower by more than 5 hPA on the day after the migraine (p = 0.009; odds ratio = 1.27).

The study demonstrated increased consumption of loxoprofen with decreased barometric pressure (p = 0.029), heavy rainfall (p = 0.002), and an increase in average humidity (p = 0.004) [90].

**Studies' Finding That Increase in Barometric Pressure Increases Headache**
Contrary to the above, a study of 20 patients performed by researchers at the University of Toronto in 2017 reported a positive association between migraine pain levels with an increase in temperature and atmospheric pressure.

Participants reported their pain level in terms of visual analogue scale (VAS) scores over a period of 14 days.

Significant positive association was reported between VAS scores and atmospheric pressure (p = 0.027).

**Studies' Finding: No Association Between Barometric Pressure and Headache**
Elcik and others analyzed headache diaries of patients that presented to EDs in the Research Triangle region of North Carolina for over a span of 7 years, and reported that there is no association between migraine headache ED visits and the magnitude of atmospheric pressure changes although they did find statistically significant differences between air mass types.

Hoffmann and others recruited 100 patients suffering from migraine with or without aura based on the ICHD-2 criteria and followed them over a year.

Thirteen percent of patients were found to be weather sensitive (13%, 95% CI = 7.1–21.2%); however, when pooled data analysis was performed, the significance was lost.

**Symptoms**
Sudden barometric pressure changes including humidity, temperature, storms, and thunder have long been believed to be triggers for migraines, but some patients have reported an association with tension headaches as well [91, 92].

Symptoms classically are somewhat different between migraine, HAH, HACE, and HAAT.

As per the ICHD-3 criteria [87], migraine is a primary headache disorder with pain attacks lasting 4–72 h which is characteristically unilateral, pulsating with moderate-to-severe intensity associated with nausea or, photophobia, and phonophobia.

HAAT is mostly unilateral with severe periocular pain and stabbing quality, lasting less than 30 min after ascent or descent is completed [58].

**Pathophysiology**

There are several theories as to how barometric pressure may cause headache. (1) Effects through spinal trigeminal nucleus: Messlinger and others found that lowering barometric pressure increased discharge rates in the spinal trigeminal nucleus of anesthetized rats.

Changes in atmospheric pressure (lowered within 8 min by a total of 40 hPa) increased discharge rates in a group of neurons in the trigeminal nucleus caudalis that receives afferent input from the cornea merging with input from the cranial dura mater [93].

This study also suggested that afferents in the inner ear, frontal sinus, or the eyeball may serve as nociceptive sensors following changes in barometric pressure [93]. (2) Effects through the sympathetic nervous system: Sato performed experiments in a rat model of neuropathic pain and reported that decreasing the atmospheric pressure (20 mmHg below the natural atmospheric pressure in 8 min in a climate-controlled room) stimulated the sympathetic nervous system and adrenal medullary hormones which in turn constrict the peripheral vessels causing tissue ischemia, lower blood oxygen levels, and lower pH [94–96]. (3) Effects of hypobaric hypoxia: Another theory is that hypobaric hypoxia, rather than the low barometric pressure, causes migraine and HAH.

The cytotoxic edema could be due to a reduction in the activity of sodium/potassium (Na/K) ATPase pumps [97, 98]. (4) Effects on sinus pressure: Another theory hypothesized was that the atmospheric pressure alters the sinus pressure triggering a headache.

**Investigations**

It is essential to perform a thorough neurological examination to screen for focal neurological deficits; the neurological exam is normal in most primary headache disorders.

In the presence of red flag symptoms, imaging may be necessary to investigate for structural causes of secondary headache disorders.

Work-up in the presence of red flags may include magnetic resonance imaging of the brain, magnetic resonance angiography or venography, and/or computed tomography of the head and sinuses.

**Treatment**

In a series of 5 patients who reported prior HAAT, all patients reported effective HAAT prevention after using various triptans 30 min before their flights [99].

Non-pharmacological treatments such as valsalva maneuvers, applying pressure to sinuses, chewing, pulling of the earlobe, and relaxation techniques are often tried, in one study by 55% of respondents with airplane headache [56].

Of 35 respondents, the investigators report response to such spontaneous maneuvers to be 46% with pressure on the headache pain, 27% with valsalva maneuver, 7% with relaxation methods, 2% with chewing, and 2% with extension of the ear lobes [56].

Migraine and other headache treatments can be tried empirically, such as acute treatment with acetaminophen or non-steroidal anti-inflammatory drugs (NSAIDs) such as ibuprofen, diclofenac, or naproxen as well as triptans and D2-antagonist antiemetics (such as promethazine, prochlorperazine, metoclopramide) for migraines attributed to barometric pressure changes.

**Limitations to Studies**

Limitations of the above studies include that most are observational using headache diaries, patient interviews, or surveys and are subject to recall bias.

There is also likely selection bias; many of the studies assessed patients in the emergency department and, as a result, may not be representative of the overall population of patients with headache, most of whom either are managed in the clinic setting or self-manage.

**Conclusion**

Migraine and other headache disorders affect billions of people worldwide.

Studies involving headache diaries and patient interviews suggest atmospheric pressure as a possible migraine trigger; however, the results of these studies are inconsistent regarding their directionality and fail to establish a strong association.

There are no evidence-based treatments at this time specifically for the prevention or treatment of headaches attributed to barometric pressure.

**Acknowledgement**

*A machine generated summary based on the work of Maini, Kushagra; Schuster, Nathaniel M. 2019 in Current Pain and Headache Reports.*

## *Headache Attributed to Aeroplane Travel: The First Multicentric Survey in a Paediatric Population Affected by Primary Headaches*

DOI: https://doi.org/10.1186/s10194-018-0939-y

**Abstract-Summary**

This multicentric survey investigates the prevalence and characteristics of Airplane Headache in children affected by primary headaches.

Patients with symptoms of Airplane Headache were recruited from nine Italian Pediatric Headache Centres.

Among 320 children suffering from primary headaches who had flights during their lifetime, 15 (4.7%) had Airplane Headache, with mean age of 12.4 years.

Our study shows that Airplane Headache is not a rare disorder in children affected by primary headaches and highlights that its features in children are peculiar and differ from those described in adults.

In children Airplane Headache prevails in females, is more often bilateral, has frequently accompanying symptoms and occurs at any time during the flight.

Further studies are needed to confirm the actual frequency of Airplane Headache in the general pediatric population not selected from specialized Headache Centres, with and without other concomitant headache condition, and to better clarify the clinical characteristics, pathophysiology and potential therapies.

Extended:

Further studies are needed in the general pediatric population to confirm the actual frequency of AH; in particular population-based studies might address the issue of analyzing AH incidence, considering a bigger sample not selected in specialized Headache Centres, with and without other concomitant headache condition, with a long-term follow-up evaluation.

## Background

Airplane headache (AH) is a relatively rare headache disorder associated only with airplane travel; in particular pain begins during taking off or landing or both [100].

The first adult case of AH was reported in 2004 [101].

There has been a steadily increase in the number of reported cases in the following years: up to now, 275 adult cases have been described in the literature [54–107] and, recently, two systematic reviews have been published [58, 108].

Most of the known cases of AH are young males.

The aim of our study is to investigate the prevalence and characteristics of AH in a large group of children suffering from primary headaches, taking into account experts' opinion about the pediatric secondary headache diagnostic criteria of ICHD-III beta [109].

## Patients and Methods

Patients with symptoms suggestive of AH were recruited from 9 Italian Pediatric Headache Centres.

Following an explanation about the study purposes, each patient was handed a structured questionnaire, aimed at obtaining all the relevant information that could clinically distinguish this peculiar disorder.

The inclusion criteria were: A. At least two episodes of headache fulfilling criterion C. B. The patient is travelling by aeroplane.

Headache has developed during the aeroplane flight.

Either or both of the following: a) Headache has worsened in temporal relation to ascent following take-off and/or descent prior to landing of the aeroplane.

b) Headache has spontaneously improved within 30 min after the ascent or descent of the aeroplane is completed.

## Results

In 7 children (46.7%) the same type of headache recurred consistently on separate flights; for those patients the pain started exclusively during landing in two, both during take-off and landing in three, during take-off in one and during cruising in one.

The attacks occurred in more than 50% of flights only in one child (n = 1/15, 6.7%); for this patient the pain started only during take-off.

The attacks occurred in less than 50% of flights in 3 patients (20%): exclusively during landing in two and also during cruising in one.

One patient reported the occasional occurrence of attacks during cruising only in the case of short-haul flights.

In three patients (20%) the attacks occurred exclusively during landing; in three patients (20%) AH started only during take-off.

Five patient (33.5%) reported headache onset during cruising.

One patient reported a reduction of pain intensity.

**Discussion**

Even though it is not possible to directly compare these data with those on AH adults recruited from the general population, it seems that AH features significantly differ between the adult and the child population in terms of several clinical features (intensity, distribution of pain, presence and type of accompanying symptoms, male to female ratio, etc.).

Differently from adults [62], no pediatric patients presented an easily recognizable postictal long-lasting mild headache phase after the AH acute attack.

Baldacci and others [103] reported a patient with AH also affected by migraine with aura: this primary headache is more rare compared to migraine without aura and episodic tension-type headache in the pediatric population.

Given the peculiar clinical features of AH in the pediatric age compared to the adult population, more attention is needed towards this form of secondary headache, for better recognition even without the concomitance of other primary headaches: therefore the next edition of the ICHD should mention this entity also for the pediatric age.

**Conclusions**

Our study shows that AH is not a rare disorder in children affected by primary headaches and highlights that features of AH in children are peculiar and differ from those described in adults.

Further studies are needed in the general pediatric population to confirm the actual frequency of AH; in particular population-based studies might address the issue of analyzing AH incidence, considering a bigger sample not selected in specialized Headache Centres, with and without other concomitant headache condition, with a long-term follow-up evaluation.

**Acknowledgement**

*A machine generated summary based on the work of De Carlo, Debora; Toldo, Irene; Tamborino, Agnese Maria; Bolzonella, Barbara; Ledda, Maria Giuseppina; Margari, Lucia; Raieli, Vincenzo; Santucci, Margherita; Sciruicchio, Vittorio; Vecchio, Angelo; Zanini, Sergio; Sartori, Stefano; Gatta, Michela; Verrotti, Alberto; Battistella, Pier Antonio. 2018 in The Journal of Headache and Pain.*

# *Primary Stabbing Headache*

DOI: https://doi.org/10.1007/s11910-019-0955-6

**Abstract-Summary**

To provide a comprehensive and updated review of the literature on primary stabbing headache.

Changes to the ICHD-3 criteria have resulted in increased sensitivity to capture primary stabbing headache (PSH).

According to the ICHD-3, the sharp stabbing pain is no longer restricted to the first division of the trigeminal nerve.

Secondary etiologies for stabbing headaches are part of the differential diagnosis of primary stabbing headache; therefore, it is reasonable to perform neuroimaging.

## Introduction

Primary stabbing headache (PSH) is a primary headache disorder that was first described by Lansche in 1964 as "ophthalmodynia periodica" [110].

The latest International Classification of Headache Disorders, 3rd edition (ICHD-3) criteria was published in 2018 and describes PSH as "transient and localized stabs of pain in the head that occur spontaneously in the absence of organic disease of underlying structures or of the cranial nerves."

## Epidemiological of Primary Stabbing Headache

Age, gender, referral bias, definition of PSH, and co-morbidity with other headache disorders appear to affect this data.

This difference may be due to referral bias and reporting bias since PSH is commonly associated with other headache disorders.

Epidemiological studies have consistently shown that in the adult population, PSH occurs more commonly in females with a female to male ratio of 1.49–6.6:1 [111, 112].

A review of PSH in children found the mean age of onset is ages 4.5–9 and unlike the female predominance in adults, there appears to be no gender predominance in children [113].

## Diagnostic Criteria of Primary Stabbing Headache

The ICHD-3 diagnostic criteria for Primary Stabbing Headache require all of A–E: data from [4] Headache Classification Committee of the International Headache Society (IHS).

No cranial autonomic symptoms C. Not fulfilling ICHD-3 criteria for any other headache disorder D. Not better accounted for by another ICHD-3 diagnosis. Due to changes in the diagnostic criteria and our understanding of primary stabbing headache over the years, previously labeled PSH or its equivalents may be excluded or other variations of headache may be included in the current ICHD-3 criteria for PSH.

The first edition of ICHD, published in 1988, referred to PSH as a idiopathic stabbing headache [114].

The new 2018 ICHD-3 diagnostic criteria are the most sensitive to capture only primary headaches causing stabbing pain.

ICHD-3 does not comment on response to indomethacin and does not limit the location of the stabbing pain to the first division of the trigeminal nerve [4].

**Clinical Features of Primary Stabbing Headache**
The clinical features of primary stabbing headache include the type of pain, duration, frequency, location, and lack of associated symptoms.

The mean duration of the pain was 1.42 s in a group of 280 migraine patients with distinct co-morbid primary stabbing headaches [115].

Previous studies on primary/idiopathic stabbing headache may have excluded patients who would now be included in the ICHD-3 criteria such as those with stabbing pain outside of the first division of the trigeminal nerve.

Triggers for PSH are not common, but a few case reports have described some potential triggers for paroxysmal stabbing pain particularly in the patients with co-morbid migraine.

Head motion, rapid alterations in posture, physical exertion, and bright lights in patients during a migraine attack appear to trigger stabbing pain in the same location as the migraine [116]; however, these triggers are an unlikely culprit in true primary stabbing headache.

**Pediatric PSH**
A recent review of ICHD-3 beta highlights that headache disorders in children have bio-psycho-social aspects that distinguish clinical presentation and management, although these specific aspects have not been elucidated for PSH [117].

Pain from PSH in children can be located in many regions, including more occipital predominance in comparison with adults [118, 119].

Pediatric PSH is less often associated with other headache types, including migraine [113, 120], but may be associated with extracephalic symptoms such as abdominal pain [121].

**Proposed Mechanism**
Current theories include irritation of trigeminal and extratrigeminal nerves and/or intermittent impairment of central pain processing leading to hyper-excitability of neurons or spontaneous synchronous discharge of neurons.

Ephaptic impulses are presumed to travel to the corresponding peripheral nerve distribution with the perception of stabbing pain [122, 123].

Other theories include dural sinus stenosis [124] and brainstem inflammation or focal demyelination [125, 126]; although these theories would suggest a secondary etiology for the stabbing headache.

**Differential Diagnosis**
The different diagnosis for PSH includes short-lasting, stab-like primary and secondary headaches, and may provisionally include probable PSH.

The diagnosis of all primary headaches must exclude secondary etiologies.

After the secondary etiologies have been considered and ruled out, the differential diagnosis of stabbing headaches is limited to primary headaches disorders.

The duration, frequency, location, presence or absence of cranial autonomic features, and triggers are used to determine the primary headache disorder.

Although PSH, like paroxysmal hemicrania and hemicrania continua, is responsive to indomethacin, these latter headache disorders have longer duration of pain and presence of cranial autonomic features, which differentiates them from PSH.

## Investigations

Recurrent stabbing headaches could be due to secondary aetiologies; therefore, neuroimaging is reasonable.

Blood work including ESR is also reasonable in patients over the age of 50 who present with stabbing pain particularly if they have additional features of giant cell arteritis [127].

## Treatment

Responsiveness to indomethacin is not specific to PSH.

Response to indomethacin is now known to vary, and some experts estimate up to 60% of patients with PSH may respond to indomethacin treatment [128].

The mechanism of indomethacin for PSH may be anti-inflammatory.

For patients with inadequate response, contraindications or intolerance to indomethacin, alternative treatment options suggested from small observational studies include other NSAIDs, such as selective COX-2 inhibitors, etoricoxib [129] and celecoxib [130], melatonin [131–135], onabotulinumtoxin A (BoNTA) [136], gabapentin [137], topiramate [124], acetazolamide [138], and nifedipine [139].

Similar to indomethacin, the mechanism of benefit from acetazolamide and topiramate may be from their effect to lower of intracranial pressure, although this remains to be studied in PSH [140, 141].

No adverse effects were reported and therefore BoNTA may be a logical treatment option for PSH.

Indomethacin is not often used in children less than age 15, but there have been some case reports of effective indomethacin treatment for two patients ages 2.5 and 5 [118].

## Conclusion

Epidemiological data on PSH will need to update to reflect this change.

Although indomethacin continues to be the main therapy for PSH, other treatment options including selective COX-2 inhibitors, melatonin, and onabotulinumtoxin A may be considered.

## Acknowledgement

*A machine generated summary based on the work of Murray, Danielle; Dilli, Esma. 2019 in Current Neurology and Neuroscience Reports.*

# *Nummular Headache: A Gender-Oriented Perspective on a Case Series from the RegistRare Network*

DOI: https://doi.org/10.1007/s10072-019-04129-2

## Abstract-Summary

Nummular headache (NH) is a rare headache disorder characterized by a small, circumscribed painful area of the scalp.

According to the gender-biased profile of certain primary headaches, we have looked further NH patients from a gender perspective.

Nineteen NH patients (11 men, 8 women) have been enrolled in the study.

No clinically evident differences between men and women have been found, including treatment prescriptions and headache resolution.

The mean time from the onset of NH to the first visit in a Headache Centre was longer in men, compared with women (13.5 vs. 0.9 years).

Headache prophylaxis with pregabalin and amitriptyline has been reported as effective in 40% and 67% of the treated patients, respectively.

NH is a primary headache clinically heterogeneous in terms of temporal patterns and pain characteristics.

Extended:

Nummular headache (NH) is a rare headache [142], with pain in a small and rounded area on the head.

According to the first 13 cases described in 2002, the area is round or oval, with a diameter ranging from 2 to 6 cm [143].

According to the current knowledge of its mechanisms, NH has been recently placed among the primary headache disorders [144].

The constitution of a registry including all patients affected by NH will both favour the future collection of observational data and increase the feasibility of clinical trials with novel treatments approaching the bedside.

## Background

Nummular headache (NH) is a rare headache [142], with pain in a small and rounded area on the head.

NH often appears in the fourth decade of life commonly as a primary disorder, but secondary forms have also been reported [145].

After the first description, several observations have been reported in full-length articles [145], contributing to increase the knowledge about NH pain.

The presence of a central mechanism behind NH has also been suggested, since it frequently coexists with other headaches, including migraine.

According to the current knowledge of its mechanisms, NH has been recently placed among the primary headache disorders [144].

We describe a series of 19 patients with NH enrolled in the RegistRare Network study, an observational retro-prospective study promoted by a collaborative group of 7 Italian Headache Centres, aimed to collect data on clinical features and pharmacological therapies.

## Methods

Patients diagnosed with NH were enrolled in a retro-prospective cohort study, including patients who visited seven tertiary Headache Centres from 1 May 2014 to 30 April 2017 [142].

A total of 15 cases were included retrospectively, of whom all were diagnosed by a neurologist or by a physician experienced in headaches.

Collected data included age, sex, marital status, employment, education, age of headache onset, headache location, pain duration, type, frequency and intensity, temporal pattern, clinical presentation and examination, diagnosis, other diseases, past and current therapies and their outcomes.

All these data are available as they are included in the set of data asked to patients during the ordinary clinical assessment at tertiary Headache Centres participating in the RegistRare network.

According to either data reported in the clinical chart for the retrospective cases or data collected prospectively, we classified the clinical response into three categories: complete response; partial response; no response.

## Results

NH patients were 11 men (M) and 8 W, each with a single painful area.

Episodic NH, defined as a headache occurring less than 15 days/month, in the 3 months before diagnosis, was diagnosed in 10 patients.

Chronic NH, a headache occurring 15 or more days/month or persistent head pain in the 3 months before diagnosis, was diagnosed in 9 patients.

The mean time from the onset of NH to the first visit in a Headache Centre was significantly longer in M than in W (13.5 vs. 0.9 years, p = 0.0586).

Each single episode of NH lasts less than 4 h in most males (n = 6, 54%) and females (n = 6, 75%), occurring mostly as a burning pain in M (n = 4, 36%) or as a stabbing or throbbing pain in W (n = 3, 27% for each symptom).

## Discussion

The main clinical features and therapeutic outcomes of the 19 patients diagnosed with NH are superimposable to those reported in other studies [145, 146].

Knowing that these data have been obtained from a low number of cases, they suggest that gender does not markedly influence the phenotype of NH patients.

NH appears to favour W, but the clinical manifestation does not look different from the male patients.

Future studies with more casuistry will clarify whether gender differences exist in NH patients, possibly observable with a larger study sample.

Gabapentin, which is recommended to treat neuropathic pain, has been already reported to be beneficial in more than 50% of patients with NH [146].

The constitution of a registry including all patients affected by NH will both favour the future collection of observational data and increase the feasibility of clinical trials with novel treatments approaching the bedside.

**Acknowledgement**

*A machine generated summary based on the work of Pellesi, Lanfranco; Cevoli, Sabina; Favoni, Valentina; Lupi, Chiara; Mampreso, Edoardo; Negro, Andrea; Russo, Antonio; Benemei, Silvia; Guerzoni, Simona. 2019 in Neurological Sciences.*

## *Sleep Disorder-Related Headaches*

DOI: https://doi.org/10.1007/s10072-019-03837-z

**Abstract-Summary**

Migraine with and without aura, cluster headache, hypnic headache, and paroxysmal hemicranias are each reported as intrinsically related to sleep.

Chronic migraine, chronic tension-type headache, and medication overuse headache may cause sleep disturbance.

The poor quality or poor duration of sleep could be a trigger of migraine attack and migraineurs with poor sleep reported a higher headache frequency.

During cluster headache, patients report a poor quality of sleep correlated with the amount of daylight.

Concerning the pathophysiology of hypnic headache, it has been hypothesized a possible role of obstructive sleep apnea in triggering nocturnal attacks: an increased number of apnea episodes has been reported in hypnic headache patients, but a lack of a temporal correlation of headache attacks with the drop of oxygen saturation has been observed.

Tension-type headache is the most common headache with sleep dysregulation (lack of sleep or oversleeping) frequently reported as a triggering factor for acute attacks: management of sleep disturbances seems crucial in this form of headache.

**Introduction**

A Korean study demonstrated the absence of significant differences concerning the sleep duration among migraine, non-migraine headache, and non-headache groups, while demonstrating an association between short-sleep duration and poor sleep quality with an increase in headache frequency among migraineurs [147].

A positive bi-directional association is reported frequently among migraine and another common sleep disorder, as RLS.

Suzuki and colleagues reported a significantly increased frequency in migraine patients of a dream-enacting behavior (DEB), a disorder classified as REM sleep behavior disorder (RBD).

The authors observed that migraine patients with DEB had severer headache-related disability and insomnia, and they pointed out to a possible association of this sleep disorder with negative emotions experienced during sleep or wakefulness, suggesting that this may reflect increased brain excitability in migraine patients due to brainstem involvement [148].

## Conclusions

Headache disorders can affect sleep.

The evaluation of sleep in headache patients in large samples and by means of objective measurements (PSG or actigraphy) could better clarify some pathophysiological aspects.

Other recent papers [149, 150] indicated that an important aspect that should be more extensively explored is the efficacy of treatments for sleep that may have positive effects on headaches.

## Acknowledgement

*A machine generated summary based on the work of Ferini-Strambi, Luigi; Galbiati, Andrea; Combi, Romina. 2019 in Neurological Sciences.*


# *New Daily Persistent Headache: A Diagnostic and Therapeutic Odyssey*

DOI: https://doi.org/10.1007/s11910-019-0936-9

## Abstract-Summary

This narrative review seeks to highlight what is known about the development of NDPH, to outline a diagnostic approach to a patient with new daily headache, and to explore management considerations and potential future therapies for patients diagnosed with NDPH.

The approach to the diagnosis and treatment of NDPH remains individualized, driven by clinical features and challenging in most cases.

Identification of patients (e.g., prediction of patients with status migrainosus destined to develop NDPH) may allow for more effective treatment.

Extended:

Future research should interrogate novel approaches to categorizing patients (e.g., based on temporal acuity) and focus on early identification of cases, which may be initially diagnosed as status migrainosus at first presentation.

## Introduction

New daily persistent headache (NDPH) is a perplexing and challenging clinical disorder, where refractory chronic head pain emerges within a single day, often in the absence of traditional chronic pain risk factors.

The disorder is recognized by the International Classification of Headache Disorders, 3rd edition (ICHD-3) as a primary headache disorder which is present for at least 3 months and has become continuous and unremitting within 24 h [4].

A history of a new daily progression of persistent headache naturally evokes the question of "what happened?"

In this narrative review, we will highlight a diagnostic approach to the patient with a new daily progression of persistent headache and explore management considerations for patients ultimately diagnosed with NDPH.

## Epidemiology and Clinical Features of NDPH

Despite the relative rarity of NDPH, it remains a commonly encountered differential diagnosis among patients presenting to specialty clinics with chronic daily headache.

In one clinic-based series of 56 patients with NDPH, 68% reported nausea, 66% photophobia, and 61% phonophobia [151].

In another series, 14 of 18 NDPH patients reported migrainous accompanying symptoms [152]; similarly, in a large pediatric series, most patients with NDPH had associated migrainous features [153].

Approximately half of patients with NDPH identify a trigger or inciting event associated with the onset of their headache.

In a clinic-based study of 97 patients with NDPH, 53% could not identify a trigger, 22% had an infection or flu-like illness, 9% had a stressful life event, 9% had a preceding surgical procedure with intubation, and 7% had another recognized trigger [154].

There has also been a case series of patients with NDPH triggered by a single Valsalva event [155].

## Clues to NDPH Pathophysiology

The same persistent headache in a patient with a history of episodic migraine might be deemed status migrainosus at 72 h, probable NDPH at 2 months, and NDPH if it remains unremitting at 3 or more months from onset.

Studies have shown that the association of non-cranial surgeries with NDPH is in cases where patients were intubated during the procedure, suggesting the possibility that hyperextension of the neck during intubation and/or extubation could predispose to the development of NDPH [153, 154].

As compared with patients with chronic migraine or chronic post-traumatic headaches, patients with NDPH are more likely to have asthma, allergies, and hypothyroidism [156].

A small case series from Brazil suggests that treating patients with panic disorder and NDPH simultaneously for both disorders can lead to a good response to treatment, perhaps indicating that there is a benefit to treating the psychiatric condition as it may improve response of headache to treatment as well [157].

## Diagnosis of NDPH: How Far Should It Go?

In evaluating a patient for NDPH, it is crucial to perform careful evaluation to rule out secondary cause for the headache, as well as primary headaches such as hemicrania continua and primary trochlear headache, which have different treatments than do NDPH.

A report of unilateral pulsatile tinnitus, or a bruit on exam, might suggest the possibility of a dural arteriovenous fistula, which has been reported to present with a unilateral NDPH-like headache, and prompt arterial imaging [158].

MRI could also potentially show evidence of sinusitis even in absence of fever or rhinorrhea; an NDPH-like headache that resolved with antibiotic therapy has been reported in two Korean patients with isolated sphenoid sinusitis on MRI without other signs/symptoms to suggest infection [159].

MRI imaging would be an appropriate evaluation for tumors that can cause new persistent headache.

Some patients may benefit from MRV or MRA imaging to evaluate for vascular causes of the headache.

### Treatment of NDPH: How Far Should It Go?

A case series of nine patients in India with post-infectious headache found that all patients had improvement with a 5-day course of IV methylprednisolone, in some cases followed with oral prednisolone, with all but two patients having near-complete improvement within 2 weeks.

In a retrospective study of 63 patients in India, 37 patients were treated with combination of steroid (IV followed by oral), sodium valproate (IV followed by oral), and tricyclic antidepressant, with or without Naprosyn, and 46% had an excellent response (less than one headache a month) and 30% had a good response (>50% reduction in headache frequency), while the remainder had a fair or poor response.

Subanesthetic doses of IV ketamine have been shown to improve symptoms in patients with migraine in a retrospective chart review, with 8 of the 14 patients with NDPH showing improvement with the treatment [160].

### Advice for Caring for Patients with NDPH

We recommend referral of patients with suspected NDPH to a headache specialist for careful review for potential secondary etiologies and for longitudinal management, anticipating a potentially refractory treatment course.

Patients with NDPH often have significant distress from their headaches.

It is important to maintain an open mind when caring for patients with NDPH.

### Conclusions

NDPH is a heterogeneous disorder defined by abrupt onset of an unrelenting headache that persists for at least 3 months and is often refractory to treatments.

A phenotypically driven approach (e.g., migraine, cervicogenic) to treatment is reasonable.

NDPH may represent a post-infectious immune/inflammatory phenomenon, which may respond to steroid treatment.

Future research should interrogate novel approaches to categorizing patients (e.g., based on temporal acuity) and focus on early identification of cases, which may be initially diagnosed as status migrainosus at first presentation.

### Acknowledgement

*A machine generated summary based on the work of Riddle, Emily J.; Smith, Jonathan H. 2019. in Current Neurology and Neuroscience Reports.*

# *Is New Daily Persistent Headache a Fallout of Somatization? An Observational Study*

DOI: https://doi.org/10.1007/s10072-021-05236-9

## Abstract-Summary

Tendency towards somatization has not been studied in NDPH patients.

In this cross-sectional study, we evaluated somatization in NDPH, chronic migraine (CM), and chronic tension type headache (CTTH) by comparing the prevalence of somatic symptom disorder (SSD, DSM-5).

We evaluated the past tendencies to somatization by comparing various characteristics of past somatic symptoms (number, duration, type, clearly remembered onset, etc.) between NDPH, CM, and CTTH.

Forty-seven patients each of NDPH and CTTH and 46 patients of CM were evaluated.

Past history of somatic symptoms was seen in 70% patients with NDPH, 15.2% CM, and 23.4% CTTH ($p < 0.001$).

Median number of past somatic symptoms was higher in NDPH.

All NDPH patients clearly remembered the onset of at least one past somatic symptom.

None of CM and CTTH patients remembered the onset of past somatic symptoms.

NDPH patients displayed significant past history of somatization.

Extended:

All NDPH patients with past somatic symptoms remembered the onset of their past symptom/s, whereas none of the patients with CM and CTTH remembered the onset of their past symptoms.

None of CM and CTTH patients reported "NDPH-like somatic symptom".

## Introduction

NDPH is characterized by persistent headache, which is daily from its onset and with the clearly remembered onset of headache (Headache Classification Committee of the International Headache Society (IHS) [161, 162].

Patients with NDPH share many headache characteristics with patients of chronic migraine (CM) and chronic tension type headache (CTTH), yet the abrupt and clearly remembered onset of headache and presence of preceding events and persistent nature makes NDPH unique [161–163].

Patients with somatization persistently remain anxious and overconcerned about their symptoms.

These features relate somatization with the clearly remembered onset and persistent nature of NDPH.

To better understand the causative relationship of somatization to NDPH, in this study, we evaluated prevalence of somatic symptom disorder [SSD, DSM-5 criteria] [164] along with past history of somatic symptoms (number, duration, type, and clearly remembered onset) among patients with NDPH and compared this with patients with CM and CTTH.

**Methods**

We assessed all patients for comorbid somatic symptom disorder (SSD) (DSM-5 criteria) (APA, 2013) [164].

We used SSD-8 to assess the burden of somatic symptoms and SSD-12 to assess the associated excessive thoughts and behaviours [165, 166].

Diagnosis of SSD requires the patient to be continuously somatic for last 6 months, yet it does not consider past discrete somatic symptoms.

We considered past somatic symptom significant if it was distressing or caused disruption in daily life and if it was associated with excessive thoughts, feelings, or behaviours.

If onset of a past symptom was clearly remembered and if the respective symptom persisted for 3 months or more, we labeled it as "NDPH-like somatic symptom" as it resembles with clinical presentation of NDPH.

The presence of somatic symptom in the past, their number, type, and presence of "NDPH-like somatic symptom" were compared among NDPH, CM, and CTTH.

**Results**

Median PHQ-9 score was higher in CTTH in comparison to CM and NDPH patients.

There was no significant difference in median GAD-7 score among NDPH, CM, and CTTH patients.

More patients with CTTH had higher moderately severe and severe PHQ-9 score as compared to NDPH and CM.

More patients with CTTH and CM had higher moderate and severe GAD-7 scores as compared to NDPH.

**Discussion**

NDPH patients had higher prevalence of past somatic symptoms as compared to patients with CM and CTTH.

All NDPH patients with past somatic symptoms remembered the onset of their past symptom/s, whereas none of the patients with CM and CTTH remembered the onset of their past symptoms.

We found a very high prevalence of SSD in patients with NDPH, CTTH, and CM as compared to previous studies [167].

To cover the downside of DSM-5 criteria for SSD, we evaluated past somatic symptoms in our patients.

DSM 5 criteria for SSD give opportunity of a diagnosis of somatization to a patient with new onset of headache without any other somatic symptom.

85.1% patients with NDPH fulfilled criteria for SSD, whereas only 70% had past history of somatic symptoms.

Nearly 15% patients had a new onset of headache fulfilled the criteria for NDPH and SSD.

**Conclusion**

Patients with NDPH display a significant tendency to somatization.

This relationship of NDPH with somatization suggests that NDPH could be an epiphenomenon of somatization.

**Acknowledgement**

*A machine generated summary based on the work of Uniyal, Ravi; Chhirolya, Rohit; Tripathi, Adarsh; Mishra, Prabhakar; Paliwal, Vimal Kumar. 2021 in Neurological Sciences.*

## *Cold Stimulus Headache*

DOI: https://doi.org/10.1007/s11910-019-0956-5

### Abstract-Summary

To provide an updated review on cold stimulus headache.

Age, type of stimulus, comorbidities, and study design but not necessarily gender appear to influence the reported prevalence of cold stimulus headache (CSH).

Different cold stimuli appear to provoke different types of CSH.

### Introduction

Cold stimulus headache is an unusual headache that can be misdiagnosed.

It is a short-lasting headache, and therefore, it is difficult to study.

The prevalence is variable depending on age, comorbidities such as migraine, speed of cold stimulus, and reporting biases.

### Definition

The latest version of the International Classification of Headache Disorder (ICHD-3) defines cold stimulus headache (CSH) as headache brought on by a cold stimulus applied externally to the head or ingested or inhaled [4].

Ice cream headache (ICH), also known as "brain freeze," and headache attributed to ingestion or inhalation of a cold stimulus are also incorporated under this definition.

The inclusion of ice cream headache and headache attributed to ingestion or inhalation of cold stimulus adds to our knowledge of this condition.

### Epidemiology

The reported prevalence of cold stimulus headache is quite variable.

Most of these studies used ice, ice water, or ice cream to trigger the cold stimulus headache while the other studies assessed the prevalence of cold stimulus headache using questionnaires [168–174].

The rate of CSH was significantly higher in students aged 10 and 14 years than their parents and teachers (62% vs 31%) in a self-administered questionnaire [173].

Cold stimulus headaches appear to be more common in migraineurs compared to tension-type headache (TTH) patients [175].

A 2016 cross-sectional epidemiological study that distributed a self-administered questionnaire to students between 10 and 14 years as well as their parents and teachers found no gender difference in the student, but the CSH rate was higher in the adult female than in the adult male groups [173].

### Diagnostic Criteria

Reprinted with permission from SAGE Publications, Ltd. A. At least two episodes of acute frontal or temporal headache fulfilling criteria B and C B. Brought on by and occurring immediately after a cold stimulus to the palate and/or posterior pharyngeal wall from ingestion of cold food or drink or inhalation of cold air C. Resolving within 10 min after removal of the cold stimulus D. Not better accounted for by another ICHD-3 diagnosis.

Reprinted with permission from SAGE Publications, Ltd. A. A single headache episode fulfilling criteria B and C B. Brought on by and occurring only during or immediately after a cold stimulus applied externally to the head or ingested or inhaled C. Resolving within 10 min after removal of the cold stimulus D. Not fulfilling ICHD-3 criteria for any other headache disorder E. Not better accounted for by another ICHD-3 diagnosis.

### Clinical Features

The location of the headache triggered by the cold stimulus is typically bilateral frontal or temporal.

The type of stimulus may influence the characteristic of the headache [174].

CSH triggered by ice water was reported to have a shorter latency, different pain character, and higher pain intensity compared to CSH triggered by ice cubes [174].

By Mages and others, ice water triggered a stabbing more than a pressing pain quality while ice cubes triggered predominately a pressing pain quality [174].

### Triggers

Ice cream, icy water, and ice cubes are common triggers studied in the literature [168–174].

Mages and others compared in a study ice cubes applied to the palate to fast ingestion of 200 mL of icy water.

They found that drinking icy water provoked CSH significantly more often than applying ice cubes to the palate (51% vs 12%) [174].

The association with speed of ingestion could potentially be explained by the fact that the ice cube cools down over a much smaller palate and tongue area compared to ice water.

### Proposed Mechanism

Local and cerebral vascular changes and direct stimulation of cold receptors are two theories.

This relates to a local vascular effect; however, changes to cerebral blood flow appear to occur in CSH [176].

Reduction in mean cerebral blood flow velocities of middle cerebral arteries on transcranial Doppler ultrasonography has been reported in patients who following cold stimulus developed a headache and not in those without a headache [176].

The difference in CSH may be related to which cranial nerves are activated.

CSH triggered by direct stimulation to the palate (innervated by the trigeminal nerve) may differ from the additional stimulation from the pharynx and esophagus (innervated by the glossopharyngeal and vagus nerve) when swallowing.

**Treatment**

There is no specific treatment for cold stimulus headache other than avoiding the triggering factors such as ice cream, ice water, and icy food.

Curling the tongue and pressing the underside against the roof of the mouth has been a method to prevent the cold stimulus headache in some people.

This appears to correspond with a report by Burkhart who suggested massaging the face in the distribution of the trigeminal nerve for 1 min prior to cryotherapy for actinic keratosis reduces incidence and severity of the headaches [177].

**Conclusion**

Age, type of stimulus, comorbidities, and study design but not necessarily gender appear to influence the reported prevalence of cold stimulus headache.

Different cold stimuli appear to provoke different types of cold stimulus headache.

**Acknowledgement**

*A machine generated summary based on the work of Chebini, Amokrane; Dilli, Esma. 2019 in Current Neurology and Neuroscience Reports.*

# References


1. Pellesi L, Cevoli S, Favoni V, Lupi C, Mampreso E, Negro A, Russo A, Benemei S, Guerzoni S. Nummular headaches: a gender-oriented perspective on a case series from the RegistRare Network. Neurol Sci. 2020;41:583–9.
2. Upadhyaya P, Nandyala A, Ailani J. Primary exercise headache. Curr Neurol Neurosci Rep. 2020;20:9. https://doi.org/10.1007/s11910-020-01028-4.
3. Gonzales-Quintanilla V, Pascual J. Other primary headaches, an update. Neurol Clin. 2019;37:871–91.
4. Headache Classification Committee of the International Headache Society (IHS). The International Classification of Headache Disorders, 3rd edition. Cephalalgia. 2018;38:1–211. https://doi.org/10.1177/0333102417738202.
5. Rabiee B, Mohammadinejad P, Kordi R, Yunesian M. The epidemiology of exertional headache in the population of Tehran, Iran. Headache. 2015;55:1225–32. https://doi.org/10.1111/head.12610. The authors assessed clinical characteristics of PEH in their large cohort and reported detailed epidemiological findings.
6. Donnet A, Valade D, Houdart E, Lanteri-Minet M, Raffaelli C, Demarquay G, et al. Primary cough headache, primary exertional headache, and primary headache associated with sexual activity: a clinical and radiological study. Neuroradiology. 2013;55(3):297–305. https://doi.org/10.1007/s00234-012-1110-0.
7. Mitsikostas DD, Ashina M, Craven A, Diener HC, Goadsby PJ, Ferrari MD, Lampl C, Paemeleire K, Pascual J, Siva A, Olesen J, Osipova V, Martelletti P, EHF Committee. European Headache Federation consensus on technical investigation for primary headache disorders. J Headache Pain. 2015;17:5. https://doi.org/10.1186/s10194-016-0596-y.
8. Tofangchiha S, Rabiee B, Mehrabi F. A study of exertional headache's prevalence and characteristics among conscripts. Asian J Sports Med. 2016;7(3):e30720. https://doi.org/10.5812/asjsm.30720.
9. van der Ende-Kastelijn K, Oerlemans W, Goedegebuure S. An online survey of exercise-related headaches among cyclists. Headache. 2012;52:1566–73. https://doi.org/10.1111/j.1526-4610.2012.02263.x.

10. Diamond S. Prolonged benign exertional headache: its clinical characteristics and response to indomethacin. Headache. 1982;22(3):96–8.
11. Halker R, Vargas B. Primary exertional headache: updates in the literature. Curr Pain Headache Rep. 2013;17:337. https://doi.org/10.1007/s11916-013-0337-8.
12. Pascual J, Gonzalez-Mandly A, Martin R, Oterino A. Headaches precipitated by cough, prolonged exercise or sexual activity: a prospective etiological and clinical study. J Headache Pain. 2008;9:259–66. https://doi.org/10.1007/s10194-008-0063-5.
13. Pascual J, Iglesias F, Oterino A, Vazquez-Barquero A, Berciano J. Cough, exertional, and sexual headache: an analysis of 72 benign and symptomatic cases. Neurology. 1996;46:1520–4.
14. Rooke ED. Benign exertional headache. Med Clin N Am. 1968;52:801–8.
15. Hanashiro S, Takazawa T, Kawase Y, Ikeda K. Prevalence and clinical hallmarks of primary exercise headache in middle-age Japanese on health check-up. Intern Med. 2015;54:2577–81. https://doi.org/10.2169/internalmedicine.54.4926. This large Japanese study addressed the clinical characteristics and epidemiology of PEH in their middle-aged population.
16. Rasmussen BK, Olesen J. Symptomatic and nonsymptomatic headaches in a general population. Neurology. 1992;42:1225.
17. Chen SP, Fuh JL, Lu SR, Wang SJ. Exertional headache—a survey of 1963 adolescents. Cephalalgia. 2008;29:401–7. https://doi.org/10.1111/j.1468-2982.2008.01744.x.
18. Wei JH, Wang HF. Cardiac cephalalgia: case reports and review. Cephalalgia. 2008;28(8):892–6. https://doi.org/10.1111/j.1468-2982.2008.01590.x.
19. Cutrer FM, Huerter K. Exertional headache and coronary ischemia despite normal electrocardiographic stress testing. Headache. 2006;46:165–7.
20. Tinel J. La cephalee a l'effort. Syndrome de distension dolourese des veines intracranienes. Medicine (Paris). 1932;13:113.
21. Doepp F, Valdueza JM, Schreiber SJ. Incompetence of internal jugular valve in patients with exertional headache: a risk factor? Cephalalgia. 2007;28:182–5. https://doi.org/10.1111/j.1468-2982.2007.01484.x.
22. Heckmann J, Hilz M, Katalinic A, Marthol H, Mück-Weymann M, Neundörfer B. Myogenic cerebrovascular autoregulation in migraine measured by stress transcranial Doppler sonography. Cephalalgia. 1998;18:133–7.
23. Headache Classification Committee of the International Headache Society (IHS). The International Classification of Headache Disorders, 3rd edn. Cephalalgia. 2018;38(1):1–211.
24. Bahra A. Secondary headache. Adv Neurosci Rehabil. 2013;3(4):14–7.
25. Practice parameter: the utility of neuroimaging in the evaluation of headache in patients with normal neurologic examinations (summary statement). Report of the Quality Standards Subcommittee of the American Academy of Neurology. Neurology. 1994;44(7):1353–4.
26. Locker TE, et al. The utility of clinical features in patients presenting with nontraumatic headache: an investigation of adult patients attending an emergency department. Headache. 2006;46(6):954–61.
27. Linn FHH, et al. Headache characteristics in subarachnoid haemorrhage and benign thunderclap headache. J Neurol Neurosurg Psychiatry. 1998;65(5):791–3.
28. Mathew NT. Indomethacin responsive headache syndromes. Headache. 1981;21(4):147–50.
29. Martins HA, et al. Headache precipitated by Valsalva maneuvers in patients with congenital Chiari I malformation. Arq Neuropsiquiatr. 2010;68(3):406–9.
30. Kato Y, et al. Cough headache presenting with reversible cerebral vasoconstriction syndrome. Intern Med. 2018;57(10):1459–61.
31. Silbert PL, et al. Benign vascular sexual headache and exertional headache. J Neurol Neurosurg Psychiatry. 1991;54:417–21.
32. Bougea A, et al. An uncommon coexistence of primary sexual, cough and exercise headaches: the first three cases from Greece. Hippokratia. 2015;19(4):369–71.
33. Pascual J, et al. Headaches precipitated by cough, prolonged exercise or sexual activity: a prospective etiological and clinical study. J Headache Pain. 2008;9(5):259–66.

34. Olesen J, Iversen HK, Thomsen LL. Nitric oxide supersensitivity: a possible molecular mechanism of migraine pain. Neuroreport. 1993;4(8):1027–30.
35. Ostergaard JR, Kraft M. Benign coital headache. Cephalalgia. 1992;12(6):353–5.
36. Frese A, et al. Triptans in orgasmic headache. Cephalalgia. 2006;26(12):1458–61.
37. Lundberg PO, Osterman PO. The benign and malignant form of orgasmic cephalgia. Headache. 1974;14(3):164–5.
38. Ducros A. Reversible cerebral vasoconstriction syndrome. Lancet Neurol. 2012;11:906–17.
39. Katz BS, Fugate JE, Ameriso SF, Pujol-Lereis VA, Mandrekar J, Flemming KD, et al. Clinical worsening in reversible cerebral vasoconstriction syndrome. JAMA Neurol. 2014;71:68–73.
40. Singhal AB, Hajj-Ali RA, Topcuoglu MA, Fok J, Bena J, Yang D, et al. Reversible cerebral vasoconstriction syndromes: analysis of 139 cases. Arch Neurol. 2011;68:1005–12.
41. Hajj-Ali RA, Furlan A, Abou-Chebel A, Calabrese LH. Benign angiopathy of the central nervous system: cohort of 16 patients with clinical course and long-term followup. Arthritis Care Res. 2002;47:662–9.
42. Chen S-P, Fuh J-L, Lirng J-F, Wang Y-F, Wang S-J. Recurrence of reversible cerebral vaso-constriction syndrome: a long-term follow-up study. Neurology. 2015;84:1552–8. This is the first prospective study which reported the recurrence rate of RCVS and risk factors for RCVS recurrence.
43. Boitet R, de Gaalon S, Duflos C, et al. Long-term outcomes after reversible cerebral vaso-constriction syndrome. Stroke. 2020;51:670–3. This prospective follow-up study of RCVS patients is consistent with Chen et al. (2015), revealing the incidence and risk factors for the recurrence of RCVS.
44. Jamali SA, Rozen TD. An RCVS spectrum disorder? New daily persistent headache starting as a single thunderclap headache (3 new cases). Headache. 2019;59:789–94. Reference 15 and 16 are studies that reported an unusual phenotype of RCVS. There were four patients in total who presented with new daily persistent headaches after RCVS onset.
45. Rozen TD, Beams JL. New daily persistent headache with a thunderclap headache onset and complete response to nimodipine (a new distinct subtype of NDPH). J Headache Pain. 2013;14:100. Reference 15 and 16 are studies that reported a unusual phenotype of RCVS. There were four patients in total who presented with new daily persistent headaches after RCVS onset.
46. García-Azorín D, González-García N, Abelaira-Freire J, et al. Management of thunderclap headache in the emergency room: a retrospective cohort study. Cephalalgia. 2021;41:711–20. https://doi.org/10.1177/0333102420981721. A recent and large retrospective cohort study on the prevalence and management of thunderclap headache among adults in the emergency department.
47. Landtblom A, Fridriksson S, Boivie J, et al. Sudden onset headache: a prospective study of features, incidence and causes. Cephalalgia. 2002;22:354–60. https://doi.org/10.1046/j.1468-2982.2002.00368.x.
48. Devenney E, Neale H, Forbes R. A systematic review of causes of sudden and severe headache (Thunderclap Headache): should lists be evidence based? J Headache Pain. 2014;15:1–18. https://doi.org/10.1186/1129-2377-15-49. A systemic review of publications on adults with thunderclap headache, until September 2009. A catalog is included of all the secondary causes reported.
49. Ravishankar K. Looking at 'thunderclap headache' differently? Circa 2016. Ann Indian Acad Neurol. 2016;19:295–301. https://doi.org/10.4103/0972-2327.186783.
50. Bo SH, Davidsen EM, Guldbrandsen P, Dietrichs E. Acute headache: a prospective work-up of patients admitted to a general hospital. Eur J Neurol. 2008;15:1293–9.
51. Nesheiwat O, Al-Khoury L. Reversible cerebral vasoconstriction syndromes. In: StatPearls. Treasure Island, FL: StatPearls Publishing; 2021.
52. Sattar A, Manousakis G, Jensen M. Systematic review of reversible cerebral vasoconstriction syndrome. Expert Rev Cardiovasc Ther. 2010;8:1417–21. https://doi.org/10.1586/erc.10.124.

53. Levinsky Y, Waisman Y, Eidlitz-Markus T. Severe abrupt (thunderclap) non-traumatic headache at the pediatric emergency department—a retrospective study. Cephalalgia. 2021;41(11–12):1172–80. https://doi.org/10.1177/03331024211014612. The only cohort study to date that examined the prevalence and characteristics of thunderclap headache in children.

54. Mainardi F, Maggioni F, Lisotto C, Zanchin G. Should aircrafts never land? Headache attributed to aeroplane travel: a new series of 140 patients. J Headache Pain. 2015;16(Suppl 1):A166.

55. Berligen MS, Mungen B. Headache associated with airplane travel: report of six cases. Cephalalgia. 2006;26(6):707–11.

56. Mainardi F, Maggioni F, Lisotto C, Zanchin G. Diagnosis and management of headache attributed to airplane travel. Curr Neurol Neurosci Rep. 2013;13(335):1–6.

57. Berligen MS, Mungen B. A new type of headache, headache associated with airplane travel: preliminary diagnostic criteria and possible mechanisms of aetiopathogenesis. Cephalalgia. 2011;31(12):1266–73. xx

58. Bui SBD, Gazerani P. Headache attributed to airplane travel: diagnosis, pathophysiology, and treatment—a systematic review. J Headache Pain. 2017;18(84):1–14. A great review article about HAAT with pooled data from prior case reports and abstracts.

59. Mainardi F, Lisotto C, Palestini C, Sarchielli P, Zanchin G. Headache attributed to airplane travel ("airplane headache"): first Italian case. J Headache Pain. 2007;8(3):196–9.

60. Headache Classification Committee of the International Headache Society (IHS). The International Classification of Headache Disorders, 3rd edition (beta version). 10.1.2 Headache attributed to aeroplane travel. Cephalalgia. 2013;33(9):750.

61. Han-Joon K, Yong-Jin C, Joong-Yang C, Keun-Sik H. Severe jabbing headache associated with airplane travel. Can J Neurol Sci. 2008;35(2):267–8.

62. Mainardi F, Lisotto C, Maggioni F, Zanchin G. Headache attributed to airplane travel ('airplane headache'): clinical profile based on a large case series. Cephalalgia. 2012;32(8):592–9.

63. Bui SBD, Petersen T, Norgaard Poulsen J, Gazerani P. Headaches attributed to airplane travel: a Danish survey. J Headache Pain. 2016;17(33):1–5.

64. Bui SBD, Petersen T, Norgaard Poulsen J, Gazerani P. Simulated airplane headache: a proxy towards identification of underlying mechanisms. J Headache Pain. 2017;18(9):1–10.

65. Ilker Ipekdal H, Karadas O, Oz O, Ulas UH. Can triptans safely be used for airplane headache? Neurol Sci. 2011;32(6):1165–9.

66. Headache Classification Committee of the International Headache Society (IHS). The International Classification of Headache Disorders (beta version). Cephalalgia. 2013;33(9):629–808.

67. Bui SB, Petersen T, Poulsen JN, Gazerani P. Simulated airplane headache: a proxy towards identification of underlying mechanisms. J Headache Pain. 2017. https://thejournalofheada-cheandpain.springeropen.com/track/pdf/10.1186/s10194-017-0724-3?site=thejournalofhead acheandpain.springeropen.com.

68. Marchioretto F, Mainardi F, Zanchin G. Airplane headache: a neurologist's personal experience. Cephalalgia. 2008;28:101.

69. Coutinho E, Pereira-Monteiro J. 'Bad trips': airplane headache not just in airplanes? Cephalalgia. 2008;28:986–7.

70. Pfund Z, Trauninger A, Szanyi I, Illes Z. Long-lasting airplane headache in a patient with chronic rhinosinusitis. Cephalalgia. 2010;30:493–5.

71. Ipekdal HI. Poster session 2, Monday 27 September. Eur J Neurol. 2010;17:351–525.

72. Cherian A, Mathew M, Iype T, Sandeep P, Jabeen A, Ayyappan K. Headache associated with airplane travel: a rare entity. Neurol India. 2013;61(2):164–6.

73. Mainardi F, Maggioni F, Lisotto C, Zanchin G. O037. Should aircrafts never land? Headache attributed to aeroplane travel: a new series of 140 patients. J Headache Pain. 2015;16(Suppl 1):A166. https://thejournalofheadacheandpain.springeropen.com/track/pdf/10.1186/1129-2377-16-S1-A166?site=thejournalofheadacheandpain.springeropen.com.

74. Grewal P, Smith JH. When headache warns of homeostatic threat: the metabolic headaches. Curr Neurol Neurosci Rep. 2017:17. https://doi.org/10.1007/s11910-017-0714-5. Good recent overall review of homeostatic headache disorders.

75. Newton HB. Neurologic complications of scuba diving. Am Fam Physician. 2001;63:2211–8.

76. Cheshire WP, Ott MC. Headache in divers. J Headache Pain. 2001;41:235–47.

77. Mainardi F, Maggioni F, Zanchin G. Aeroplane headache, mountain descent headache, diving ascent headache. Three subtypes of headache attributed to imbalance between intrasinusal and external air pressure? Cephalalgia. 2017;38:1119–27. Paper discussing the significance of airplane headache and possible correlation with diving ascent headache.

78. Hochachka PW, Monge C. Evolution of human hypoxia tolerance physiology. Adv Exp Med Biol. 2000;475:25–43.

79. Xiong J, Lu H, Wang R, Jia Z. Efficacy of ibuprofen on prevention of high altitude headache: a systematic review and meta-analysis. PLoS One. 2017;12(6):e0179788. https://doi.org/10.1371/journal.pone.0179788.

80. Lipman GS, Jurkiewicz C, Winstead-Derlega C, Navlyt A, Burns P, Walker A, et al. Day of ascent dosing of acetazolamide for prevention of acute mountain sickness. High Alt Med Biol. 2019; https://doi.org/10.1089/ham.2019.0007.

81. Ulrich S, Nussbaumer-Ochsner Y, Vasic I, Hasler E, Latshang TD, Kohler M, et al. Cerebral oxygenation in patients with OSA: effects of hypoxia at altitude and impact of acetazolamide. Chest. 2014;146(2):299–308. https://doi.org/10.1378/chest.13-2967.

82. Salazar H, Swanson J, Mozo K, White AC Jr, Cabada MM. Acute mountain sickness impact among travelers to Cusco, Peru. J Travel Med. 2012;19(4):220–5. https://doi.org/10.1111/j.1708-8305.2012.00606.x.

83. Casikar V, Mujica E, Mongelli M, Aliaga J, Lopez N, Smith C, et al. Does chewing coca leaves influence physiology at high altitude? Indian J Clin Biochem. 2010;25(3):311–4. https://doi.org/10.1007/s12291-010-0059-1.

84. Bui SBD, Gazerani P. Headache attributed to airplane travel: diagnosis, pathophysiology, and treatment—a systematic review. J Headache Pain. 2017:18. https://doi.org/10.1186/s10194-017-0788-0.

85. Bui SB, Petersen T, Poulsen JN, Gazerani P. Headaches attributed to airplane travel: a Danish survey. J Headache Pain. 2016;17:33. https://doi.org/10.1186/s10194-016-0628-7.

86. Burdack-Freitag A, Bullinger D, Mayer F, Breuer K. Odor and taste perception at normal and low atmospheric pressure in a simulated aircraft cabin. Journal für Verbraucherschutz und Lebensmittelsicherheit. 2011;6:95–109.

87. The International Classification of Headache Disorders. 3rd edn. Cephalalgia. 2013;33(9):629–808.

88. Prince PB, Rapoport AM, Sheftell FD, Tepper SJ, Bigal ME. The effect of weather on headache. Headache. 2004;44:596–602.

89. Mukamal KJ, Wellenius GA, Suh HH, Mittleman MA. Weather and air pollution as triggers of severe headaches. Neurology. 2009;72:922–92.

90. Ozeki K, Noda T, Nakamura M, Ojima T. Weather and headache onset: a large-scale study of headache medicine purchases. Int J Biometeorol. 2015;59:447–51.

91. Spierings ELH, Ranke AH, Honkoop PC. Precipitating and aggravating factors of migraine versus tension-type headache. Headache. 2001;41:559–64.

92. Turner LC, Molgaard CA, Gardner CH, Rothrock JF, Stang PE. Migraine trigger factors in a non-clinical Mexican-American population in San Diego county: implications for etiology. Cephalalgia. 1995;15:523–30.

93. Messlinger K, Funakubo M, Sato J, Mizumura K. Increases in neuronal activity in rat spinal trigeminal nucleus following changes in barometric pressure—relevance for weather-associated headaches? Headache. 2010;50:1449–63.

94. Sato J. Possible mechanism of weather related pain. Jpn J Biometeorol. 2003;40:219–24.

95. Sato J, Morimae H, Seino Y, Kobayashi T, Suzuki N, Mizumura K. Lowering barometric pressure aggravates mechanical allodynia and hyperalgesia in a rat model of neuropathic pain. Neurosci Lett. 1999;30:21–4.
96. Sato J. Weather change and pain: a behavioral animal study of the influences of simulated meteorological changes on chronic pain. Int J Biometeorol. 2003;47:55–61.
97. Kallenberg K, Bailey DM, Christ S, et al. Magnetic resonance imaging evidence of cytotoxic cerebral edema in acute mountain sickness. J Cereb Blood Flow Metab. 2007;27:1064–71.
98. Houston CS. Incidence of acute mountain sickness at intermediate altitudes. JAMA. 1989;261:3551–2.
99. Ipekdal HI, Karadas O, Oz O, Ulas UH. Can triptans safely be used for airplane headache? Neurol Sci. 2011;32:1165–9.
100. Titlić M, Demarin V. Airplane headaches-two new cases and a review of the literature. Acta Med Croatica. 2008;62:229–31.
101. Atkinson V, Lee L. An unusual case of an airplane headache. Headache. 2004;44:438–9.
102. Evans RW, Purdy A, Goodman SH. Airplane descent headaches. Headache. 2007;47(5):719–23.
103. Mainardi F, Lisotto C, Maggioni F. Headache attributed to airplane travel: three new cases with first report of female occurrence and classifying criteria. J Headache Pain. 2007;8(Suppl):12.
104. Baldacci F, Lucetti C, Cipriani G, Dolciotti C, Bonuccelli U, Nuti A. Airplane headache' with aura. Cephalalgia. 2010;30(5):624–5.
105. Kararizou E, Anagnostou E, Parskevas GP, Vassilopoulou SD, Naoumis D, Kararizos G, et al. Headache during airplane travel ("airplane headache"): first case in Greece. J Headache Pain. 2011;12(4):489–91. xxx.
106. Bui SB, Petersen T, Poulsen JN, et al. Headaches attributed to airplane travel: a Danish survey. J Headache Pain. 2016;17:50.
107. Purdy RA. Airplane headache—an entity whose time has come to fly? Cephalalgia. 2012;32:587–8.
108. Nierenburg H, Jackfert K. Headache attributed to airplane travel: a review of literature. Curr Pain Headache Rep. 2018;22:48.
109. Ozge A, Abu-Arafeh I, Gelfand AA, et al. Experts' opinion about the pediatric secondary headache diagnostic criteria of ICHD-III beta. J Headache Pain. 2017;18:113.
110. Lansche RK. Ophthalmodynia periodica. Headache. 1964;4:247–9.
111. Sjaastad O, Pettersen H, Bakketeig LS. The Vågå study, epidemiology of headache. The prevalence of ultrashort paroxysms. Cephalalgia. 2001;21:207–15.
112. Pareja JA, Ruiz J, de Isla C, al-Sabbah H, Espejo J. Idiopathic stabbing headache (jabs and jolts syndrome). Cephalalgia. 1996;16(2):93–6.
113. Hagler S, Ballaban-Gil K, Robbins MS. Primary stabbing headache in adults and pediatrics: a review. Curr Pain Headache Rep. 2014;18(10):450.
114. Classification and diagnostic criteria for headache disorders, cranial neuralgias and facial pain. Headache Classification Committee of the International Headache Society. Cephalalgia. 1988;8(Suppl 7):1–96.
115. Piovesan EJ, Kowacs PA, Lange MC, Pacheco C, Piovesan LRM, Werneck LC. Prevalence and semiologic aspects of the idiopathic stabbing headache in a migraine population. Arq Neuropsiquiatr. 2001;59(2A):201–5.
116. Selekler HM, Komşuoğlu S. The relationship of stabbing headaches with migraine attacks. Agri. 2005;17(1):45–8.
117. Özge A, Faedda N, Abu-Arafeh I, Gelfand AA, Goadsby PJ, Cuvellier JC, Valeriani M, Sergeev A, Barlow K, Uludüz D, Yalın OÖ, Lipton RB, Rapoport A, Guidetti V. Experts' opinion about the primary headache diagnostic criteria of the ICHD-3rd edition beta in children and adolescents. J Headache Pain. 2017;18:109. https://doi.org/10.1186/s10194-017-0818-y.
118. Myers KA, Smyth KA. Preadolescent indomethacin-responsive headaches without autonomic symptoms. Headache. 2013;53(6):977–80.

119. Mukharesh LO, Jan MM. Primary stabbing "ice-pick" headache. Pediatr Neurol. 2011;45(4):268–70.
120. Victorio MC. Uncommon pediatric primary headache disorders. Pediatr Ann. 2018;47(2):e69–73.
121. Kakisaka Y, Ohara T, Hino-Fukuyo N, Uematsu M, Kure S. Abdominal and lower back pain in pediatric idiopathic stabbing headache. Pediatrics. 2014;133(1):e245–7.
122. Fuh JL, Kuo KH, Wang SJ. Primary stabbing headache in a headache clinic. Cephalalgia. 2007;27(9):1005–9.
123. Selekler HM, Budak F. Idiopathic stabbing headache and experimental ice cream headache (short-lived headaches). Eur Neurol. 2004;51(1):6–9.
124. Montella S, Ranieri A, Marchese M, De Simone R. Primary stabbing headache: a new dural sinus stenosis-associated primary headache? Neurol Sci. 2013;34(Suppl 1):S157–9.
125. Ergun U, Ozer G, Sekercan S, Artan E, Kudiaki C, Ucler S, et al. Headaches in the different phases of relapsing-remitting multiple sclerosis: a tendency for stabbing headaches during relapses. Neurologist. 2009;15(4):212–6.
126. Rampello L, Malaguarnera M, Rampello L, Nicoletti G, Battaglia G. Stabbing headache in patients with autoimmune disorders. Clin Neurol Neurosurg. 2012;114(6):751–3.
127. Rozen TD. Brief sharp stabs of head pain and giant cell arteritis. Headache. 2010;50(9):1516–9.
128. Chua AL, Nahas S. Ice pick headache. Curr Pain Headache Rep. 2016;20(5):30.
129. O'Connor MB, Murphy E, Phelan MJ, Regan MJ. Primary stabbing headache can be responsive to etoricoxib, a selective COX-2 inhibitor. Eur J Neurol. 2008;15(1):e1.
130. Piovesan EJ, Zukerman E, Kowacs PA, Werneck LC. COX-2 inhibitor for the treatment of idiopathic stabbing headache secondary to cerebrovascular diseases. Cephalalgia. 2002;22(3):197–200.
131. Rozen TD. Melatonin as treatment for idiopathic stabbing headache. Neurology. 2003;61(6):865–6.
132. Leite Pacheco R, de Oliveira Cruz Latorraca C, Adriano Leal Freitas da Costa A, Luiza Cabrera Martimbianco A, Vianna Pachito D, Riera R. Melatonin for preventing primary headache: a systematic review. Int J Clin Pract. 2018;72(7):e13203.
133. Gelfand AA, Goadsby PJ. The role of melatonin in the treatment of primary headache disorders. Headache. 2016;56(8):1257–66.
134. Gelfand AA. Melatonin in the treatment of primary headache disorders. Headache. 2017;57(6):848–9.
135. Bermudez Salazar M, Rojas Ceron CA, Arana Munoz RS. Prophylaxis with melatonin for primary stabbing headache in pediatrics: a case report. Colomb Med. 2018;49(3):244–8.
136. Piovesan EJ, Teive HG, Kowacs PA, Silva LL, Werneck LC. Botulinum neurotoxin type-A for primary stabbing headache: an open study. Arq Neuropsiquiatr. 2010;68(2):212–5.
137. Franca MC Jr, Costa AL, Maciel JA Jr. Gabapentin-responsive idiopathic stabbing headache. Cephalalgia. 2004;24(11):993–6.
138. Ranieri A, Topa A, Cavaliere M, De Simone R. Recurrent epistaxis following stabbing headache responsive to acetazolamide. Neurol Sci. 2014;35(Suppl 1):181–3.
139. Jacome DE. Exploding head syndrome and idiopathic stabbing headache relieved by nifedipine. Cephalalgia. 2001;21(5):617–8.
140. Godoy DA, Rabinstein AA, Biestro A, Ainslie PN, Di Napoli M. Effects of indomethacin test on intracranial pressure and cerebral hemodynamics in patients with refractory intracranial hypertension: a feasibility study. Neurosurgery. 2012;71(2):245–57; discussion 57–8.
141. Celebisoy N, Gokcay F, Sirin H, Akyurekli O. Treatment of idiopathic intracranial hypertension: topiramate vs acetazolamide, an open-label study. Acta Neurol Scand. 2007;116(5):322–7.
142. Lupi C, Evangelista L, Favoni V, Granato A, Negro A, Pellesi L, Ornello R, Russo A, Cevoli S, Guerzoni S, Benemei S. Rare primary headaches in Italian Tertiary Headache Centres: three year nationwide retrospective data from the RegistRare Network. Cephalalgia. 2018;38:1429–41.

143. Pareja JA, Caminero AB, Serra J, Barriga FJ, Barón M, Dobato JL, Vela L, Sánchez del Río M. Nummular headache: a coin-shaped cephalalgia. Neurology. 2002;58:1678–9.
144. Headache Classification Committee of the International Headache Society. The International Classification of Headache Disorders. Cephalalgia. 2018;38:1–211.
145. Cuadrado ML, Lòpez-Ruiz P, Guerrero AL. Nummular headache: an update and future prospects. Expert Rev Neurother. 2018;18:9–19.
146. Martins IP, Abreu L. Nummular headache: clinical features and treatment response in 24 new cases. Cephalalgia Rep. 2018;1:1–8.
147. Song TJ, Yun CH, Cho SJ, Kim WJ, Yang KI, Chu MK. Short sleep duration and poor sleep quality among migraineurs: a population-based study. Cephalgia. 2018;38:855–64.
148. Suzuki K, Miyamoto T, Miyamoto M, Suzuki S, Watanabe Y, Takashima R, Hirata K. Dreamenacting behaviour is associated with impaired sleep and severe headache-related disability in migraine patients. Cephalalgia. 2013;33:868–78.
149. Long R, Zhu Y, Zhou S. Therapeutic role of melatonin in migraine prophylaxis: a systematic review. Medicine (Baltimore). 2019;98(3):e14099.
150. Palacios-Ceña M, Wang K, Castaldo M, et al. Variables associated with the use of prophylactic amitriptyline treatment in patients with tension-type headache. Clin J Pain. 2019;35:315–20.
151. Li D, Rozen TD. The clinical characteristics of new daily persistent headache. Cephalalgia. 2002;22(1):66–9.
152. Meineri P, Torre E, Rota E, Grasso E. New daily persistent headache: clinical and serological characteristics in a retrospective study. Neurol Sci. 2004;25(Suppl 3):S281–2.
153. Kung E, Tepper SJ, Rapoport AM, Sheftell FD, Bigal ME. New daily persistent headache in the paediatric population. Cephalalgia. 2009;29(1):17–22.
154. Rozen TD. Triggering events and new daily persistent headache: age and gender differences and insights on pathogenesis-a clinic-based study. Headache. 2016;56(1):164–73. This is a retrospective cohort demonstrating a similar age- and sex-profiles irrespective of triggering events, suggesting the possibility of common susceptibility factors. Further, patients developing NDPH following a surgical procedure are all required endotracheal intubation, suggesting cervicogenic mechanisms.
155. Rozen TD. New daily persistent headache (NDPH) triggered by a single valsalva event: a case series. Cephalalgia. 2018; https://doi.org/10.1177/0333102418806869.
156. Bigal ME, Sheftell FD, Rapoport AM, Tepper SJ, Lipton RB. Chronic daily headache: identification of factors associated with induction and transformation. Headache. 2002;42:575–81.
157. Peres MF, Lucchetti G, Mercante JP, Young WB. New daily persistent headache and panic disorder. Cephalalgia. 2011;31(2):250–3.
158. Garza I. Images from headache: a "noisy" headache: dural arteriovenous fistula resembling new daily persistent headache. Headache. 2008;48(7):1120–1.
159. Lee J, Rhee M, Suh ES. New daily persistent headache with isolated sphenoiditis in children. Korean J Pediatr. 2015;58(2):73–6.
160. Pomeroy JL, Marmura MJ, Nahas SJ, Viscusi ER. Ketamine infusions for treatment refractory headache. Headache. 2017;57(2):276–82.
161. Uniyal R, Paliwal VK, Anand S, Ambesh P. New daily persistent headache: an evolving entity. Neurol India. 2018;66:679.
162. Li N, Wang J, Huang Q, Tan G, Chen L, Zhou J. Clinical features of new daily persistent headache in a tertiary outpatient population. Headache. 2012;52:1546–52.
163. Rozen TD. New daily persistent headache: an update. Curr Pain Headache Rep. 2014;18:431.
164. American Psychiatric Association. Diagnostic and statistical manual of mental disorders. 5th ed. Washington, DC: American Psychiatric Publishing; 2013.
165. Gierk B, Kohlmann S, Kroenke K, Spangenberg L, Zenger M, Brähler E, Löwe B. The somatic symptom scale-8 (SSS-8): a brief measure of somatic symptom burden. JAMA Intern Med. 2014;174:399–407.

166. Toussaint A, Murray AM, Voigt K, Herzog A, Gierk B, Kroenke K, Rief W, Henningsen P, Löwe B. Development and validation of the somatic symptom disorder-B criteria scale (SSD-12). Psychosom Med. 2016;78:5–12.
167. Uniyal R, Paliwal VK, Tripathi A. Psychiatric comorbidity in new daily persistent headache: a cross-sectional study. Eur J Pain. 2017;21:1031–8.
168. Raskin NH, Knittle SC. Ice cream headache and orthostatic symptoms in patients with migraine. Headache. 1976;16(5):222–5.
169. Mattsson P. Headache caused by drinking cold water is common and related to active migraine. Cephalalgia. 2001;21(3):230–5.
170. Kaczorowski M, Kaczorowski J. Ice cream evoked headaches (ICE-H) study: randomised trial of accelerated versus cautious ice cream eating regimen. BMJ (Clin Res Ed). 2002;325(7378):1445–6.
171. Fuh JL, Wang SJ, Lu SR, Juang KD. Ice-cream headache—a large survey of 8359 adolescents. Cephalalgia. 2003;23(10):977–81.
172. de Oliveira DA, Valenca MM. The characteristics of head pain in response to an experimental cold stimulus to the palate: an observational study of 414 volunteers. Cephalalgia. 2012;32(15):1123–30.
173. Zierz AM, Mehl T, Kraya T, Wienke A, Zierz S. Ice cream headache in students and family history of headache: a cross-sectional epidemiological study. J Neurol. 2016;263(6):1106–10.
174. Mages S, Hensel O, Zierz AM, Kraya T, Zierz S. Experimental provocation of 'ice-cream headache' by ice cubes and ice water. Cephalalgia. 2017;37(5):464–9. Updated experiment that describes different characteristics of the cold stimulus headache based on the type of cold stimulus.
175. Selekler HM, Erdogan MS, Budak F. Prevalence and clinical characteristics of an experimental model of 'ice-cream headache' in migraine and episodic tension-type headache patients. Cephalalgia. 2004;24(4):293–7.
176. Hensel O, Mages S, Kraya T, Zierz S. FV 3 Functional transcranial Doppler (fTCD) during cold-induced pain in the oral cavity and ice cream headache. Clin Neurophysiol. 2017;128(10):e306–7. Cerebral vascular changes documented on transcranial doppler in this study in patients given a cold stimulus and reporting a cold stimulus headache but not those without the headache.
177. Burkhart CG, Burkhart CN. Ice cream headaches with cryotherapy of actinic keratoses. Int J Dermatol. 2006;45(9):1116–7.

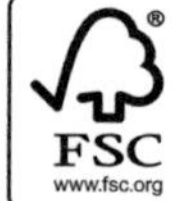

MIX
Papier aus verantwortungsvollen Quellen
Paper from responsible sources
FSC® C105338

www.fsc.org

If you have any concerns about our products,
you can contact us on
ProductSafety@springernature.com

In case Publisher is established outside the EU,
the EU authorized representative is:
**Springer Nature Customer Service Center GmbH
Europaplatz 3, 69115 Heidelberg, Germany**

Printed by Libri Plureos GmbH
in Hamburg, Germany